Women and COVID-19

Women and COVID-19: A Clinical and Applied Sociological Focus on Family, Work and Community focuses on women's lived experiences amid the pandemic, emphasising migrant labourers, ethnic minorities, the poor and disenfranchised, the incarcerated, and victims of gender-based violence, to explore the impact of the pandemic on women.

The COVID-19 pandemic highlighted and exacerbated pervasive gender inequalities in homes, schools, and workplaces in the developed world and the Global South. Female workers, particularly those from poor or ethnic minority backgrounds, were often the first to lose their jobs amidst unprecedented lay-offs and economic uncertainty. National lockdowns and widespread restrictions blurred the boundaries between work and home life and increased the burden of domestic work on women within patriarchal societies. This so-called 'new normal' in everyday life also exposed women to increased levels of gender-based violence and the likelihood of contracting COVID-19 due to overcrowding. This edited volume includes contributions from leading applied and clinical sociologists working and living in Asia, Africa, Europe, and the Americas and gives a global overview of the impact of the pandemic on women. Each chapter adopts an applied and clinical sociological approach in analysing gendered vulnerabilities. The volume innovatively uses personal accounts, including narratives, interviews, autoethnographies, and focus group discussions, to explore women's lived experiences during the pandemic.

This edited collection will greatly interest students, academics, and researchers in the humanities and social sciences with an interest in gender and the impact of the COVID-19 pandemic.

Mariam Seedat-Khan is Professor of Sociology at the University of KwaZulu-Natal, South Africa, where she is head of the clinical sociology postgraduate programme. She is also a visiting professor at Taylor's University, Malaysia, vice president-elect of the Association for Applied and Clinical Sociology (AACS) and an executive member of the Clinical Sociology Research Committee (RC46) of the International Sociological Association (ISA). She is an NRF-rated researcher and certified clinical sociologist who explores applied and clinical teaching and learning disabilities. She is the author of *Domestic Workers and Socialisation* *in South Africa* (2009) and co-editor of *Sociology: A South African Perspective* (2016).

Johanna O. Zulueta is Professor of Sociology at Toyo University, Japan. She is also a visiting professor at Taylor's University, Malaysia, and a member of the steering committee of the Philippine Migration Research Network (PMRN). Her research explores issues of gender, ethnicity, and immigration in East and Southeast Asia. She is the author of *Transnational Identities on Okinawa's Military Bases: Invisible Armies* (2020), and *Okinawan Women's Stories of Migration: From War Brides to Issei* (Routledge, 2022), and editor of *Thinking Beyond the State: Migration, Integration, and Citizenship in Japan and the Philippines* (2018) and co-editor of *Japan: Migration and a Multicultural Society* (2014).

The COVID-19 Pandemic Series

This series examines the impact of the COVID-19 pandemic on individuals, communities, countries, and the larger global society from a social scientific perspective. It represents a timely and critical advance in knowledge related to what many believe to be the greatest threat to global ways of being in more than a century. It is imperative that academics take their rightful place alongside medical professionals as the world attempts to figure out how to deal with the current global pandemic, and how society might move forward in the future. This series represents a response to that imperative.

Series Editor: *J. Michael Ryan*

Titles in this Series:

COVID-19 and Social Change in Spain
Edited by Carlos de Castro, Andrés Pedreño and Marta Latorre

COVID-19: Cultural Change and Institutional Adaptations
Edited by J. Michael Ryan

COVID 19: Individual Rights and Community Responsibilities
Edited by J. Michael Ryan

COVID 19: Surviving a Pandemic
Edited by J. Michael Ryan

Pandemic Pedagogies
Teaching and Learning during the COVID-19 Pandemic
Edited by J. Michael Ryan

COVID-19 in Brooklyn
Everyday Life During a Pandemic
Jerome Krase and Judith DeSena

The Pandemic in Britain
COVID-19, British Exceptionalism and Neoliberalism
Sean Creaven

Women and COVID-19
A Clinical and Applied Sociological Focus on Family, Work and Community
Edited by Mariam Seedat-Khan and Johanna O. Zulueta

Women and COVID-19

A Clinical and Applied Sociological Focus on
Family, Work and Community

**Edited by Mariam Seedat-Khan and
Johanna O. Zulueta**

Routledge
Taylor & Francis Group

LONDON AND NEW YORK

First published 2024
by Routledge
4 Park Square, Milton Park, Abingdon, Oxon OX14 4RN

and by Routledge
605 Third Avenue, New York, NY 10158

Routledge is an imprint of the Taylor & Francis Group, an informa business

British Library Cataloguing-in-Publication Data
A catalogue record for this book is available from the British Library

ISBN: 978-1-032-21175-6 (hbk)
ISBN: 978-1-032-21177-0 (pbk)
ISBN: 978-1-003-26713-3 (ebk)

DOI: 10.4324/9781003267133

Typeset in Times New Roman
by Deanta Global Publishing Services, Chennai, India

This edited volume is dedicated to the women academics that came before, academics that were lost to COVID-19 and a legacy of women that will come after.

Contents

PART VII
Conclusion: Interventions and Change 287

Figures

Tables

List of Abbreviations

4IR	Fourth Industrial Revolution
ALT	Assistant Language Teacher
ANM	Auxiliary Nurses and Midwives
APEDFI	Associação de Pessoas com Doença Falciforme de Ilhéus
ASHA	Accredited Social Health Activists
CHW	Community health worker
CIEYA	Centre for Integrated Education Youth and Adults
CLAIR	Council of Local Authorities for International Relations
CNA	Certified Nursing Assistant
CNI	National Immigration Council
DV	Domestic Violence
DVA	Domestic Violence and Abuse
FENAFAL	Federation of Associations of People with Sickle Cell Disease of Brazil
GBV	Gender-Based Violence
HCP	Healthcare practitioner
HHA	Home Health Aid
IPV	Intimate Partner Violence
JET	Japan Exchange and Teaching
MCO	Movement Control Order
NRPF	No Recourse to Public Funds
SA	South Africa
SCD	Sickle cell disease
UK	United Kingdom
USA	United States of America

Notes on Contributors

Favour Atinuke Akindele obtained a BSc (Hons) degree in Sociology from Landmark University, Kwara State, Nigeria, and proceeded to the University of Ibadan where she obtained a Master's degree in Sociology. Her research interests include gender, intimate partner violence, reproductive health, and domestic abuse.

Shoba Arun, Manchester Metropolitan University, is a Reader in Sociology and Head of the Research Centre for Applied Social Sciences (RCASS) Research Cluster at Manchester Metropolitan University. As an economic sociologist, she has substantial research experience on comparative and international socio-economic inequalities, with seminal and key scholarship on social and gender inequalities and migration.

Alicja Blada-Edgeley works as a trauma therapist in a private practice in Cheshire, UK. She dedicated her master's research to Polish women affected by domestic abuse in the UK. Alicja is passionate about work with people impacted by domestic violence and abuse. She also works closely with a local domestic abuse charity where she delivers trauma therapy to women.

Amber Blake is a postgraduate researcher in the Department of Sociology and Social Anthropology at Stellenbosch University, South Africa. Her research revolves around the sociology of work and social inequality and investigates women's experiences working in the Global South from a feminist perspective.

Benedicte Brahic is a senior lecturer in Sociology at Manchester Metropolitan University (United Kingdom) where she co-convenes the Migration and Interdisciplinary Global Studies (MIGS) research group. Her research interests concern the intersections of gender and bordering in migratory and educational contexts. Her more recent work explores the impact of uncertain migratory contexts and citizenship status on female migrants and their families in Brexit Britain and during the Covid-19 pandemic. She is the Principal Investigator for the Global Challenges Research Fund project 'Higher Educational Attainment Inequalities and Single Parent families in South Africa (HEAPS): differences by region, gender, and race'.

Edwin Carlos is a School Psychology PhD student at the Berkeley School of Education, University of California, Berkeley. He is a second-generation Filipino American from Renton, Washington, and graduated with a Bachelor of Arts in Psychology and a minor in education from Stanford University in 2020. His research focuses on the ethnic–racial identity attitudes of Filipino

Americans, and he works with Dr Frank Worrell on his research with the Cross-Ethnic Racial Identity Scale.

Viviane Letícia Silva Carrijo holds a PhD in Applied Linguistics and Language Studies from PUC-SP, São Paulo, Brazil. She works as a Portuguese language teacher, a textbook author, and an individual consultant at the United Nations Educational, Scientific and Cultural Organization (UNESCO) in partnership with the São Paulo Department of Education, focusing on didactic material for the Education of Youth and Adults in the Languages and Technologies area.

Elaika Janin Celemen is a Community Health Sciences student at the University of California Los Angeles Fielding School of Public Health fulfilling a Master of Public Health. She immigrated from the Philippines at age 8 to the United States and currently resides in Los Angeles, CA. She received her BA in Psychology and minor in Neuroscience from the University of Portland, Oregon in 2019. She works with Dr. Valerie Francisco-Menchavez on the CARE Project, which focuses on the work conditions of Filipino caregivers. Elaika's research focus is on health promotion among the Asian American immigrant community through health education and awareness of local public health resources.

Loreen Chikwira is an academic and researcher who has led projects working with various statutory and voluntary, community, and faith organisations on tackling inequalities working in partnership with local communities. Loreen is currently working as a researcher in the policy directorate at the King's Fund. Her role includes working with colleagues across the organisation to plan, design and deliver projects on a wide range of issues related to health and social care policy and practice. Her interests lie in how intersectional approaches are employed in implementing policies and addressing health inequalities. She is also interested in how voices of minority ethnic women can be brought to the fore of social policy and practice, focusing on using inclusive research methods.

Maria Noemia das Neves Conceição is a municipal civil servant working as a community health agent in Ilhéus-BA, Brazil (1999–2014), coordinator of the Association of People with Sickle Cell Disease of Ilhéus, Brazil [Associação de Pessoas com Doença Falciforme de Ilhéus – APEDFI] (2014 to the present) and health counsellor in Ilhéus Municipal Council, Brazil (2019 to the present).

Quraisha Dawood is a brand research manager of Independent Institute of Education Varsity College. She received her PhD in Sociology from the University of Kwa-Zulu Natal in 2016. She is a member of the International Sociological Association (RC 52) and the Development Studies Association. Her interests lie in intersectionality and informal employment. She has recently published *Stirring the Pot*, based on her Master's thesis on 'madams and maids.'

Flávia Alessandra de Souza has a degree in Social Sciences from the Universidade Estadual Paulista Júlio de Mesquita Filho (2001), a master's degree in Social Sciences from the Federal University of São Carlos (2004), and a doctorate in Sociology from the Federal University of São Carlos (2008), with an internship PhD at the University of Pittsburgh (PA, USA, 2007). She was a guest lecturer at the University of New York City – the City University of New York, John Jay College of Criminal Justice, Department of Latin American and Latina/o Studies (NY, USA, 2009). She has been Adjunct Professor of Sociology based in the Department of Philosophy and Human Sciences (DFCH) at the State University of Santa Cruz (UESC), Ilhéus-BA, Brazil, since 2009.

Iraiza de Souza Pereira has a degree in Social Science from Federal University of Recôncavo da Bahia – UFRB (2022). She is a translator, doula and teacher of Sociology in the State of Bahia, Brazil. She is also a member of the Black Feminist Collective Angela Davis in Bahia.

Joyce Suellen Lopes Dias has a master's degree in Applied Linguistics from PUC – São Paulo. Specialist in Education for Diversity, with degrees in Letras and Pedagogy. Member of the Research Group – LACE. Acting as a municipal São Paulo Middle school principal and English teacher at Santa Cruz school at the night courses.

Khayaat Fakier is Prince Claus Chair of Equity and Development (2021–2023) at the International Institute for Social Studies at Erasmus University in the Netherlands. Her research interest is in unpaid care for humans and other than humans. Her latest publication is a co-edited book titled *Marxist-Feminist Theories and Struggles Today: Essential Writings on Intersectionality, Labour and Ecofeminism* published in 2021 by ZED Books. She is a member of the Department of Sociology and Social Anthropology at Stellenbosch University, where she teaches and supervises the sociology of work and feminist sociology.

Tricia Abigail Santos Fermin is Assistant Professor at the Centre for Language Education, Josai International University in Japan. She received her Sociology PhD (2014) from the Graduate School of Human Sciences, Osaka University. Broadly, her research focuses on gender and sexual politics in Japan and Southeast Asia, cultural studies, and the sociology of education. She has published on the globalisation of fujoshi and otaku culture, most recently 'BL Coupling in a Different Light: Filipino Fans Envisioning an Alternative Model of Intimacy' in *Queer Transfigurations: Boys Love Media in Asia* (University of Hawai'i Press, 2022). Her current research focuses on the pedagogical contributions of Filipino Assistant Language Teachers in Japanese language classrooms and the issues they face as foreign migrant workers in Japan.

Valerie Francisco-Menchavez is Associate Professor in the Department of Sociology and Sexuality Studies at San Francisco State University. Her book entitled, *The Labour of Care: Filipina Migrants and Transnational Families in the Digital Age* (2018), explores the dynamics of gender and technology of care work and intimacy in Filipino transnational families in the Philippines and the United States. Currently, she is writing a book about Filipino migrant workers' mental and physical health outcomes while working in the understudied industry of caregiving to the elderly, especially under the COVID-19 pandemic.

Jayanathan Govender is faculty in the School of Social Sciences, University of KwaZulu-Natal, Durban, South Africa. He researches public policy, inequality studies, clinical sociology, BRICS sociology and COVID-19. His affiliations are: South African and International Sociological Associations; Visiting Fellow, Jawaharlal Nehru Institute of Advanced Studies, Jawaharlal Nehru University, New Delhi; Visiting Fellow, Shivaji University, Kolhapur; Guest Lecturer, Department of Sociology and Social Work, University of Mumbai; Visiting Professor and Faculty Advisor, Chandigarh University, Punjab.

Thomas Gumbo is an academic supervisor for fourth-year social work students in the School of Applied Human Sciences at the University of KwaZulu-Natal, Durban. His area of interest is advancing the rights of children and women in society.

Ujjwala Gupta is a Doctorate in Development Studies and a Public Health faculty member at Yenepoya (Deemed to be University) at Mangalore in Karnataka, India. She has over a decade of research experience in community-based family planning and maternal and child health. Gupta is a member of the International Sociological Association-ISA. She is the recipient of the prestigious International Fellowships- Shastri Indo Canada Doctoral Research Fellowship and the Policy Communication fellowship- Population Reference Bureau (USAID).

Kim Heyes, Department of Nursing, Manchester Metropolitan University, Manchester, is Senior Lecturer of Health and Social Justice in the Department of Nursing at Manchester Metropolitan University. Her primary research is around gender-based abuse and mental health.

Daniela Jauk-Ajamie is a Certified Clinical Sociologist (CCS) and Assistant Professor for Sociology and Criminal Justice at the University of Akron, Ohio. After a Master's in Sociology in her home country Austria, she completed her doctoral work in Sociology as a Fulbright student at the University of Akron/OH, specialising in Qualitative Research Methodologies and Sociology of Deviance and Gender Studies. She has taught and published in Europe and the US and returned to Akron permanently in 2017. She worked as an applied sociologist, initiated a pilot project for women, and researched horticultural sociological interventions in community corrections.

Alabi Oluwatobi Joseph is a Global Excellence Stature Postdoctoral Research Fellow at the Department of the Sociology University of Johannesburg. His research interests span gender and sexuality, family and reproductive health; poverty and inequality; education; and youth and development. He has taught at the Department of Sociology, University of KwaZulu-Natal, Durban, and the Centre for General Education at the Durban University of Technology, South Africa. Alabi has over 15 academic publications in international peer-reviewed journals like *Global Public Health, Sage Open, International Journal of Gambling Studies, Journal of Medical Sciences, Alternation,* and *Contemporary Perspective in Family Research,* among others. He has also published several book chapters.

Kezia Lewins is an experienced researcher with a demonstrated history of working in higher education and health settings. Skilled especially in sociology, data collection, and analysis (qualitative and quantitative). Strong lecturing professional with a PhD degree focused on race and gender-based transformation from the University of the Witwatersrand, Johannesburg. Works with healthcare professionals, families, and patients to support those with and affected by chronic illnesses and COVID-19.

Fernanda Coelho Liberali is a teacher educator, researcher, and professor at the Pontifical Catholic University of São Paulo, in the Language Sciences and Philosophy Department, in the Program of Postgraduate Studies in Applied Linguistics and Language Studies, in the Postgraduate Program in Education: Education of Educators, and in the Postgraduate Program in Education: Curriculum. She holds a degree in Languages from the Federal University of Rio de Janeiro, a master's and a doctorate degree in Applied Linguistics and Language Studies from the Pontifical Catholic University of São Paulo, and three postdoctoral degrees from the University of Helsinki, from the Berlin Freie Universität, Germany and from Rutgers University, USA.

Takunda Mathathu is a longstanding member of the Golden Key International Honour Society. His humanitarian work in ecological citizenship frameworks, gender, and natural disasters has contributed to an outstanding study under Professor Seedat-Khan. His area of study includes gender, natural disasters, domestic violence, and developmental issues. He is currently a part-time Development Studies lecturer at the University of Mpumalanga.

Wan Puspa Melati is an Associate Professor and Head of Department at Taylor's University, Malaysia. She holds a PhD in Sociology and Anthropology from International Islamic University Malaysia (IIUM). She completed her MSc in Sociology from the University of Oxford, UK (Oxford) and her BA in Sociology and Psychology from the University of San Francisco, US (USF). Identifying herself as a Clinical Sociologist and passionate about the community, Wan Puspa Melati has worked with both local and international NGOs and managed grassroots empowerment programmes for various target groups. This includes community work with single mothers, children of low-income households, abused women and children, juvenile delinquents, transgender individuals, senior citizens, and the deaf community.

Marjorie L. Naidoo holds Bachelor of Economics (Hons) and MPhil Sustainable Development Cum Laude degrees from Stellenbosch University. Her thesis, 'Exploring the Contribution of Design to a Sustainable City,' addressed the intersection of Design and Urbanism, Environmental Ethics, Political Economics, Complexity, and Sustainability. During a career in Communications and Public Relations, she served in seven non-government institutions – the subject matter ranging from the Wool Industry to Iron and Steel to Tourism to Telecommunications; and finally the Craft and Design sector. She has taught Transdisciplinary Design in Transition at the postgraduate level since 2015 and has co-supervised several masters' theses.

Chenicheri Sid Nair is currently Executive Dean and the Dean of Learning, Teaching and Student Experience at the Victorian Institute of Technology (VIT), Australia. In his role, he is responsible for the strategic directions, the learning, teaching, student experience, and quality matters of the Institution.

His research focuses on quality in the Australian higher education system, classroom, and school environments, and the implementation of improvements from stakeholder feedback. He has extensive lecturing experience in the applied sciences in Canada, Singapore, and Australia. He is an international consultant in quality and evaluations in higher education.

Chloe Janelle Punsalan is a fourth-year undergraduate student majoring in Psychology, with an emphasis on clinical psychology and Asian American and Asian Diaspora Studies at the University of California, Berkeley. After graduating, she hopes to enter into a PsyD program. Through her experiences as a second-generation Filipina American and her extensive research experiences, she has developed a passion for learning about how ethnic, racial, and cultural influences can affect psychosocial and identity development. Some of her research interests include bicultural identity development, role/identity conflict, and mental health disparities in Asian Americans.

Kalai Vaani Rajandram is a Senior Lecturer in the School of Liberal Arts and Sciences at Taylor's University, Malaysia. Her areas of study span across teacher education, literature in English, and narrative reality. Her expertise is in Narrative Ethnography and Netnography. Her interest lies in exploring social realities and how these not only facilitate the construction of gender, identity, and culture but also promote the understanding of newer forms of social cohesion and integration.

Aradhana Ramnund-Mansingh acquired her PhD in 2019 from the University of KwaZulu-Natal, South Africa. Her study *explored the link between institutional culture and women's career trajectories in academia.* She is a prolific writer and has been acclaimed as an exemplary scholar, publishing a series of book chapters and five scientific journal articles within a year of completing her PhD. Dr Mansingh is a valuable member of the Association for Applied and Clinical Sociology (AACS), the International Sociological Association, and the South African Board for People Practices (SABPP).

Usha Rana, PhD, is Assistant Professor of Sociology and Social Work at the Dr Harisingh Gour Central University (A Government Central University), Sagar, Madhya Pradesh, India. She is a sociology academic specialising in sexual studies and gender studies and has more than ten years of teaching and research experience. She has published more than 30 articles in reputed national and international peer-reviewed journals/conferences, including SCI/Scopus-indexed journals published by Inderscience, Springer, Elsevier, and Cambridge. In addition, she also serves as a reviewer for many SCI/Scopus journals. She has delivered lectures as a speaker at various national and international workshops. Professor Rana is an active member of the International Sociological Association, Indian Sociological Society, and Women's Indian Association, among others. Dr Rana completed her master's and doctorate in Sociology from Jiwaji University, Gwalior, Madhya Pradesh, India, and Dr Harisingh Gour Central University, respectively.

Mariam Seedat-Khan, Certified Clinical Sociologist (CCS), is a certified clinical sociologist at the University of KwaZulu-Natal in Durban, South Africa.

She is a member of the UKZN-Imbokodo, a steering committee of women in leadership. In 2020, she was named a UKZN phenomenal. She is the SMART founder – Simply Managing Academic Related Tasks developed to assist students with learning disorders. She is an executive member of the International Sociological Association ISA RC-46 Clinical Sociology, South African Sociological Association (SASA) Working Group Convener Clinical Sociology; a board member of the Association for Applied and Clinical Sociology (AACS) a member of the Canadian Sociological Association (CSA). Professor Seedat-Khan is a visiting professor at Taylor's University in Malaysia.

Upasana Singh is the Academic Leader and a Senior Lecturer in the Discipline of Information Systems and Technology at the University of KwaZulu-Natal, Westville Campus, in Durban, South Africa. She has been appointed Adjunct Senior Lecturer at the Victorian Institute of Technology, Australia. She has a keen interest in Educational Technologies and has served as the lead researcher in a number of international research projects on Digital Teaching, Learning, and Assessment. She is the convener and Chair of the International Conference on Digital Teaching, Learning and Assessment (digiTAL 2K). Dr Upasana Singh completed her Fellowship in 'Teaching Advancement in Universities' (TAU), from the Council of Higher Education in 2019.

Daniela Aparecida Vieira holds a PhD and a master's degree in Italian Language, Literature and Culture from the University of São Paulo. She has a degree in Portuguese and Italian languages and their respective literature from the same university. She also has a postgraduate degree in Portuguese from the Pontifical Catholic University of São Paulo (PUC-SP). She developed postdoctoral research in Applied Linguistics at PUC-SP from 2018 to 2020. She has been teaching Portuguese and Italian since 2005. She has been teaching Portuguese to Haitians at CIEJA Perus since 2019.

Rashmi Watson has been an educator for 25 years and currently leads assessment and teaching development in the Medical School at the University of Western Australia. She has a keen interest in leadership development and provides consultancy in this area often applying an Appreciative Inquiry (strengths-based approach). Some of her recent publications include experiences during COVID-19 (academic female leadership, remote teaching and working from home and academic integrity). She has a background in appreciative inquiry and facilitation, which strengths leadership capability. Her publications focus COVID-19 on women leaders in academia, and virtual teaching that intersect the domestic space.

Johanna O. Zulueta is Professor at the Faculty of Sociology of Toyo University, Japan. She received her A.B. in Social Sciences from the Ateneo de Manila University and her PhD in Sociology from Hitotsubashi University as a Japanese Ministry of Education scholar. Presently, she is part of the Steering Committee of the Philippine Migration Research Network (PMRN). Her main research interest is on migrations in East Asia, looking at ethnicity, gender, citizenship, home, and ageing. She recently published a monograph titled *Okinawan Women's Stories of Migration: From War Brides to Issei* (Routledge, 2022).

Series Foreword

We are very pleased to introduce *Women and COVID-19: A Clinical and Applied Sociological Focus on Family, Work and Community. Applied Sociology* refers to research for practical purposes, and *Clinical Sociology* focuses on the analysis of and intervention in problematic situations in order to improve the quality of all lives and the planet as a whole. Clinical sociology also often involves applied research.

As clinical sociologists, we have long been involved in topics such as human rights, environmental justice, whistleblowing, the protection of children in armed conflict, mandatory retirement of older adults, and the central inclusion of women and girls. Therefore, we very much looked forward to reading the contributions to this volume.

Women and COVID-19 analyses the situation of women during a global health crisis. The chapters cover very different topics in several regions of the world as well as at least ten countries – Zimbabwe, South Africa, India, Brazil, the United States, Nigeria, Malaysia, Japan, Australia, and the United Kingdom. The editors of the volume – Mariam Seedat-Khan and Johanna O. Zulueta – asked authors to document and analyse how people adapted to a **new normal** in their lives. The authors show how the new normal 'intensified gender-based and intimate partner violence' and focus on the urgent need to prioritise dealing with women's vulnerability. The editors emphasise that since COVID-19, the 'challenges, risks, inequalities, and marginalization' usually facing women have become more difficult for women.

We certainly support the editors' call for a solution-driven approach to dealing with these critical issues. We look forward to the development of clinical sociology programmes and initiatives that seek to dramatically reduce or eliminate the identified problems through a combination of analysis and intervention. Research should allow the direct voices of community members to be heard, and policymakers need to be involved at every step to make sure that they hear those community voices. The involvement of representatives of foundations and government agencies could help in providing any needed resources to ensure the participation of women from different backgrounds and communities of all sizes in the development of interventions as well as the evaluation and monitoring of initiatives.

Tina Uys, DLitt et Phil, CCS

Professor, University of Johannesburg (South Africa); Vice President of the Clinical Sociology division (RC46) of the International Sociological Association; Co-editor of *Clinical Sociology for Southern Africa* as well as the *Clinical Sociology Review*; and former President of the South African Sociological Association, as well as a former Vice President of National Associations of the International Sociological Association.

Jan Marie Fritz, PhD, CCS

Professor, University of Cincinnati (USA) and Distinguished Visiting Professor, University of Johannesburg (South Africa); Executive Committee Member of the International Sociological Association (ISA); UN representative for the ISA to the United Nations (New York City); and a former ISA. Vice President for Finance; Editor of the *Clinical Sociology* book series for Springer; and a member of the Steering Committee of the US Environmental Protection Agency's National Environmental Justice Advisory Council.

Acknowledgements

The editors and authors recognise the devastation that women, families, work-spaces, and communities have experienced amid COVID-19. The resilience is evident in the narratives. Families and communities have provided the impetus for this book. COVID-19 lived experiences, fatalities, and economic, political, and social disruption have redirected a global future. Clinical and applied sociologists are recognised for their commitment to social change during an unprecedented time. Heartfelt thanks are extended to the women who supported and encouraged this edited volume. We acknowledge Professors Tina Uys (South Africa), Jan Marie Fritz (USA), Emma Porio (Philippines), and the team of academic peer reviewers, all of whom challenged our thinking and writing. Thank you to our families, work-spaces, friends, and communities that carried the authors as we worked tirelessly to assemble this edited volume. This edited volume is a product of the international research network for applied and clinical sociology. The editors remained committed to the vision of bringing women's lived experiences to life from scholars across the globe.

1 Women and COVID-19

A Clinical and Applied Sociological Focus on Family, Work, and Community

Mariam Seedat-Khan and Johanna O. Zulueta

About the Book

Women and COVID-19: A Clinical and Applied Sociological Focus on Family, Work and Community examines the surreptitious arrival of the COVID-19 global pandemic. This trans- and inter-continental co-authored edited book demonstrates an inclusive global approach with a shift towards scientific scholarship prioritising the intersections between the Global South and the Global North. This collaborative initiative paves the way for scholars to recognise and highlight universal rights and responses to the human condition across the globe. Change agents and clinical and applied scientists are engaged in multi- and interdisciplinary research in gender, family and community, work, to improve the human condition. The unprecedented scientific value of this volume is underscored by the presentation and formulation of clinical and applied models that offer academically rigorous interventions at local, national, and global levels.

Edited Volume

This edited volume includes contributions from leading applied and clinical sociologists working and living in East Asia, Africa, Europe, the United Kingdom, North and South America, and India. This book contributes significantly to this burgeoning field of clinical sociology, offering first-hand pandemic experiences and social implications for vulnerable women worldwide. We deliver innovative scientific scholarship via narratives, interviews, and auto-ethnographies and focus group discussions that highlight and understand the plight of women in the context of a global pandemic. The volume will offer personal accounts to explore women's lived experiences with various methodologies, augmenting the socially constructed realities of inequality and injustice worldwide. Each chapter adopts an applied or clinical sociological approach to analyse gendered vulnerabilities that intersect family work, community, and pandemic implications. This edited volume is the first clinical and applied sociology volume that has concentrated on clinical interventions and applied developments in countries across the globe with a gendered, family, and community focus amid COVID-19. A total of 38 authors have contributed significantly to this edited volume, with 32 women authors, of whom 20 are from the Global South, 12 from the Global North and 6 male authors (Table 1.1).

DOI: 10.4324/9781003267133-1

Table 1.1 Author demographics

Country	South authors	North authors	Total authors	Women	Men
Brazil	South		7	7	–
South Africa	South		8	7	1
United Kingdom		North	5	5	–
United States of America		North	5	4	1
Malaysia	South		3	3	–
Japan		North	2	2	–
Australia		North	2	1	1
India	South		2	2	–
Nigeria	South		2	1	1
Zimbabwe	South		2	-	2
Total	23	14	38	32	6

Source: Authors' own.

Universal Scholarship

Clinical and Applied Sociologists, have focussed on the impact of COVID-19, this book adopts a global clinical focus on family, work, and community framed within scientific methods. The authors include a few men. However, women authors from Australia, Japan, South Africa, the United Kingdom, the United States, Malaysia, Brazil, India, Nigeria, and Zimbabwe have delivered research findings. The scientific scholarship offers significant value to applied social scientists, change agents, clinical sociologists, practitioners, and sociotherapists in the North and the South. The intersecting disciplinary practitioners include educators, criminologists, environmentalists, psychologists, linguists, economists, industrial sociologists, social workers, information technologists, public health specialists, public policy academics, public administration experts, and certified clinical sociologists working towards effective and sustained change amid COVID-19. The intended beneficiaries include researchers, practitioners, and clinicians to support scientific and social interventions to advance applied and clinical sociology research projects, academic programmes, and professional development workshops. The edited series offers ongoing global interventions, intersecting multidisciplinary perspectives from researchers across the globe.

Citizen Scientists

SARS-CoV-2 has forced innovation, reconfiguring the role and function of researchers and academics in knowledge creation to support interventions. Expertise, skills, and proficiencies contribute to specialists critical to engaging indigent sectors of societies. The citizen science approach draws intersecting groups of people to solve complex pandemic emergent social conditions from lived experiences. Formulating contextual Global South and North resolutions to systemic institutional prejudices that proliferate social problems is essential for establishing universal rights. Aimed at forms of constructive social interventions, clinical sociologists aim to assist in the analyses of significant problems via the construction of alternative social systems, serving the well-being of all persons equally, with consent, guided by specific groups confronting significant social problems.

Global COVID-19 Responses

The devastating global impact of the COVID-19 pandemic commanded the cooperation between the country-specific ministries of communications, public service sectors, and the Department of Health's Institute of Communicable Diseases to promote COVID-19 health education. The establishment of a country-specific COVID-19 Ministerial Advisory Committee was lawfully founded in March 2020 with key objectives to support the Health Ministers' guidelines on mitigating the transmission of the unfamiliar life-threatening SARS-CoV-2 novel virus. The World Health Organization (WHO) collaborated with leading academics and clinical specialists to offer empirical evidence on COVID-19. The global team established accessible online WhatsApp helplines and news portals to offer important health communication data. The overarching aim of the collaboration was to mitigate the risk of inaccurate news, misinformation, and panic. Global traditional media and social media platforms led the campaign promoting COVID-19 health education messages.

The New Normal

Authors from across the globe document social scientific research as people have tried adapting to a **new normal** in everyday life. The new normal enforced unfamiliar professional work–life contexts, obscuring work and home-life boundaries. The new normal forced unskilled workers into unemployment, underemployment, and escalated poverty. Public and private businesses, travel, factory, service and entertainment sectors, schools and universities, and the health and pharmaceutical sectors experienced dire economic and resource strife. The implications of a new normal intensified gender-based and intimate partner violence. Women directly confronted multiple intersecting roles – overload augmented by pandemic protocol and a new normal. COVID-19 set in motion a series of social scientific initiatives that led to the development of clinical interventions and multidisciplinary applied sociological models. Interventions and models responded globally to family modifications, work configurations, and familial contexts.

Community Responses

Responses in rural, urban, developed, and underdeveloped, north and south, wealthy and poor communities, increased pre-existing skewed gendered, race, class, and geographic inequalities. The global community was by no means prepared for the surreptitious arrival of the COVID-19 global pandemic. The forced responses led to the creation of global and county-specific pandemic safety protocols.

Pandemic Protocol

Pandemic protocol and legislation saw lockdowns in cities and countries across the globe. The significant impact of the pandemic has culminated in adverse socio-economic realities for vulnerable women from the Global South and the Global North, who grapple with employment and food insecurity. Financial setbacks have impacted migrant labourers, whose vulnerable position culminated in the loss of livelihood and repatriation. Migrants from rural areas largely live in urban slums, an already vulnerable group, occupying overcrowded makeshift homes with inadequate access to sanitation and electric power. Their living arrangements and weak economic position increase their risk of contracting COVID-19. Their cramped lockdown COVID-19 living conditions expose women to increased levels of gender-based violence. This volume focuses on women's lived experiences amid the pandemic, emphasising migrant labourers, ethnic subgroups, the poor and disenfranchised, the incarcerated, and victims of gender-based violence. An increasing set of scientific articles have confirmed pervasive gender inequalities in homes, schools, and workplaces. Alongside national lockdowns, international travel bans, and unprecedented lay-offs, women workers from indigent backgrounds were the first to lose their income. The contributions in this volume prioritise women's vulnerability and experiences from the Global South and the Global North.

Clinical and Applied Sociology

Clinical and applied sociologists develop interventions to create scientifically rigorous methodologies to support change agents' work of improving individuals, families, communities, gender, race, class, north, south, cultural, and geographically diverse societies. Generating new COVID-19 scientific scholarship documents an important unfolding history in the field of sociology and human society.

Chapter Preview

A brief introduction to each chapter, located across seven thematic categories, offers an overview of *Women and COVID-19*, clearly outlining conceptual formulations of the clinical focus on family, work, and community. The daunting task of identifying seven thematic categories was by no means an easy undertaking. The editors considered the intersections with country contributions and geographic locations to help determine the same.

Key Themes

Seven key themes encompass clinical and applied sociology and outline advances in applied and clinical practice across the globe. Themes include gender-based violence, health, work, education, migration, adversity and resilience, and reflections on COVID-19 interventions and change. Each part of the book provides detailed scholarship, narratives, and case studies from the developed Global North and developing Global South.

Part I: Gender-Based Violence

COVID-19 intensified gender-based violence and intimate partner violence (IPV) across the globe; free of prejudice, women experienced violence across race, class, and geographic locations. Natural disasters increase women's vulnerability in the Global South.

The authors of Chapter 2 explore intimate partner violence (IPV) experiences of pregnant women in Ibadan North, Oyo State, Nigeria. Systemic patriarchal structures influence behavioural patterns intensified by COVID-19, deepening inequality, and vulnerability to IPV. COVID-19 lived experiences and coping mechanisms provide a framework for the qualitative phenomenological lens that considers ten pregnant women and five healthcare workers' experiences. Galtung's framework of violence measures the ways in which social structures enhance IPV and the effect of cultural ideologies on legitimising and normalising IPV, with limited access to support. The burden of IPV on pregnant women intensifies their physical, emotional, and mental burden affecting the unborn child's life. The intersecting threats of SARS-CoV-2, IPV, and pregnancy mandated an innovative public health response to ensure unhindered access to medical and psychosocial support during times of crisis.

Gender-based violence (GBV) experiences of Zimbabwean rural women flood victims deliver lived realities of dire social conditions, as exposed in Chapter 3. Notwithstanding natural disasters and climate change, GBV is a human rights violation, systemic in disrupting rural women's safety in Zimbabwe. COVID-19 intensified global cases with Zimbabwean women facing complexities from the Tokwe–Mukosi floods. This chapter explores GBV, COVID-19, and rural flood disaster gendered between 2017 and 2021. In 2020, twelve in-depth interviews and two focus group discussions were conducted at Chingwizi temporary shelter. Victims of the Tokwe–Mukosi flood share their lived experiences and relocation to temporary shelters. The findings revealed systemic patriarchy, gendered typecasts, and socially constructed cultural realities that subjugate women, increasing GBV. Systemic gendered prejudicial governance and customary law escalated GBV, with unsympathetic effects on agriculture, income, and education exacerbating women's social vulnerability. The study underscores the urgency to mainstream clinical interventions that mitigate gender risk and establish safety management in global natural disasters and pandemic crisis studies. Mandated critical gender transformative clinical interventions are required to reframe prejudicial, oppressive GBV bearings on rural women in Zimbabwe.

Part II: Health

COVID-19 has exposed the divide between the developed and developing world. The reality of care in South Africa is offered from an autoethnographic lens to specifically identify women and COVID-19 care. COVID-19 provided challenging contexts for qualitative researchers. Engaging with public policy in scientific spaces has become essential for clinical sociologists. Chapter 4 discusses the gendered dynamics and intersectional effects of COVID-19 care. It reflects on the work of sociologists in under-resourced clinical settings in Gauteng, South Africa. The chapter offers autoethnographic reflections on practices and person-centred care. Understanding vulnerable peoples' healthcare needs, families, and communities as an embryonic COVID-19 narrative, the syndemic brings a broad range of human experiences in a quest for change. Consideration is given to the COVID-19 context, which has necessitated new public and professional relations for clinical sociologists.

The women's community health workforce is the backbone of India's healthcare delivery system, which plays a significant proactive role in combating the COVID-19 crisis, as explained in Chapter 5. Their lived professional hardships compound their vulnerable position. Secondary data and narratives from women community health workers explore first-hand pandemic experiences. India's infection rate worsens among community workers. Risk mitigation, global safety protocol, and transmission reduction are made real by the role of women community healthcare workers in India. Extended working hours, inadequate payment, increasing fatigue, and higher workloads impact work–life balance well-being. The chapter suggests a gendered policy and health delivery approach to reduce women's vulnerabilities among healthcare workers in India.

Chapter 6 is based on face-to-face meetings with APEDFI pre-COVID-19, physical APEDFI databases, public access Facebook page, and activity records. Black Brazilian feminist avant-garde intellectuals identify racial, gender, and class disadvantages; resistance; and protagonist, drawing on intersectional adversities. The Brazilian association of people with sickle cell disease (APEDFI) sociologically deconstructs black women in Ilhéus amid COVID-19. APEDFI's mobilisation of black women with sickle cell disease (SCD) led to the first COVID-19 vaccines for adults with SCD on 4 May 2021.

COVID-19 and its impact on transnational obligations intensify Filipino caregivers' mental health consequences, as illustrated in Chapter 7. Migrant care workers understand the precarious nature of caregiving. COVID-19 working conditions in the United States of America among Filipina elder caregivers exacerbated preexisting mental health conditions. Internalising gendered roles, Filipina caregivers' personal health and well-being are relegated in favour of family demands in the US and the Philippines. This mixed-methods study relies on 56 Filipino caregivers working in the San Francisco Greater Bay Area. Data from 32 interviews explored gendered and psychosocial impacts of fear, isolation, and migrant anxiety work in harsh conditions amid the pandemic. Migrants' transnational obligations expressed fear of COVID-19 negative risk to work and financial responsibilities. Multifaceted transnational obligations, intersections, and psychosocial impacts on Filipina caregivers require urgent attention.

Part III: Work

Case studies and research from South Africa systematically deconstruct the impact of COVID-19 on women cashiers in supermarkets, addressing social distancing protocol and the increasing dehumanisation of labour in a virtual context of affective labour. Chapter 8 focuses on the interactions between supermarket cashiers and customers in a coastal town in South Africa in 2020. COVID-19 restrictions mandated 'socially distant' contact. Qualitative in-depth telephone interviews explored lived experiences of women cashiers during the lockdown. The chapter examines contradictory work experiences, and theoretical insights towards understanding frontline workers amid COVID-19. Sociability measured by race, age, and gender was identified among customers. Cashiers worked closely throughout global lockdowns, increasing COVID-19 cross-infections. The findings suggest that women cashiers engaged in emotional and affective labour while interacting with customers.

In Chapter 9, Malaysian scholars chronicle the lived realities of Indonesian domestic helpers in Malaysian households, augmenting the women behind the success of professional and successful women. Malaysian urban women's multiple personal and professional roles intensified amid the pandemic, and career demands, home-schooling, and chores increased. Indonesian women's financial insecurity resulted in their exploitation, meeting employers demands for cheap domestic labour. The emotional and soci-economic impacts on Indonesian women was made worse by unreasonable working hours, This Chapter uncovered the challenges of migrant Indonesian domestic helpers' wages during the pandemic and responses to crisis away from home. The narrative ethnography framework reflects on realities activated, produced, organised, and transmitted via a social constructivist lens. The situational and interactional terrains of narratives unearthed embedded ideologies of power relationships highlighting acculturation.

Physically compromised Deaf women in Malaysia receive a vital focus with narratives on their unspoken truths, experiences, and challenges amidst the COVID-19 pandemic in Chapter 10. The impact of COVID-19 adopts an intersectional lens to consider marginalised deaf women. Qualitative data, with ten semi-structured interviews with Deaf Malaysian women, provides insight into lived experiences and COVID-19 challenges. Gender, disability, marital status, occupational status, socio-economic status, and social capital are scrutinised. The lived experiences of Deaf women have been categorised into (1) communication during the pandemic; (2) financial constraints and well-being; (3) socialising and social support; and (4) interpersonal conflict. The need for a sensitised hearing world and policymakers to action fundamental via inclusive citizen science approaches to manage COVID-19 sustained challenges.

Part IV: Education

Australian and South African scholars merge to deliver an intellectual evaluation providing an African perspective on work, health, vulnerabilities, and lived realities of women in the academy. Chapter 11 underscores the career progression and intrinsic motivation among women during COVID-19.

Female academics' COVID-19 experiences in higher education institutions (HEIs) have transformed academics' work–life balance. The chapter explores

African, female career progression, workload, and motivation at the onset of COVID-19 providing data from HEI in Africa. Decision-makers would be wise to capitalise on future data to sustain, integrate, and support women in the academy. The chapter relies on a larger study that examined gender gaps, disparities, biases, and unique hardship experiences. HEIs must institute supportive frameworks for female academics' significant knowledge contribution.

The impact of COVID-19 on school policies for assistant language women teachers in Japan provides critical identification of the implication on language. Chapter 12 considers the impact of Japanese school policies and COVID-19 responses on foreign women assistant language teachers (ALT). The chapter considers health data collected via semi-structured interviews with eight Filipino JET (Japan Exchange and Teaching programme)-employed ALTs via Zoom from February to March 2021. Data were analysed using an inductive thematic approach. Results demonstrate the sustained pandemic has not endangered ALTs' livelihood and immigration status in Japan. The pandemic has exacerbated pre-existing problems of marginal positionality in Japanese education systems, increasing their vulnerability to mental health. This chapter highlights online and digital media platforms to improve well-being.

Lone mothers' increased difficulties with COVID-19's educational impact analysed in the Global South deliver a clinical intervention. The separatist South African (SA) history impacts work, family, and community unreservedly, intersecting women's education and economic position. Fractured African families in SA constitute 30% of children raised by lone mothers. Chapter 13 capitalises on the experiences of vulnerable, indigent lone mothers' ability to access social capital to support educational success for their children. Despite minimum wage, migrant labour, and reliance on surrogate caregivers, COVID-19 has orphaned 82,000 children impacting education. A secondary desktop approach included a review of scientific studies between 2019 and 2021. The results are analysed thematically, underpinned by intersectionality and the social construction of reality.

Part V: Migration

The analysis and in-depth narratives highlighting migrant Brazilian women's memories during the pandemic times make a remarkable effort to reframe gendered migrant histories. Chapter 14 discusses the educational perspective of Brazilian women educators and Haitian women students during the pandemic. It departs from necro education, limited access, and those that struggle without government and legal support. The necropolitical context is considered to identify the vulnerability of women. Women's narratives enhance the subversive force of remembering. This overcoming of presentism through access via community is examined. Minorities' understanding of secular oppression is extracted methodologically, with questions to enhance the narratives' power to share pandemic events. Two teachers, one principal, and three students form the basis of multimodal analyses of women's wealth and virtues on surviving adversity, with hope amid oppression.

In Chapter 15, scholars from the United Kingdom (UK) consider the impact of COVID-19 on policy and support services for migrant women. Significant intersections of GBV document women's experiences in semi-rural marginalised areas. The significant increase in the migrant population in rural England has generated service delivery resources, knowledge, and skill challenges that compromise migrant support. The Cheshire East rural region case study scrutinises marginalised migrant women's needs and poor community support. An autoethnographic analysis informed by women authors diversifies minority ethnic migrant positions as professionals. Data from non-profit organisation workshop examines the challenges of third-sector organisations supporting victims of Domestic Violence and Abuse (DVA) during the pandemic. Recognising that the case study does not apply to all rural areas of England, it provides an opportunity to explore migrant women's rural experiences and the challenges. Intersectionality serves as a critical tool to examine support services' response to intersections of gender, ethnicity, immigration status, culture, and religion, in developing services and policies to support migrants experiencing DVA. The chapter offers policy recommendations considering service providers' support for migrant women.

Still, within the United Kingdom, the question of 'whose cost?' is measured against vulnerable female migrants with no recourse to public funds (NRPF) during COVID-19, intensifying women's precarious position within a stratified society that continuously excludes their dispossession. This is further explored in Chapter 16 of this volume. According to Section 115 of the Immigration and Asylum Act 1999, the NRPF policy prevents migrants from accessing state-funded benefits. The UK Home Office's hostile environment policies, guided by NPRF policy, problematise the life of UK migrants. This resulted in migrant families' precarity and poverty, turning solely to charitable organisations for support. NRPF policy criticisms intensified amid COVID-19 resulting in two prominent legal precedents. This chapter explores the pervasive ramifications of NRPF policy on female migrants' lives, increased poverty, homelessness, illegal work, exploitation, declining physical and mental health, and GBV. Locating NRPF policy within the nexus of migration, race, and gender subordination, authors identify oppressive interlocking systems and structures, reinforced by COVID-19.

Part VI: Adversity and Resilience

The reality of resilience building is propelled by adversity and women's lived experiences, as seen in Chapter 17. Women living behind bars in the United States of America (USA) unearth a hidden and vulnerable population in pandemic times. The USA is the largest global incarcerator of women and girls. The author identifies limited scholarship on women prisoners, building an ethnographic analysis drawing on observations from a women's gardening programme in residential correctional communities in the USA–Midwest. The gardening project is a clinical intervention, addressing women's complaints about poor food quality and idle time. The findings suggest poor COVID-19 safety protocol, apathy from criminal justice employees, limited social support, and declining nutrition. The call is to embrace feminist clinical sociology and community gardening for respite, healthy nutrition, and agency for women.

The unprecedented burden made worse by the digital divide between the Global North and the Global South is highlighted in Chapter 18, on bread or data. The hard choices between education and food security are presented in a narrative that delivers the realities of the online teaching transition during COVID-19 in South Africa (SA). The pandemic has imposed histrionic conversion on time-honoured university traditions. Typically, an auditorium with students and academics promotes discourse, however, a socially constructed university has innumerable systems signified by synchronous and asynchronous teaching, delivering virtually a new normal demanding expeditious transformation to safeguard innovative teaching frameworks. The study examines the significant online pedagogical teaching enhancements. This qualitative desktop approach examines the bearing of online teaching at universities in South Africa. The analysis facilitates an understanding of virtual education, delivering clinical intermediations, cogitating COVID-19, intricacies, challenges, and opportunities. The chapter concludes with a clinical model that identifies SA risks with responses to challenges.

Part VII: Conclusion – Reflections on COVID-19 Interventions and Changes

The conclusion begins with reconstruction, rebuilding, and renewal of South African and Indian applied scholars by delivering a new clinical sociology for a post-COVID-19 world, as mapped out in Chapter 19. Training and professionalisation of clinical and applied sociology require urgent development in developing countries. At best, social work professionals were trained in medical sociology methods over the years. COVID-19, understood as a poly-pandemic, provided the intellectual window for the urgency of advancing the discipline of clinical and applied sociology. The methods and applications in a multidisciplinary context offer significant value. Theoretical foundations rest on the socio-medical crisis interventions recommended by the World Health Organization (WHO) and government-led task teams for COVID-19 safety protocol. The theories of crisis interventions (development crises, situational crises, and existential crises), transdisciplinary theory, and intersectionality scrutinise a poly-pandemic. The method of disciplinary analysis facilitates the establishment of a new clinical sociology, which is informed by poly-pandemic lessons. The current state of clinical and applied sociological methods and applications is ably suited for crises and therapeutic interventions at the levels of individuals and groups and micro-levels. However, at higher national and global levels, the methods and applications cannot measure up appropriately, mandating change and significant contextual modification. The development of new clinical and applied sociological methods and applications can serve global governance, programmes, and policy through the cooperation of clinical sociologists globally.

In Chapter 20, the editors conclude with a brief critical evaluation of a gendered pandemic world in which intersections of family, work, and community have played a critical role in pushing women to the edge amid the COVID-19 global pandemic. The clinical focus of this edited volume is by no means accidental. The social problems highlighted draw on institutions that sustain unequal family structures, systemic patriarchy in workspaces, and the exclusion of vulnerable women in communities across the globe.

Conclusion

The introductory chapters preview the 19 chapters, strategically segmented into seven universal themes carefully crafted to highlight clinical and applied sociological research, practice, and interventions resulting from pandemic responses. The edited series offers credence to the reality of women living on the edge, which was made worse by COVID-19. The clinical focus offers change agents and public policy specialists opportunities to effect change and improve the social condition of women, family, work, and community.

Part I
Gender-Based Violence

2 Intimate Partner Violence in Pandemic Times

The Experiences of Pregnant Women in Ibadan North, Oyo State, Nigeria

Alabi Oluwatobi Joseph and Akindele Favour Atinuke

Background

Intimate partner violence (IPV) is the psychological, emotional, physical, and/or economic abuse by a current or former partner; it also includes stalking and sexual abuse (Stylianou, 2018; Davila, Johnson, and Postmus, 2021). IPV is experienced across race, gender, sexual orientation, sociocultural, and religious class. IPV is relatively prevalent across communities and social classes, but factors that cause vulnerability include economic instability, unsafe household, inadequate access to social support, and other forms of marginalisation prevalent within societies (Gillum, 2019; Turell, Brown, and Herrmann, 2018; Sabri et al., 2020). Economic dependence is argued in literature as a major factor precipitating IPV; reliance on an abusive partner for livelihood or economic sustenance usually puts the victim at the mercy of the abuser, especially in situations where there are no economic alternatives. As such, the economic meltdown or disruption that accompanied the COVID-19 pandemic complicated relationships and exposed partners in abusive relationships to more abuse.

Lockdowns became necessary during the COVID-19 pandemic across many countries, as a measure to curtail and control the spread of the coronavirus. Consequently, this period witnessed an increased occurrence of domestic violence in intimate spaces (Fawole, Okedare, and Reed, 2021; UN Women, 2020b). Social isolation and movement restrictions confined victims and aggressors or potential aggressors within the same spaces with little or no opportunity to escape abuse or seek support. Exacerbating the spate of IPV at this period were income loss, inability to pay for housing and food, and stress, among other factors (Wood et al., 2022; Alnas-Smiley et al., 2020). As a result of the peculiarity of this period, fleeing abuse to safety became practically impossible.

Scholars argue that there was a surge in IPV cases globally because of the COVID-19 lockdown (Fraser, 2020; UN Women, 2020a). The UN Women (2020a) brief on COVID-19 and ending violence against women and girls reported that Singapore, France, and Cyprus experienced a 33%, 30%, and 25% increase,

DOI: 10.4324/9781003267133-3

respectively, in IPV cases during the lockdown. Also, spikes in IPV cases and housing demand were reported in Brazil, Germany, Canada, Italy, Spain, the United Kingdom, and the United States (UN Women, 2020a; Graham-Harrison et al., 2020). IPV is argued to have increased during the lockdown to about 56% in Nigeria (Fawole, Okedare, and Reed, 2021). A UN Women (2020b) report on the nature of gender-based violence in Nigeria during the COVID-19 pandemic noted that in the first two weeks of the lockdown (4–17 May 2020) IPV cases spiked from 346 to 794. It is important to note that these are reported cases; meanwhile, most cases of IPV in Nigeria are unreported for various sociocultural, geographical, and economic reasons (Cullen, 2020). Through this period of global uncertainty, women and children particularly in abusive intimate spaces are faced with multiple burdens. Hence, IPV-related experiences of pregnant women in the Ibadan–North area of Oyo State, Nigeria, were investigated and documented through this study.

Intimate Partner Violence and COVID-19 Pandemic: Severity and Prevalence

IPV is a global social problem that poses serious threats to the physical, mental, and social well-being of victims (Gama et al., 2021). IPV is reported by Evans, Lindauer, and Farrell (2020) to be experienced by one in every four women and ten men in the United States, respectively (and argued to be majorly perpetuated by men against women in heterosexual relationships and sometimes same-sex relationships (Lyons and Brewer, 2021; Brink et al., 2021). Beyond the narrative that men are the major perpetrators of IPV, some scholars argue that abuse in intimate relationships irrespective of the form is strongly connected to a dominant power structure and sociocultural normativity (Antai, 2011; Vyas and Jansen, 2018; Mondal and Paul, 2021; Sanger and Lynch, 2018). For instance, part of the arguments advanced for the underreporting of male abuse is the social stigma men often face when they lodge an official complaint of abuse by women (Demars, 2022; Nelson, 2019). Hence, abuse is more structural than gender-related; it is deeply understood when examined in relation to power structures and dynamics of marginalisation within societies (economic, sociocultural, political, etc.). There is also evidence in literature that male victimisation increased during the COVID-19 lockdown period (Ghimire et al., 2020; Jetelina, Knell, and Molsberry, 2021; Lausi et al., 2021).

Studies show that there is a possibility of an increased occurrence and prevalence of IPV in the face of crisis and disasters (Cannon et al., 2021; Brink et al., 2021; Lyons and Brewer, 2021; Nakyazze, 2020) such as hurricanes, economic meltdown, and pandemic such as COVID-19. A 10.4% increase in IPV prevalence was reported in Tunisia (Sediri et al., 2020; Lausi et al., 2021). Nakyazze (2020) argued that there is an increase in reported IPV cases across Africa even though the reported cases and prevalence statistics do not totally mirror the severity of the phenomenon. However, data from South Africa reported that there were over 87,000 incidents of gender-based violence (including IPV) in the first week of the lockdown (Masweneng, 2020).

Several studies have argued that IPV did not just remain prevalent through the COVID-19 pandemic, its severity and spate became alarming, especially in the first phase of the pandemic (Nakyazze, 2020; Masweneng, 2020). Many of these studies have been conducted as online surveys considering the lockdown measures, as well as the social distancing rules that became necessary because of the coronavirus pandemic. Gosangi et al. (2021) attempted to understand the severity of IPV during the pandemic (11 March 2020 and 3 May 2020) in comparison with the previous three years (2017, 2018, and 2019) at a large urban academic medical centre located in the north-eastern United States. Findings from this study show that IPV incidences during the COVID-19 pandemic were 1.8-fold higher than those in 2017–2019; there were 28 serious injuries (such as through strangulations, stab injuries, or use of weapons) during the period of observation compared to the 16 serious injuries reported between 2017 and 2019; and the number of white IPV victims surged from 26% recorded between 2017 and 2019 to 65% in 2020.

In an Ethiopian study examining the IPV experiences of women of reproductive age, under psychological, physical, and sexual violence categories, findings revealed that one-quarter of the study population had experienced IPV either in the form of insults, intimidation, attack on self-esteem (psychological violence), slapping, objects being thrown at victims (physical violence), and sexual intercourse under duress (sexual violence) (Gebrewahd, Gebremeskel, and Tadesse, 2020). This is like the findings of a Bangladesh study by Hamadani et al. (2020) which also reported women experiencing similar variants of IPV. In another study conducted in the United States, Jetelina, Knell, and Molsberry (2021) show that 18% (from 2,441) of the target population indicated experiencing IPV, the majority of whom mentioned that their experiences included screaming and insults. The study further revealed that men experienced IPV more than women in the study, which may be because of sexuality or the prevalence of IPV among them, especially male minority couples in the United States and very consistent with the argument presented above that abuse is usually more connected to relations of power (economic, social, political, cultural, among others) within intimate spaces. The study also revealed that about 17% of the participants who experienced IPV experienced an escalation of IPV, compared to 54% who asserted that victimisation remained the same, and 30% who affirmed that there was a reduction in IPV experiences during the pandemic. The study also recognised the relativity in physical victimisation among those that screened positive for IPV, as this worsened and improved significantly. While respondents reported that victimisation remained the same during the pandemic, they noted that physical and sexual victimisation became significantly increased as a result of stay-at-home measures put in place to curb the spread of the COVID-19 virus.

Ghimire et al. (2020) on interpersonal violence in Nepal found that 49% of the study respondents experienced only verbal violence, and 4% of the respondents experienced only physical violence, while 47% of the respondents experienced both verbal and physical violence. On the other hand, 43% of the study respondents admitted to committing verbal violence, 8.9% admitted to committing physical violence, while 48.5% have committed different forms of violence. The study also found men to be more of a victim than a perpetrator, making women less of a victim in this case. Sediri et al. (2020) equally observed that emotional abuse was the most experienced form of violence by women, followed by economic violence and physical violence. The study equally revealed that nearly all women who experienced IPV did not seek assistance, and those who experienced emotional abuse never reported it. The study reported a significant correlation between variants of violence during the lockdown and an increased rate of depression, anxiety, and stress among respondents.

Fawole, Okedare, and Reed (2021), in a study conducted in Nigeria, found that of all seven identified cases of IPV, there existed four forms of violence: psychological, physical, economic, and sexual violence. Their experiences included threats to be evicted from their houses, while two out of the victims were locked outside their apartments in the middle of the night by their partners. In addition, victims reported experiencing IPV that disrupted their sources of income, as well as victimisation when seeking custody of their children.

Findings from literature show that IPV is a serious social problem that affects women and men alike and continues to expose victims to various forms of injury and even death in some cases. While there are several literatures that have investigated the effects of IPV on women across the globe, thus establishing a pattern that women are often the victims in most cases, this study argues that often abuse within intimate spaces is brewed in relations to power structures – social, cultural, economic, and political. Approaching the investigation of IPV, particularly through this lens, broadens the scope of analysis and deepens the criticality of investigation.

Johan Galtung's Violence Triangle in the Context of Intimate Partner Violence

Galtung developed a framework (1967, 1990) for understanding violence; he explained violence in three interrelated dimensions – direct violence, structural violence, and cultural violence (see Figure 2.1).

Direct violence as depicted above is the most common type of violence. It often deploys physical force, for example, physical assault and killing, but can also include verbal or psychological behaviours that can cause humiliation, trauma, anxiety, or stress. Galtung (1969, p. 167) believes

> structural violence exists when some groups, classes, genders, nationalities, etc. are assumed to have, and in fact do have, more access to goods, resources, and opportunities than other groups, classes, genders, nationalities, etc., and this unequal advantage is built into the very social, political and economic systems that govern societies, states and the world.

Structural violence is woven into the complex interaction between various social systems of society. Societies are made up of systems and these systems form part of the functional (or dysfunctional) whole that fosters societal sustenance or existence. As such, these social systems create complex relationships of power that manifest in access to resources, decision-making, and opportunities. Galtung believes that these structures of society can result in the marginalisation or discrimination of certain groups or identities. This marginalisation is often a result of an interplay

DIRECT VIOLENCE

VISIBLE

INVISIBLE

CULTURAL VIOLENCE   STRUCTURAL VIOLENCE

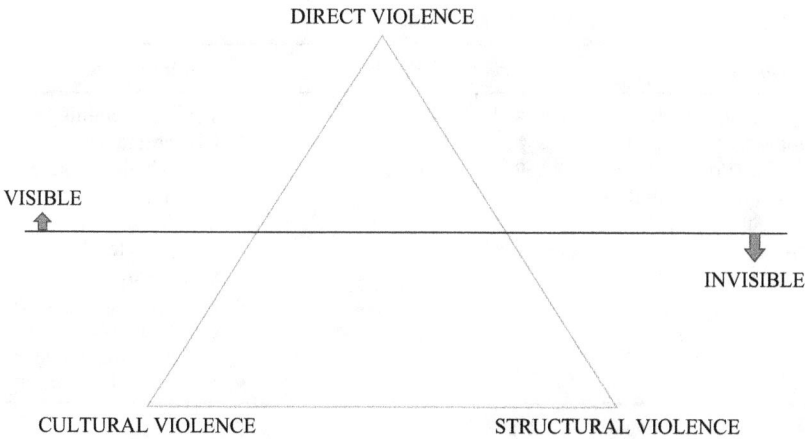

Figure 2.1 Galtung's violence triangle

of diverse factors like complex and intentional manipulation and orchestration of systems. He believes that this type of violence is usually not intended because it arises from the actions of certain groups within society trying to profit from the working of social systems, and as such he used the term 'social injustice' to describe structural violence. Without special attention to the intricacies of social systems and their implications on the lives of people, it becomes difficult to see the manifestations of structural violence.

Galtung describes cultural violence as the ideas, values, mores, and beliefs that are used to legitimise or normalise the direct and structural forms of violence. According to Galtung (1990, p. 292),

the study of cultural violence highlights the way in which the act of direct violence and the fact of structural violence are legitimised and thus rendered acceptable in society. One-way cultural violence works is by changing the moral colour of an act from red/wrong to green/right or at least to yellow/acceptable.

This form of violence includes prevailing stereotypes and prejudices existing in society that have been internalised, normalised, and used in everyday interactions.

Galtung suggests that these three forms of violence feed and reinforce each other; while direct violence is visible and common, structural, and cultural violence is not apparently visible in society. Therefore, contextualising and understanding IPV through this lens require critically explicating not just the direct consequences of abuse within intimate spaces but highlighting the structural factors that make these abuses possible and the various cultural ideologies that legitimise and normalise abuse (Table 2.1).

Table 2.1 Direct, structural, and cultural violence

Direct violence	Structural violence	Cultural violence
• Physical abuse – hitting, slapping, throwing objects • Emotional/psychological abuse – insults, humiliation, intimidation, attack on self-esteem • Sexual abuse	• Patriarchy • COVID-19 pandemic • Religion	• Toxic masculinity • Discriminatory widowhood practices • Discriminatory inheritance practices • Religious teachings on submission • Discriminatory gender role socialisation and performance languages • Subservient femininity

Source: Researcher's compilation (2022).

Structural violence in this context occurs in those social and cultural institutions that perpetuate abuse through the normalisation of dangerous ideas bordering on discrimination and marginalisation; it also includes ideas that discourage reporting abuse like in the case of epistemic barriers that discourage reporting intimate abuse among men because of stigma and social judgement. Hence, the structural violence perpetuated by institutions such as religion and patriarchy does not just normalise the abuse of women, it discourages men from reporting abuse (emphasis on culture and its normative ideas of masculinity). Contextually, COVID-19 and the hard lockdown was a structural process that exposed several women and some men to abuse; the peculiarities of this public health emergency confined abusers and victims within the same physical spaces with very little or non-existent help, and this offers some insight into why cases of IPV significantly surged during this period. While direct violence is an event occurring in time, structural violence is a complex ongoing process and cultural violence is more enduring because culture takes a gradual process to transform.

Methodology

Location of the Study

The study's location is important given its potential influence on the unique features of individual cases (Thorne, 2013). Ibadan is an ancient city in the Southwestern part of Nigeria, predominantly habited by the Yoruba people of Western Nigeria. The historically indigenous city has gradually transformed into a multicultural and multi-ethnic urban settlement boasting a vibrant economic system that attracts migrants from every part of the country. The proximity of the city to Lagos, as well as its cheaper livelihood (transport, housing, food, among others), makes it a desirable location. Specifically, the study areas are the University College Hospital (UCH), Ibadan, and Adeoyo Maternity Teaching Hospital in the Ibadan North Local Government Area of Oyo State. Participants were pregnant women (married and unmarried) registered and attending the Antenatal Care programme and healthcare workers.

Research Design

A phenomenological research design was adopted for this study. Creswell (2007) argued that phenomenology helps understand a social issue from the perspective of those experiencing or that have experienced it. It provides first-hand information in the understanding and analysis of social phenomena. Creswell (2007) notes that phenomenology is best suited for research that is concerned with understanding the common and shared experiences of several individuals about a phenomenon. Because it was important to bring to the fore the IPV-related experience of pregnant women during the COVID-19 lockdown, phenomenology became an appropriate research method.

Population of the Study

The population of the study constituted ten women (married and unmarried) attending antenatal care programmes at the University College Hospital (UCH), Ibadan, and Adeoyo Maternity Teaching Hospital in Ibadan and five healthcare workers. As emphasised by Johnson and Christensen (2010, p. 239), when researchers sample, 'they study the characteristics of a subset (called the sample), to understand the characteristics of the larger group (the population).' The sample thus gives the researcher a manageable size to examine, analyse, and understand to make inferable opinions about the nature of a problem affecting the general population.

Sampling Technique

A purposive sampling procedure was adopted for this study. In purposive sampling, researchers utilise their own judgement about which participants will be chosen. The purposive sampling technique was used to select participants based on their availability, as well as their readiness to participate in this study. The inclusion criteria are that the participant must be pregnant, in an intimate relationship, above the age of 18, and must be willing and available for the interview.

Data Collection

In-depth interviews were used to collect data from the participants with the aid of a semi-structured interview guide. An in-depth interview is a face-to-face (mostly long) interview conducted to obtain a deep understanding of a subject (Showkatand Parveen, 2017). Through this in-depth interview, participants' perceptions of patterns, prevalence, and effects of IPV on pregnant women in Ibadan North of Oyo State were adequately captured. Patients who met the inclusion criteria were identified and approached with the help of the staff (nurses and administrative officers) at the research locations. The study's aims and objectives were explained to the identified participants, and they were given some time to think about it before getting back to the researchers to express their interest. Some noted they were not interested immediately, a couple collected the information sheet and promised to reach out and some others indicated interest immediately. After drawing up a list of all the participants interested in the study, we agreed on a convenient time, and all interviews were carried out on the premises of the hospitals. Before every interview, the aim and objectives were explained to the participants, they were given an informed consent sheet and they were reminded that the consent to participate could be withdrawn at any point during the interview. The interviews lasted between 40 and 75 minutes.

Data Analysis

Several stages of data reading and coding were adopted to identify the themes and emerging patterns in participants' narratives for discussion in this study. These stages are re-reading the transcribed data for familiarisation; identifying, and labelling the themes that were jotted in the first phase, which were later used to develop major themes; themes were checked according to the participants' statements; and the main themes were separated from the sub-themes (Pretorius et al., 2011).

Ethical Considerations

Ethical approval was obtained from the ethics committees of the Oyo State Ministry of Health. Written informed consent was obtained from each participant at the beginning of each interview. Also, pseudonyms were assigned while writing this report to ensure the anonymity of the participants.

Results

The findings of this study show that the occurrence of IPV became more prevalent during the COVID-19 lockdown for various reasons including limited/restricted movement regulations, little/no access to formal and informal support networks, and a strained socio-economic climate. As such, pregnant women through the pandemic and specifically during the hard lockdown were exposed to multiple challenges – the threat of a deadly virus, challenges of gestation, and exposure to IPV without/with limited help (Table 2.2).

Intimate Partner Violence Incidents, Types, and Effects

Although the lockdown measure was not completely implemented in Ibadan, especially for economic reasons, findings from this study show that all study participants had experienced IPV in varying degrees, particularly during the first and second waves of COVID-19 when there was a hard lockdown across the country. The prevalence of IPV amongst all study participants shows its endemic nature within the study locale. Some of the violence/abuse common in the narratives of

Table 2.2 Variables

Variables	Numbers	Percentage (%)
Age group	6	40
• 18–25	9	60
• 26–40		
Level of education	2	13.3
• No formal education	4	26.7
• Secondary school	9	60
• Tertiary		
Employment status	9	60
• Employed	6	40
• Unemployed		
Marital status	11	73.3
• Married	4	26.7
• Single		
Income	2	13.3
• 0–₦ 25,000	9	60
• ₦ 25,000–₦ 50,000	4	26.7
• ₦ 50,000–₦ 100,000		

Source: Researcher's compilation (2022).

participants include physical assault, emotional, verbal, and sexual abuses. One of the participants recounted her experience and described it thus:

> Yes, my husband has assaulted me before, and I think this is an act of wickedness towards your partner. He often verbally abuses me and sometimes slaps me depending on how angry he was at the time, and all these happened more during that lockdown because he was always at home, and I don't know but it seems he just get angry unnecessarily.
>
> (IDI/Adeoyo maternity hospital/2021)

Another participant corroborated this:

> My husband is hot tempered, he slaps and hits me at the slightest provocation, and I get scared that he will kill me. But I do report to family, and they usually talk to him, and they tell me to be patient with him and be prayerful.
>
> (IDI/UCH/2021)

From the foregoing, physical incidence of IPV was an occurrence that was quite common throughout the pandemic, and in most cases, women are the victims of this abuse. This physical form of violence can be as severe as slaps, being hit, being beaten with objects like a belt, which causes scars and/or bruises on the victim's body. Triggering some of this incidence is the use of hard drugs, abuse of alcohol, stress often because of financial incapacitation, and toxic ideas of masculinity often looking to feast on power. Another type of abuse that was very prevalent in participants' narratives is verbal abuse. From the narratives, it also occurs in public spaces often causing embarrassment and potentially damage to a person's self-esteem. One of the participants described:

> I consider intimate partner violence as constant fighting between husband and wife. For me I think is verbally because my husband shouts at me a lot even in public. This usually affects me emotionally and often affects my self-esteem.
>
> (IDI/UCH/2021)

Multiple occurrences of situations where a person is publicly embarrassed usually take a negative toll on such individuals and can result in the loss or reduction in self-esteem, which will subsequently affect the personality, as well as the adequate functioning of such individuals. Another prevalent type of IPV is sexual abuse. One of the participants mentioned that:

> I often suffer sexual abuse from my husband; he doesn't know when someone is tired or that you are even pregnant that he should take it easy, all he wants is sex without care or understanding of your condition. He wants it whenever he likes even when I am not in the mood and has threatened to bring in another woman if I refuse him.
>
> (IDI/Adeoyo maternity hospital/2021)

Another participant recounted her experience and how it affected her pregnancy:

> The violence affected my last baby because he pushed me, and I fell on my stomach and started bleeding. So, based on this kind of experience, I will not want to be pregnant again because I don't want to experience losing a baby again except, I know he has changed and won't hit me again.
>
> (IDI/UCH/2021)

IPV has severe physical, mental, emotional, and health implications for victims. From the narrative above, physical abuse of a pregnant woman could lead to complications, loss of the baby, and severe health outcomes for the woman. Touching on abuse and its implication, another participant mentioned that 'there are days I missed clinic because my eyes were swollen, I did not want people to see it and ask what happened and I will feel shame to say (IDI/Adeoyo maternity hospital/2021).' One of the participants reiterated that the emotional and physical abuse of pregnant women by their partner affects gestation:

> As we know that any pregnant woman should be taken care of physically, emotionally, financially. There have been cases of beating that led to miscarriages and made us to deliver the baby before time because of the severity

of the case. And on these occasions, their husbands don't follow them for treatment.

(KII/Adeoyo maternity hospital/2021)

The effects of IPV on pregnant women, the foetus, and intimate relationships are complex and can be damaging; however, women in this context bear the brunt of these incidences. As such, it is important not just to understand this epidemic, but to implement workable frameworks to abate its spate. It is important to note that while the incidences discussed in this chapter as shared by participants are alarming, they only represent a fraction of the spate of IPV not only in Ibadan North but in Oyo State and Nigeria at large. Cases are usually not reported to both formal and informal networks of support because of shame and the normative (often dangerous) idea that an intimate relationship is a private affair between a man and woman that does not require the interference of a third party. Expressing this line of thought, one of the participants mentioned:

> I think it happens a lot, but only a few cases are being reported because many don't like to talk about it, and one cannot deny IPV occurrences. Sometimes, during our interaction with pregnant women, we get to know the real issues, and when we probe further, many of them do not want to talk about it. Some will just be sobbing helplessly.

(KII/UCH/2021)

Narratives of participants in this study bring to the fore the severity of IPV. We argued that the hard lockdown because of the COVID-19 pandemic exposed pregnant women to abuse with very limited or no support networks. The most common types of IPV experienced by participants are physical, emotional, verbal, and sexual abuses. We brought to the fore the factors triggering some of these abuses which include alcohol abuse, use of hard drugs, and toxic ideas about masculinity.

Surviving the Shadow Pandemic: Pregnant Women's IPV Coping Strategies

The previous section has indicated and discussed the various forms of intimate partner violence that pervaded the lives of pregnant women in the Ibadan North Local Government Area. To survive and conquer these epidemics (COVID-19 and IPV), these women adopted different coping strategies – survival tools. Nevertheless, certain factors mediate between their experience of IPV and the coping strategies they adopt. A crucial observation from the study is that these women in many cases do not report their experiences to any formal authority, but only to informal authority, and have expressed their dissatisfaction with the outcomes of the reports made. However, they have adopted various personal strategies during their plight of being abused. These include prayers, crying, and make-up to cover their scars. One of the participants noted:

I don't report to anyone because I don't want people to laugh at me and I don't want anything that will annoy my husband more. I also did not like the response I got when I reported the issue first few times, he beat me, so I decided to talk to God instead. People that you think will speak sense to him will tell you to watch your behaviour, your husband is the head of the home, you must be submissive, don't do anything that will anger him. Really? I was really shocked, so he is apparently justified to hit me, I am obviously the problem.

(IDI/UCH/2021)

The narrative above actually captures the thought of most of the participants in this study, they have come to accept that IPV is part of the ordeal they must deal with in intimate relationships – fate, a burden to bear. Hence, their surest hope is to continue to pray that God changes their partner and that they have the strength to prevail and overcome this plight. One of the participants said:

I pray about my husband every day and I believe God can still change my husband and he will love me more. More so, my children are there as my source of joy. So, I have nothing to worry about. He will change some day but for now I keep crying, enduring the pain, wearing makeup to cover the scars so people won't notice and praying fervently that God changes him.

(IDI/UCH/2021)

These strategies that were adopted by married women were perceived as a means of comfort to them, as they believe that they have found themselves in a helpless situation, and have completely accepted their fate, hoping that their partner will change someday. In addition, another strategy that was adopted, though on behalf of the victim (by their partners), has been to take actions such as taking their wives out, or purchasing items for them, in a bid to make up for their actions. This suggests that the perpetrators are aware that their actions are untoward and unwarranted, prompting them to make up for such misdeeds, but they tend to persist in committing those terrible acts. It is important to state that these coping strategies do not necessarily keep women from abuse; rather it helps them endure and stay with the abuser, it is dangerous and potentially damaging to the physical, mental, and emotional well-being of the victims.

Discussion of Findings

This study provides evidence of IPV among pregnant women during the COVID-19 hard lockdown, and this is consistent with findings in literature that there is usually a high occurrence of violence in times of disaster or crisis (Krahé and Berger, 2013; Graham-Harrison et al., 2020). Pregnant women's experiences of IPV as explained in this chapter are complicated by the restriction of movement and/or confinement of people within their households (Fawole, Okedare, and Reed, 2021). IPV has severe implications for the reproductive, physical, and mental health of the victims and the common effects from participants' narratives include preterm birth, induced abortion, low birth weight, maternal/infant mortality, suicidal ideation, placental abruption, miscarriage, depression, and pelvic pains. This implies that aside from the poor state of health infrastructure contributing to poor gestation outcomes and maternal/ infant mortality in Nigeria, IPV plays subtle but significantly dangerous roles.

The strategies adopted for survival as described by participants in this study are very personal, ranging from prayers to crying, resort to fate, support from friends, understanding family members, and religious institutions, and in very rare instances support from health professionals and police. Interestingly, there is a normalised but dangerous ideology about intimate abuse that participants in this study connected to what is arguably masculinity's innate tendency to be aggressive and violent. Further probing revealed that most participants believe 'men will be men,' and this means they are naturally violent and aggressive: a perception of problematic male behaviours (varying and complex forms of masculinities) that have been argued in literature to (re)produce domestic violence (Thacker, 2019; Parkhill and Ray, 2020).

This study also revealed that most of the victims of IPV do not report abuse or seek help because of various normative ideas about marriage, relationships, gender roles, specifically a recurring acceptance of masculinity as innately aggressive and toxic. This type of masculinity is one that is understood to (re)produce itself through normative sociocultural practices and gender expectations that are often limiting for women, and justification for gender-based violence within the patriarchal system of power. These epistemic barriers to reporting IPV-related abuses are very consistent with arguments made in the literature (Hardyns et al., 2020; Nandakumar, 2018). Victims do not trust the justice system, and there is a deep sense of distrust for the formal and informal support systems available because most often they feel the significance of abuse is downplayed. This distrust is fuelled by a feeling of shame and embarrassment that comes from opening up about abuse. Also, because of the restrictions on movement during the hard lockdown, seeking help from health services, police, and community-support groups might not have been feasible.

Limitation and Recommendation for Future Research

It is important to put into consideration methodological limitations in the interpretation of the findings of this study. Its scope, locale, and sociocultural context are significant factors that could potentially influence the narratives of participants as shared and analysed. The participants were recruited from selected (accessible) antenatal care centres in Ibadan North, and this might have hindered the chances of recruiting marginalised participants who might not be able to afford healthcare. Also, this study did not account for the roles that age, income, and education, among several other socio-economic variables, might play in the experience of IPV among pregnant women in the study location. More studies are required to highlight marginalised pregnant women's experiences of IPV as well as the roles that age, education, and income could play in this.

Conclusion and Recommendations

This study examined IPV experiences of pregnant women in Ibadan North during the COVID-19 pandemic lockdown in 2020. The findings revealed that IPV is prevalent among pregnant women in the study location during the pandemic with a degree that might be higher than usual with very limited support because of the regulations implemented to curb the spread of the deadly coronavirus.

Participants in this study (pregnant women particularly) were burdened by multiple challenges throughout this period; they described how they had to cope with the demands of gestating in the face of restricted movement where access to medical help through antenatal programmes was limited. This alone was mentally and physically draining for these women. To them, it was normative to access the medical and social support that antenatal clinics provided on a weekly basis, but with the COVID-19 pandemic and the attendant public health policy consequence, some of them barely made it to antenatal once in a month and it implicatively created concern for their safety and that of their pregnancy.

Also, participants explained how being trapped in the home with an abusive partner because of the hard lockdown complicated the already precarious situation, exposed them to repeated abuse, and increased their level of anxiety. Further, this chapter highlighted and critically discussed the most common types of abuse pregnant women in the study location reported. They include physical (including sexual), emotional, and verbal abuses that are (re)produced and sustained through cultural and structural violence and complicated by the peculiarities of the COVID-19 pandemic.

The effect of abuse during pregnancy could be very damaging as it could affect the reproductive, mental, and physical well-being of the woman. As such, it is important to put in place multilevel (formal and informal support, national, state, local government, and community-based) support systems to tackle abuse. These systems of support will have to be designed in a way that they will remain functional and accessible during times of crisis to continually provide support.

Organisations supporting women experiencing or exposed to abuse should work closely with community-based networks (clinics, market women associations, diverse artisan associations, among others) to increase their reach to victims (including potential), and these organisations must be strongly supported with funding that remains in the long term and not just bails out in the face of an emergency. It is important that technologies such as responsive-free SMS service for reporting abuse, support WhatsApp groups, and other online tools are leveraged in an attempt to provide better support systems for victims of abuse. Cost-effective mobile phones can be provided for women without access to phones or the internet. Helplines, psychosocial support, and online counselling should be implemented and popularised. It is not only during times of crisis that these support systems should be utilised, but they should also be normalised so the stigma of reporting abuse is reduced.

Sociocultural and religious beliefs (re)producing and/or legitimising the subordination of women need to be addressed; targeted campaigns aimed at reorienting the populace, especially men about problematic male behaviours that often promote aggression, dominance, and abuse among several others must be initiated. Campaigns through religious institutions, government parastatals, private organisations, and labour unions sensitising people about abuse, highlighting the facts and dangers of IPV as well as domestic violence, and encouraging people to take positive steps like sharing care responsibilities at home and within neighbourhoods must be pursued nationally.

References

Alnas-Smiley, K., Huey, M., Valmores, N. and Moni, S. (2020). Impact of coronavirus on services to survivors of intimate partner violence: A look at my sister's house. *Journal of Asian American Studies, 23*(3), pp. 407–419.

Antai, D. (2011). Controlling behavior, power relations within intimate relationships and intimate partner physical and sexual violence against women in Nigeria. *BMC Public Health, 11*(1), pp. 1–11.

Brink, J., Cullen, P., Beek, K. and Peters, S.A. (2021). Intimate partner violence during the COVID-19 pandemic in Western and Southern European countries. *European Journal of Public Health, 31*(5), pp. 1058–1063.

Cannon, C.E., Ferreira, R., Buttell, F. and First, J. (2021). COVID-19, intimate partner violence, and communication ecologies. *American Behavioral Scientist, 65*(7), pp. 992–1013.

Creswell, J.W. (2007). *Qualitative inquiry and research design: Choosing among five approaches* (2nd ed.). Los Angeles: Sage Publications.

Cullen, C. (2020). Method matters: Underreporting of intimate partner violence in Nigeria and Rwanda. World Bank Policy Research Working Paper (9274).

Davila, A.L., Johnson, L. and Postmus, J.L. (2021). Examining the relationship between economic abuse and mental health among Latina intimate partner violence survivors in the United States. *Journal of Interpersonal Violence, 36*(1–2), pp. 287–310.

Demars, R. (2022). *Male victims of interpersonal abuse: How to best break the barriers and toxic masculinity men encounter when seeking services and suggested guidelines for agencies when offering services to men.* Seminar paper presented at the University of Wisconsin-Platteville.

Evans, M.L., Lindauer, M. and Farrell, M.E. (2020). A pandemic within a pandemic— Intimate partner violence during Covid-19. *New England Journal of Medicine, 383*(24), pp. 2302–2304.

Fawole, O.I., Okedare, O.O. and Reed, E. (2021). Home was not a safe haven: Women's experiences of intimate partner violence during the COVID-19 lockdown in Nigeria. *BMC Women''s Health, 21*(1), pp. 1–7.

Fraser, E. (2020). *Impact of COVID-19 pandemic on violence against women and girls.* UKAid VAWG Helpdesk Research Report, 284.

Galtung, J. (1967). Theories of peace. *A Synthetic Approach to Peace Thinking.* Oslo: International Peace Research Institute, pp. 1–251.

Galtung, J. (1969). Violence, peace, and peace research. *Journal of Peace Research, 6*(3), pp. 167–191.

Galtung, J. (1990). Cultural violence. *Journal of Peace Research, 27*(3), pp. 291–305.

Gama, A., Pedro, A.R., Leote de Carvalho, M.J., Guerreiro, A.E., Duarte, V., Quintas, J., Matias, A., Keygnaert, I. and Dias, S. (2021). Domestic violence during the COVID-19 pandemic in Portugal. *Portuguese Journal of Public Health, 38*(1), pp. 32–33.

Gebrewahd, G.T., Gebremeskel, G.G. and Tadesse, D.B. (2020). Intimate partner violence against reproductive age women during COVID-19 pandemic in Northern Ethiopia 2020: A community-based cross-sectional study. *Journal of Open Access BioMed Central, 17*(152), pp. 4–6.

Ghimire, C., Acharya, S., Shrestha, C., ,KC P., Singh, S. and Sharma, P. (2020). Interpersonal violence during the COVID-19 lockdown period in Nepal: A descriptive cross-sectional study. *Journal of Nepal Medical Association, 58*(230), pp. 751–757.

Gillum, T.L. (2019). The intersection of intimate partner violence and poverty in Black communities. *Aggression and Violent Behavior, 46*, pp. 37–44. https://doi.org/10.1016/j.avb.2019.01.008.

Gosangi, B., Park, H., Thomas, R., Gujrathi, R., Bay, C.P., Raja, A.S., Seltzer, S.E., Balcom, M.C., McDonald, M.L., Orgill, D.P. and Harris, M.B. (2021). Exacerbation of physical intimate partner violence during COVID-19 pandemic. *Radiology, 298*(1), pp. E38–E45.

Graham-Harrison, E., Giuffrida, A., Smith, H. and Ford, L. (2020). Lockdowns around the world bring rise in domestic violence. *The Guardian, 28*.

Hamadani, J.D., Hasan, M.I., Baldi, A.J., Hossain, S.J., Shiraji, S., Bhuiyan, M.S.A., Mehrin, S.F., Fisher, J., Tofail, F., Tipu, S.M.U. and Grantham-McGregor, S. (2020). Immediate impact of stay-at-home orders to control COVID-19 transmission on socioeconomic conditions, food insecurity, mental health, and intimate partner violence in Bangladeshi women and their families: An interrupted time series. *The Lancet Global Health, 8*(11), pp. e1380–e1389.

Hardyns, W., Keygnaert, I., Ponnet, K. and Vandeviver, C. (2020). Partner and domestic violence during the COVID-19 crisis. *Freedom From Fear, 2020*(16), pp. 48–55.

Jetelina, K.K., Knell, G. and Molsberry, R.J. (2021). Changes in intimate partner violence during the early stages of the COVID-19 pandemic in the USA. *Injury Prevention, 27*(1), pp. 93–97.

Johnson, B. and Christensen, L. (2010). *Educational research: Quantitative, qualitative, and mixed approaches* (4th ed.). Los Angeles: Sage Publications.

Krahé, B. and Berger, A. (2013). Men and women as perpetrators and victims of sexual aggression in heterosexual and same-sex encounters: A study of first-year college students in Germany. *Aggressive Behavior, 39*(5), pp. 391–404.

Lausi, G., Pizzo, A., Cricenti, C., Baldi, M., Desiderio, R., Giannini, A.M. and Mari, E. (2021). Intimate partner violence during the COVID-19 pandemic: A review of the phenomenon from victims' and help professionals' perspectives. *International Journal of Environmental Research and Public Health, 18*(12), pp. 1–17.

Lyons, M. and Brewer, G. (2021). Experiences of intimate partner violence during lockdown and the COVID-19 pandemic. *Journal of Family Violence*, pp. 1–9. https://doi.org/10.1007/s10896-021-00260-x.

Masweneng, K. (2020). Gender based violence complaints hit 87,000 so far in lockdown, as cop arrested for allegedly raping wife. Available at: https://www.timeslive.co.za/news/south-africa/2020-04-03-gender-based-violence-complaints-hit-87000-so-far-in-lockdown-as-cop-arrested-for-allegedly-raping-wife/.

Mondal, D. and Paul, P. (2021). Associations of power relations, wife-beating attitudes, and controlling behavior of husband with domestic violence against women in India: Insights from the National Family Health Survey–4. *Violence against Women, 27*(14), pp. 2530–2551.

Nakyazze, B. (2020). Intimate partner violence during the COVID-19 pandemic: An impending public health crisis in Africa. *The Anatolian Journal of Family Medicine, 3*(2), pp. 92–94.

Nandakumar, M. (2018). *Pathologizing abuse: Examining public health approaches to addressing intimate partner violence in Canada* (Masters Dissertation at York University).

Nelson, M. (2019). *Traditional gender roles: The culture of toxic masculinity and the effect on male rape victims* (Masters Dissertation at Bridgewater State University).

Parkhill, M.R. and Ray, T.N. (2020). *The role of masculinity in the perpetration of relationship violence.* Los Angeles: Sage Publications.

Pretorius, G., Chauke, P.A. and Morgan, B. (2011). The lived experiences of mothers whose children were sexually abused by their intimate male partners. *Indo-Pacific Journal of Phenomenology, 11*(1), pp. 1–14.

Sabri, B., Hartley, M., Saha, J., Murray, S., Glass, N. and Campbell, J.C. (2020). Effect of COVID-19 pandemic on women's health and safety: A study of immigrant survivors of intimate partner violence. *Health Care for Women International, 41*(11–12), pp. 1294–1312.

Sanger, N. and Lynch, I. (2018). 'You have to bow right here': Heteronormative scripts and intimate partner violence in women's same-sex relationships. *Culture, Health & Sexuality, 20*(2), pp. 201–217.

Sediri, S., Zgueb, Y., Ouanes, S., Ouali, U., Bourgou, S., Jomli, R. and Nacef, F. (2020). Women's mental health: Acute impact of COVID-19 pandemic on domestic violence. *Archives of Women's Mental Health, 23*(6), pp. 749–756.

Stylianou, A.M. (2018). Economic abuse experiences and depressive symptoms among victims of intimate partner violence. *Journal of Family Violence, 33*(6), pp. 381–392.

Thacker, L. (2019). *The danger of 'no': Rejection violence, toxic masculinity and violence against women* (Doctoral dissertation, Eastern Kentucky University).

Thorne, S. (2013). Interpretive description. In T. Beck (Ed.), *Routledge international handbook of qualitative nursing research* (pp. 295–306). London: Routledge.

Turell, S.C., Brown, M. and Herrmann, M. (2018). Disproportionately high: An exploration of intimate partner violence prevalence rates for bisexual people. *Sexual and Relationship Therapy, 33*(1–2), pp. 113–131.

UN Women. (2020a). Issue brief: COVID-19 and ending violence against women and girls. Available at: https://perma.cc/G48D-BVCU.

UN Women. (2020b). Gender-based violence in Nigeria during the COVID-19 crisis: The shadow pandemic.

Vyas, S. and Jansen, H.A. (2018). Unequal power relations and partner violence against women in Tanzania: A cross-sectional analysis. *BMC Women's Health, 18*(1), pp. 1–12.

Wood, L., Schrag, R.V., Baumler, E., Hairston, D., Guillot-Wright, S., Torres, E. and Temple, J.R. (2022). On the front lines of the COVID-19 pandemic: Occupational experiences of the intimate partner violence and sexual assault workforce. *Journal of Interpersonal Violence, 37*(11–12), pp. NP9345–NP9366.

3 COVID-19 and Gender-Based Violence

Experiences of Zimbabwean Flood Victims

Takunda Mathathu, Mariam Seedat-Khan, and Thomas Gumbo

Introduction

Gender-based violence (GBV) violates fundamental human rights, expressing toxic masculinity and varying prevalence in societies globally. GBV encompasses sexual threats, exploitation, domestic violence, sexual assaults, prostitution, female genital mutilation, and trafficking that increase morbidity (Mashiri and Mawire, 2013). GBV affects the victim's self-esteem and hinders the attainment of countries' developmental goals. Dlamini (2021: 584) argued, 'violence against girls and women undermines countries' achievements of at least the first six of the eight United Nations Millennium Development Goals.' GBV impacts victims and impedes socio-economic progression despite initiatives. The onset of COVID-19 deepened women's vulnerability acting as a catalyst for GBV. State lockdowns restricted movements accelerating existing GBV. Sharma and Borah (2020: 2) contend 'domestic abuse is acting like an opportunistic infection, flourishing in the conditions created by the pandemic.' The surge of GBV globally saw UN Women (2020) identify COVID-19 as a GBV catalyst, conceptualising it as 'the shadow pandemic' (UN Women, 2020). GBV is dubbed a pandemic within COVID-19, confining women with abusers (Safe, 2020), limiting police access. Perpetrators' proximity to victims of GBV and intimate partner violence (IPV) is characterised by co-dependent relationships (Van Raemdonck, Seedat-Khan, and Raeymackers, 2017). Public and private systemic patriarchy in dowry systems increases GBV. Partnerships intended to offer security increases victims' vulnerability (Made and Nyakujarah, 2015). Women are stripped of agency and refuge and quarantined with frequent violence. Separation from supportive networks, isolation, and natural disasters disrupts normative lifestyles, increasing GBV (Sharma and Borah, 2020). Temporary shelters and lockdown COVID-19 protocol increased vulnerability. UN Women estimated 736 million women experienced some form of GBV increase in 2020–2022 (UN Women, 2021). Zimbabwe reported a 69.5% increase in IPV between March 2020 and June 2020 (Safe, 2020). Chitando (2020) reported that the National Musasa GBV NGO hotline registered 10,000 cases, a huge increase from the 500 incidences recorded pre-COVID-19. We contend that COVID-19 and natural disasters disproportionately affected rural women, exacerbating GBV and inequality (Agarwal, 1997).

DOI: 10.4324/9781003267133-4

Women's Disaster Vulnerability

Women are disadvantaged socially, economically, and culturally, making them highly vulnerable to COVID-19 and disasters. Social vulnerability intersects with gender inequalities, reducing women's social and economic capital to respond to natural disasters (Armas and Gavris, 2013; Matiza, 2021). Characteristics that include age, health, income, housing, and employment determine women's socially constructed vulnerability. Azad, Hossain, and Nasreen, (2013: 192) argue that 'the patriarchal nature of society, the position of women, their needs and capabilities' places women in a further vulnerable state than men. Exposure demographics and socio-economic contexts determine communities' susceptibility to natural disasters (Berkes, 2007; Solangaarachchi, Griffin and Doherty, 2012). De Silva and Jayathilaka's (2014) study on flood risks in Sri Lanka asserted women's disaster vulnerability embedded in cultural processes. Normative sociocultural patterns perpetuate disparities to sustain susceptibility (Ciampi Gell, Lasap, and Turvill, 2011). Nabegu's (2014) study on flooding in Kano, Nigeria, reported that gendered roles influenced fatalities, indicating 72% of women and 28% men died during flooding. All indicators demonstrate that gender dynamics in society curtails women's capability to respond to disasters effectively. GBV increased amid the pandemic in the Global South. Sharma and Borah (2020: 3) found that the lockdown COVID-19 protocol prompted a global recession creating a climate that 'can fuel violence.' GBV and COVID-19 within a post-flood Zimbabwean context mandated urgent humanitarian aid. Intersections indicated the prioritisation of gender-inclusive clinical interventions to mitigate GBV risk and secure financial food, human security, and relief access for rural women. Interventions prioritising rural women must establish access to facilitate COVID-19 screening and access to treatment.

Simultaneously occurring, COVID-19 and flooding forced a state of disaster, made worse by psychological and financial insecurity that caused the proliferation of GBV in shelters. A systematic review of natural disaster literature established that 'one in five refugee and displaced women experience violence' (Sommer, Likindikoki, and Kaaya, 2013: 154). GBV is pervasive in post-flood Zimbabwe with displaced women's vulnerability to violence heightened by a gender-blind temporary shelter. Baig and Sharif (2013), Djalante; Thomalla, Sinapoy, and Carnegie (2012); Rabbani, Rahman, and Mainuddin (2009); and Horton (2012) indicate incidents of abuse, violence, and rape increased during tsunami and floods in Sri Lanka, Indonesia, Thailand, Bangladesh, and India (Emmar, 2017). Azad, Hossain, and Nasreen (2013) report that 58% of participants stated that they were harassed daily by their husbands. Data was validated by a key informant who verified daily increases of GBV in temporary camps (Azad, Hossain, and Nasreen, 2013). Fisher (2010: 908) noted that 'domestic violence was considered by most of the respondents to be the most prevalent and sustained form of post-disaster violence against women in all provinces that were affected by the tsunami disaster.' Reyes and Lu (2016) reported a rise in cases of sexual harassment in temporary shelters for disaster victims. Likewise, Nguyen and Rydstrom (2018) found intensifying GBV incidences after typhoon Haiyan in Vietnam and the Philippines, where 'women were subjected to violence in the home by their partner and also in the public realm' (Nguyen and Rydstrom, 2018: 56). Distressing GBV victim paradox denies women agency 'if they decide or are forced by their partner to stay home, they risk the danger of enduring or escalating violence and if they can leave, they risk exposure to COVID-19, a highly infectious and dangerous virus' (Kofman and Garfin, 2020: 2; Chamorro-Premuzic and Wittenberg-Cox, 2021). GBV exacerbated disaster-induced unemployment and the loss of household property and possessions.

Fisher (2010: 906) noted 'disaster affected communities endure considerable loss, stress, trauma and disruption to everyday life of the household including family responsibilities and income generation.' A study conducted in Bangladesh showed that men physically abused their wives due to financial difficulties. For instance, 'one mother said that her husband did not want to hear anything about the family, when she was talking about how much rice was needed, her husband suddenly became angry and kicked her' (Biswas et al., 2010: 6). These findings are consistent with Demettriades and Esplen's (2010: 135) argument that 'the experiences of poverty, a decline in food security and livelihood opportunities can also cause considerable stress for men given the social expectation that they have to provide economically for the household.' Wisner (1998) argued that there is a correlation between expected gender roles and the impacts of floods, by illustrating how the loss of families' possessions often leads to tensions and GBV within families.

Theoretical Framework

The capability approach offers a comprehensive guide to understand gender gaps, enabling researchers to avoid generalisation of women's lived experiences in a patriarchal post-flood, COVID-19, and rural geography context. The capability approach provides the foundations for an accurate analysis. The framework traverses notions of intersectionality theory which argues how several systemic oppressions increase GBV (Cho, Crenshaw, and McCall, 2013). Intersectionality advances individuals at varied socio-economic classes, stratified along class, race, and gender intersections (Raza, 2017; Carbado and Harris, 2019). Gopaldas (2013: 90) and Poole et al., (2020) stated, 'theory of intersectionality refers to the interactivity of social identity structures such as race, class and gender in fostering life experience, especially experiences of privilege and oppression.' Santos and Toomey (2018) note that an intersectionality lens helps understand overlapping systems of oppression. Class and status intersections determine women's vulnerability to flood disasters, GBV, and COVID-19.

Zimbabwean rural women's lived experience demonstrates higher poverty levels than urban women showing that 'human behaviour and functioning is not the same for every individual' (Teater, 2010: 75). Exploring women's post-flood vulnerability relies on the capability framework propounded by Sen (1979) as cited in Tyupa, (2011). The capability approach is a theoretical framework 'discipline that gives a central role to the evaluation of a person's achievements and freedoms in terms of his or her actual ability to do the different things a person has reason to value doing or being' (Sen, 2009: 16; Robeyns,2017). The capability approach offers a rich understanding of the gendered flood experiences to evaluate inequality and poverty. Applying the notions of functioning and capabilities was crucial in denoting how rural women residing in substandard emergency shelters governed by norms constraining their capabilities to live a life of value. Flood victims denied functionings and capabilities limited by exclusion. Capabilities framework assessed the distribution of socio-economic resources, access, and opportunities that enhanced meaningful satisfaction. Inadequate amenities compromise the realisation of capabilities, intensifying women's socio-economic vulnerability. Women failed to access equitable treatment, limiting successes, intensifying poverty, and marginalisation. Women's safety and security rights are compromised and aggravated by poorly designed accommodation structures in Tokwe–Mukosi. Mobile unisex toilets located outside compromise privacy and safe access with frequent GBV reports. Temporary shelters intensify mental and emotional health impacting women realising capabilities.

Methodology

The study employed an inductive qualitative approach, underpinned by an interpretive perspective. This form of research focuses on examining human behaviour in its natural context through the participants' viewpoints, which originate from field contacts (Babbie and Mouton, 2007; Ponelis, 2015). The emphasis is on eliciting meanings and interpretations from the participants' words, allowing for a better understanding of their social reality. Interpretivism facilitates a rigorous grasp of natural disasters and gendered complexities within the Zimbabwean context (Creswell, 2009). To this end, the two focus group discussions and 12 in-depth interviews conducted using open-ended questions enabled the researchers to document the lived experiences of women residing in the flood-stricken Tokwe–Mukosi area.

Research Site

The study was conducted in Chingwizi, a temporary camp located adjacent to the Tokwe–Mukosi area within Masvingo Province, Region IV in Zimbabwe. The Tokwe–Mukosi dam is constructed at the confluence of two rivers, the Tokwe and Mukosi, earning its name (Chazireni and Chigonda, 2018). The area is a semi-intensive agricultural region, with an average annual rainfall of 300–600 mm (Chazireni and Chigonda, 2018). The region's varying seasons increase flooding and seasonal droughts. In January and February 2014, the Tokwe–Mukosi region recorded 850 mm of rain, with detrimental after-effects. Tarisayi (2015) indicated that 2014 rains caused flooding displacing 6,000 families from 12 villages. At the outset, 80% of rural flood victims were transferred to the Chingwizi temporary camp (Chendume, 2016). Effects of intensified flooding were specifically evident among women's well-being and quality of life. Hove (2016) and Tarisayi (2018) found that cultural and systemic patriarchy marginalised women.

Sample

Purposive and snowballing sampling techniques were used to select the 12 women affected by the Tokwe–Mukosi floods. Purposive sampling is a technique to recognise data-rich cases and optimise limited resources (Patton, 2002). Locating and selecting respondents or groups offers lived intelligence about personal GBV experiences (Bless, Higson-Smith, and Sithole, 2013). On the other hand, snowball sampling is when the researcher requests participants to identify others in a similar situation (De Vos, Strydom, Fouche, and Delport, 2002). In turn, the identified persons are requested to identify others with similar characteristics who may also potentially make up the study sample. The snowballing strategy is applied to this inquiry as the targeted participants were difficult to locate because of the stigma associated with GBV. The two methods were selected to obtain responses relevant to the study from participants who had first-hand knowledge and a vested interest in the topic.

Data Collection

A triangulation strategy was used to collect data. According to Terre Blanche and Durrheim (1999: 128), 'triangulation helps researchers to home in on a correct understanding of phenomenon by approaching it from several different angles.' Furthermore, triangulation allows for a thorough understanding of phenomena. It provides more than one data collecting source to ensure rigour, reliability, validity, and good quality are reached during data collection operations (Patton, 2002). Consequently, data was collected through focus group discussions, in-depth interviews, and participant observation to explore gender-specific challenges confronting rural women living in temporary shelters in a post-flood disaster context. A focus group interview schedule guided the focus group discussions. The focus group guided in-depth data collection, employing open-ended questions, which did not strictly adhere to a pre-designed plan. An audio recorder was used to collect knowledge from focus groups and interviews. Data was transcribed verbatim, to maintain fair, valid, and reliable analysis. Research instruments were translated and made available in Shona and English. While participants all spoke and understood English, Shona was their first language, which required the use of the back-translation technique.

Analysis

Thematic analysis of the data was undertaken. Ibrahim (2012: 40) reinforces that 'thematic content analysis is a type of qualitative analysis used to analyse classifications and present themes or patterns that relate to the data.' Moreover, it greatly illustrates the data and deals with diverse subjects via interpretations (Boyatziz, 1998). Trustworthiness was ensured through credibility, transferability, dependability, and confirmability. Data triangulation, peer review, persistent observation, and reflexivity were also employed. Transferability was maintained by providing rich accounts of the context, sample size, sample strategy, demographic, interview procedure, and excerpts from the guide. To ensure dependability, a pilot test was conducted with a population similar to the main study. And to fulfil the task of confirmability, an audit trial which included process notes, observation notes, audio recordings, and transcripts was maintained. The study was steered by key ethical considerations: human participant's protection, informed consent, voluntary participation, protection from harm and privacy, anonymity, and confidentiality. Before commencing the research study, the researchers obtained ethical approval from the Humanities and Social Sciences Research Ethics Committee at the University of KwaZulu-Natal, South Africa. Permission to conduct research in the Chingwizi temporary camp was obtained via a gatekeeper's letter from the local authority.

GBV, Floods, and COVID-19 Intersections

Families in disaster-affected communities face significant losses and disruption in their daily lives, including family responsibilities and income generation, all of which fuel GBV. Given the social expectation that males contribute economically to the household, a loss in food security and livelihood prospects can generate significant stress for men. The high prevalence of GBV in the aftermath of floods has been exacerbated by the COVID-19 pandemic as highlighted by participants in the current study. Pandemic data demonstrates that all forms of GBV and IPV have intensified. Participants highlighted that:

> There is patriarchal dominance by men over women in the camp. Our needs as women are not taken seriously and we are left to suffer from emotional, physical, and sexual abuse from men. This has increased dramatically because of COVID-19 as most of the men in the camp are no longer working and they tend to vent their frustrations on women.
>
> (Chipo Dumba)

> GBV in the camps is a daily occurrence as most women are being beaten by their husbands because men here are struggling to sustain their families, and women tend to feel the full brunt of men's joblessness as they are beaten when asking for money for the upkeep of the family. Men's livelihood sources were disrupted by COVID-19 and as women we are left to suffer the consequences of both floods and COVID-19.
>
> (Kundai Zondo)

It is impossible to secure employment in the aftermath of floods, making women become scapegoats for venting their frustrations. Loss of income-generating sources during the pandemic escalated economic vulnerability and pervasive poverty within poor households. In turn, socio-economic adversity triggered by absent livelihoods intensified IPV and increased domestic conflict over familial care and support. Limited economic opportunities and resources left male bread-winners frustrated and emasculated. Pandemic protocol to mitigate transmission resulted in psychological and socially disruptive GBV and IBV trauma intensified by 75% between March and June 2020 (Ocha, 2020). Another consequence of the COVID-19 pandemic is that concerns around mental health and substance abuse have grown significantly.

> My husband has become a drug addict and also, he is always drunk. I think he is using these drugs to relieve stress because he has not worked since the outbreak of COVID-19 pandemic. You can tell he is annoyed and every small thing in the house triggers him to beat me, I am now afraid of living with him, I fear that he will kill me one day, but I don't have anywhere to go as the government said we are not allowed to move, we must stay in the tents.
>
> (Tsitsi Nyamayemombe)

> Men in the camp are aggravated by their inability to provide for their families which drives them to beat their women and children. The restrictions from COVID-19 have made it difficult for men to find employment in the sur-rounding communities. Men tend to roam around the camp without any plan as they are not permitted to go anywhere, leading to frustrations which are then passed to women. My husband is always moody and I remember one time he beat me when I asked money to buy vegetables, he told me that he was not a bank that printed money.
>
> (Mutsawashe Gumbojena)

> When a disaster occurs, some people develop PTSD (post-traumatic stress disorder and this affects men mostly as they no longer have the money to pro-vide for their families. My husband never drank beer when we were married and before the floods happened. But all that changed when we started staying in Chingwizi temporary camp, you could tell that he was always contemplat-ing. That is when he started drinking the cheap traditional beer and always when he came home drunk, he always started a fight, and he would beat me. I think he is beating me out of frustrations, and I am just being used as a scape-goat for him to deal with what we have gone through because of these floods. To make matters worse there is now COVID-19, and we are forced to stay together as there are restrictions meaning that my husband can't even go to the nearest town to look for temporary work and this again has made things worse at home and has contributed to the abuse I am receiving.
>
> (Tarisai Chimuti)

These findings confirm the assertion that GBV is a profound and widespread prob-lem in the aftermath of floods and is exacerbated by COVID-19 restrictions imposed by the government of Zimbabwe. Women are more vulnerable to GBV after a disas-ter (floods, COVID-19) due to disruptions in communities and services, poor living conditions, and loss of livelihoods. The impact of COVID-19 lockdown restrictions has exacerbated GBV for women who are already victims of floods in Zimbabwe. The imposition of mandatory COVID-19 restrictions and lockdown in Zimbabwe resulted in an increase of GBV incidences within the Chingwizi camp. For most participants, these restrictions meant they were always close to their abusive partners.

Before COVID-19 came my husband was working in Chiredzi town and he will spend three months away working and will only come for a few days and this meant that I will not see him most of the time. But when the government said that no one is allowed to go out and we should stay indoors it meant that my husband was home all the time and, in a way, I believe this frustrated him and he started drinking traditional beer sold in the camp and is always drunk and he occasionally beats me and the children. We lived in constant fear of him.

(Tatenda Dzapasi)

Most men were not always around the camp as they worked in the surrounding towns and most of them lived at their workplaces (like those working as security guards). Traditionally, men working in the sugarcane fields around Chiredzi town rarely came home, only did so on special occasions. But now all that changed when the Zimbabwean government closed the country through lockdown because of COVID-19. These men were forced to come back to Chingwizi camp, and they were now confined with their families.

(Sarudzai Kutsva)

These findings indicate that GBV against women and girls in Zimbabwe is linked to the COVID-19 pandemic and the steps made to contain and mitigate the virus. Deplorably, Zimbabwe's already high levels of GBV were further exacerbated by the imposition of the lockdown restrictions. In addition, COVID-19 increased women's vulnerability to sexual abuse in the Chingwizi camp. Zimbabwe's state-mandated lockdown resulted in many men failing to secure employment in Chiredzi and Masvingo located close to the Chingwizi temporary camp.

Overcrowding

Men roamed the camp aimlessly increasing the risk of sexual violence, intensified by inadequate security and overcrowding.

I really don't feel safe at all in this camp as most men are now idle because of COVID-19. Whenever I go to the toilet or to bath, I fear that I will be sexually abused as there are incidences, I have heard of women being victims of sexual assault in those toilets at night or even during the day. This camp is not good at all for women and young girls as it exposes us to rape. There should be tight security in the camp to make sure that women are safe to go to the toilets anytime they wish that they need to do.

(Nyasha Nyambuya)

This place is not at all sensitive to the needs of women and is a haven for GBV and sexual abuse. The place is overcrowded now as people are no longer allowed to move or relocate anywhere because of the COVID-19 lockdown. We live in this one tent together with our children. Due to COVID-19 regulations they (children) are always with us, making it impossible for married couples to make love because there is no privacy anymore. This then leads to frustrations and anger from the men in the camp. Consequently, men vent-out these frustrations on their women. I remember my husband wanted to have sex with me in the presence of my children in the afternoon as he said they will not hear anything, but I was not comfortable having sex with him in the children's presence and he slapped me and scolded me. This is a problem that most women are facing in this camp.

(Pauline Nzenza)

GBV is a big issue in the temporary camp as there is too much tension. The floods have caused considerable depression emanating from the pressures prevalent and surrounding the camp. Overcrowding in the tents has caused tempers to flare and unnecessary arguments and fights in the household due to lack of sex. There is no privacy to have sex for married partners as the children are always around because schools closed because of COVID-19. Hence, most camp men are traumatised and let their frustrations and depression manifest in GBV.

(Samantha Madzorera)

The living conditions in the camp acted as a catalyst for the sexual abuse of women. For instance, basic amenities like toilets are far away from where the women slept, and it is difficult for women to access these toilets at night as they feared being raped. Natural disasters and pandemics increase women's vulnerabilities and susceptibility to sexual exploitation and violence. These vulnerabilities are exacerbated by a cultural environment that sees disproportionately high rates of sexual harassment of girls and women by men. Mittal and Singh (2020) found that simultaneous pandemic and natural disasters led to unprecedented levels of economic and food insecurity. Chingwizi camp women remained silent on increasing GBV, influenced by cultural notions confining GBV to private domains. Rural women were silenced and unable to access authorities to file and report violence. Silence and the lack of social networks sustain GBV, and the failure to report it continues to maintain the culture of violence. Women residing at Chingwizi were dissociated from community support systems.

I suffered without having anyone to talk about the abuse I am receiving from my husband. I did not know what to do as we were not allowed to go out because of COVID-19 and I had no one to tell even my family which is very far away in Masvingo. I cannot travel because I heard there are soldiers and police everywhere and you will be arrested for travelling during COVID-19, so I just suffered in silence and most of the time I cry, if only I had someone to talk about this abuse. My husband sometimes takes advantage of this by continuously beating me because he knows I have no one to talk about this.

(Chipo Dumba)

I think the government did not think through this lockdown because we don't have any police near us and if we want to report anything we have to travel to Chiredzi which is very far. And now most women are being beaten by their husbands. Still, they cannot travel to Chiredzi to go and report because the government is not allowing anyone to travel because of COVID, so it means most women had to endure the abuse at the hands of their husbands with nowhere to report this abuse. Even if you want to make a call to the police you can't do that because this camp does not have network for phones.

(Tsitsi Nyamayemombe)

I was abused by my husband in every aspect, he would beat me, scold me and even rape me sometimes and I wanted to leave him but I couldn't because I didn't know where to go. I remember when we moved here there were many NGOs that helped women who were abused but now, I heard they were all based in the neighbouring towns, and I could not travel because it was not allowed by the government to travel during COVID. These NGOs could have helped me leave my husband and give me and my children safe shelter to live but because of COVID I had to stay with him under the same tent without anywhere to seek help.

(Nyembesi Muroyi)

COVID-19 lockdowns, safety protocols, and quarantines intended to reduce virus proliferation. Coinciding natural disasters foisted women into temporary camps. Intersecting complexities increased isolation, unemployment, abuse, and control that were free from public scrutiny and were pardoned from punitive penalties. SAFE (2020) verified the fact that women were subjected to intensified forms of GBV and IPV during the COVID-19 national lockdown.

Conclusion

Undoubtedly, COVID-19-mandated safety protocols heightened GBV among rural Zimbabwean women displaced by flooding and subject to pandemic disaster management. Intersecting factors increased women's GBV vulnerability. The paucity of rigorous gender-directed, natural disaster, pandemic, and Global South scholarship is a substantive knowledge limitation. COVID-19 and GBV have disconnected women from access to fundamental universal human rights and the right to life. The findings demonstrate a globally pervasive GBV proliferation with long-term consequences that demand urgent intervention. Legislation, universal GBV declarations, recovery, and survival resources for victims are lacking. Efforts to abate GBV and operationalising policy must take precedence to restore women's agency.

References

Agarwal, B. (1997). 'Bargaining' and gender relations: Within and beyond the household. *Feminist Economics*, *3*(1), pp. 1–51.

Armas, I. and Gavris, A. (2013). Social vulnerability assessment using spatial multi-criteria analysis (SEVI model) and the social vulnerability index (SOVI model)–a case study for Bucharest, Romania. *Natural Hazards and Earth System Sciences*, *13*(6), pp. 1481–1499.

Azad, A.K., Hossain, K.M. and Nasreen, M. (2013). Flood-induced vulnerabilities and problems encountered by women in northern Bangladesh. *International Journal of Disaster Risk Science*, *4*(4), pp. 190–199. [Online] Available at: https://link.springer.com/article/10.1007/s13753-013-0020-z [Accessed 8th May 2022].

Babbie, E. and Mouton, J. (2007). *The practice of social research*. Cape Town: Oxford University Press.

Baig, M.N. and Sharif, R. (2013). Gender perspective considerations in disasters like earthquakes and floods of Pakistan. *International Journal of Humanities and Social Sciences*, *7*(6), pp. 1520–1523.

Berkes, F. (2007). Understanding uncertainty and reducing vulnerability: Lessons from resilience thinking. *Natural Hazards*, *41*(2), pp. 283–295. [Online] Available at: https://oxfordre.com/naturalhazardscience/view/10.1093/acrefore/9780199389407.001.0001/acrefore-9780199389407-e-275 [Accessed 8th May 2022].

Biswas, A., Rahman, A., Mashreky, S., Rahman, F. and Dalal, K. (2010). Unintentional injuries and parental violence against children during flood: A study in rural Bangladesh. *Rural and Remote Health*, *10*(1), pp. 1–12.

Bless, C., Higson-Smith, C. and Sithole, S. (2013). *Social research methods: An African perspective* (5th ed.). Cape Town: Juta.

Boyatzis, R.E. (1998). *Transforming qualitative information: Thematic analysis and code development*. California: Sage Publications.

Carbado, D.W. and Harris, C.I. (2019). Intersectionality at 30: Mapping the margins of anti-essentialism, intersectionality, and dominance theory. *Harvard Law Review*, *132*(8), pp. 2193–2239.

Chamorro-Premuzic, T. and Wittenberg-Cox, A. (2021). *How the pandemic increased domestic abuse and sexual violence*. [Online] Available at: https://www.forbes.com/sites/tomaspremuzic/2021/03/27/how-the-pandemic-increased- [Accessed 18th May 2022].

Chazireni, E. and Chigonda, T. (2018). The socio-economic impacts of dam construction: Case of Tokwe Mukosi in Masvingo Province, Zimbabwe. *European Journal of Social Sciences Studies*, *3*(2), pp. 209–218.

Chendume, P. (2016). *Investigating the impact of development-induced displacements on rights of the people: The case of Tokwe Mukosi Dam construction*. Unpublished Master's thesis, National University of Science and Technology, Bulawayo. [Online] Available at: https://jamba.org.za/index.php/jamba/article/view/592/980 [Accessed 7th May 2022].

Chitando, M. (2020). Narrowing the 'physical distance' between public health policies and gender: An analysis of government responses to COVID-19 in Zimbabwe and South Africa. *African Journal of Governance and Development*, *9*(1), pp. 352–366.

Cho, S., Crenshaw, K. and McCall, L. (2013). Toward a field of intersectionality studies: Theory, applications, and praxis. *Signs*, *38*, pp. 785–810.

Ciampi, M.C., Gell, F., Lasap, L. and Turvill, E. (2011). *Gender and disaster risk reduction: A training pack*. Britain: Oxfam. [Online] Available at: https://wrd.unwomen.org/practice/listing-toolbox/gender-and-disaster-risk-reduction-training-pack [Accessed 7th May 2022].

Creswell, J.W. (2009). *Research design: Qualitative, quantitative, and mixed methods approach.* California: Sage Publications.

Demetriades, J. and Esplen, E. (2010). The gender dimensions of poverty and climate change adaptation. In *Social dimensions of climate change: Equity and vulnerability in a warming world*, 133–143. [Online] Available at: https://www.ipcc.ch/apps/njlite/srex/njlite_download.php?id=6380 [Accessed 17th May 2022].

De Silva, K. and Jayathilaka, R. (2014). Gender in the context of disaster risk reduction: A case study of a flood risk reduction project in the Gampaha District in Sri Lanka. *Procedia Economics and Finance, 18*(1), pp. 873–881. [Online] Available at: https://giwps.georgetown.edu/resource/gender-in-the-context-of-disaster-risk-reduction-a- [Accessed 8th May 2022].

De Vos, A.S., Strydom, H., Fouche, C.B. and Delport, C.S.L. (2002). *Research at grassroots: For the social sciences and human service profession.* Pretoria: Van Schaik. [Online] Available at: http://ijds.org/Volume10/IJDSv10p535-550Ponelis0624.pdf [Accessed 18th May 2022].

Djalante, R., Thomalla, F., Sinapoy, M.S. and Carnegie, M. (2012). Building resilience to natural hazards in Indonesia: Progress and challenges in implementing the Hyogo framework for action. *Natural Hazards, 62*(3), pp. 779–803. [Online] Available at: https://www.sei.org/publications/building-resilience-to-natural-hazards-in-indonesia -progress-and-challenges-in-implementing-the-hyogo-framework-for-action/ [Accessed 18th May 2022].

Dlamini, N.J. (2021). Gender-based violence, twin pandemic to COVID-19. *Critical Sociology, 47*(4–5), pp. 583–590.

Emmar, A. (2017). *Glacier retreat and Glacial Lake Outburst Floods (GLOFs).* [Online] Available at: https://doi.org/10.1093/acrefore/9780199389407.013.275 [Accessed 8th May 2022].

Fisher, S. (2010). Violence against women and natural disasters: Findings from post-tsunami Sri Lanka. *Violence against Women, 16*(8), pp. 902–918.

Gopaldas, A. (2013). Intersectionality 101. *Journal of Public Policy and Marketing*, 32(1), pp. 90–94.

Horton, L. (2012). After the earthquake: Gender inequality and transformation in post-disaster Haiti. *Gender and Development*, 20(2), pp. 295–308.

Hove, M. (2016). When flood victims became state victims: Tokwe Mukosi, Zimbabwe. *Democracy and Security, 12*(3), pp. 135–161.

Ibrahim, M. (2012). Thematic analysis: A critical review of its process and evaluation. *West East Journal of Social Sciences, 1*(1), pp. 39–47.

Kofman, Y.B. and Garfin, D.R. (2020). Home is not always a haven: The domestic violence crisis amid the COVID-19 pandemic. *Psychological Trauma: Theory, Research, Practice, and Policy, 12*(1): S199. [Online] Available at: https://psycnet.apa.org/fulltext /2020-37317-001.pdf [Accessed 18th May 2022].

Made, P.A. and Nyakujarah, L. (2015). *SADC gender protocol 2015 barometer–Zimbabwe.* Johannesburg: Gender Links. [Online] Available at: https://genderlinks.org.za/wpcontent /uploads/imported/articles/attachments/20418_chap11baro2014zim_climatrev.pdf [Accessed 18th May 2022].

Mashiri, L. and Mawire, P.R. (2013). Conceptualization of gender-based violence in Zimbabwe, Midland state. *International Journal of Humanities and Social Science, 3*(15), pp. 94–103.

Matiza, V.M. (2021). Human factor development and the displacement of affected communities at Tugwi – Mukosi Dam in Zimbabwe. *African Identities*, (1), pp. 1–9.

Mittal, S. and Singh, T. (2020). Gender-based violence during COVID-19 pandemic: A mini-Review. *Frontier Global Women's Health, 1*(1), pp. 4

Nabegu, A.B. (2014). Morphologic response of a stream channel to extensive sand mining. *Research Journal of Environmental and Earth Sciences, 6*(2), pp. 96–101.

Nguyen, H. and Rydstrom, H. (2018). Climate disaster, gender, and violence: Men's infliction of harm upon women in the Philippines and Vietnam. *Women's Studies International Forum,* 71(1), pp. 56–62.

Ocha. (2020). *Zimbabwe cluster status: Protection (Gender-based violence).* [Online] Available at: https://reports.unocha.org/en/country/zimbabwe/card/2XxB9GOV93/ [Accessed 18th May 2022].

Patton, M.Q. (2002). Two decades of developments in qualitative inquiry: A personal, experiential perspective. *Qualitative Social Work, 1*(3), pp. 261–283.

Ponelis, S.R. (2015). Using interpretive qualitative case studies for exploratory research in doctoral studies: A case of information systems research in small and medium enterprises. *International Journal of Doctoral Studies, 10*(1), pp. 535–550. [Online] Available at: http://ijds.org/Volume10/IJDSv10p535-550Ponelis0624.pdf [Accessed 18th May 2022].

Poole, S.M., Grier S.A., Thomas, K.D., Sobande, F., Ekpo, A.E., Torres, L.T., Addington, L.A., Weekes-Laidlow, M. and Henderson, G.R. (2020). *Race, diversity, and inclusion.* [Online] Available at: https://www.ama.org/research-articles-diversity-race-inclusion/ [Accessed 18th May 2022].

Rabbani, M., Rahman, A. and Mainuddin, K. (2009). Women's vulnerability to water-related hazards: Comparing three areas affected by climate change in Bangladesh. *Waterlines, 28*(3), pp. 235–249.

Raza, H. (2017). Using a mixed method approach to discuss the intersectionalities of class, education, and gender in natural disasters for rural vulnerable communities in Pakistan. *Journal of Rural and Community Development, 12*(1), pp. 128–148.

Reyes, D.D. and Lu, J.L. (2016). Gender dimension in disaster situations: A case study of flood prone women in Malabon city, Metro Manila. *International Journal of Disaster Risk Reduction,* (15), pp. 162–168.

Robeyns, I. (2017). *The capability approach: An interdisciplinary approach.* [Online] Available at: https://www.suz.uzh.ch/dam/jcr:bd248fa2-70ca-483f-9d52-dad8c2aafe7d/19%20I%20Robeyns%202017%20The%20Capability%20Approach.pdf [Accessed 18th May 2022].

Safe. (2020). *Violence against women and girls during the COVID-19 crisis in Zimbabwe: Analysis of practice-based data from women's coalition of Zimbabwe, stopping abuse and female exploitation (SAFE) Zimbabwe technical assistance facility.* [Online] Available at: http://www.adultrapeclinic.org.zw/wp-content/uploads/2020/09/SAFE-Report-on-Gender-Based-Violence-Data-in-Zimbabwe-during-C19-for-publication-with-logo.pdf [Accessed 18th May 2022].

Santos, C.E. and Toomey, R.B. (2018). Integrating an intersectionality lens in theory and research in developmental science. *New Directions for Child and Adolescent Development,* (161), pp. 7–15. [Online] Available at: https://jyd.pitt.edu/ojs/jyd/article/view/859 [Accessed 18th May 2022].

Sen, A. (2009). *The idea of justice.* London: Allen Lane.

Sharma, A. and Borah, S.B. (2020).Covid-19 and domestic violence: An indirect path to social and economic crisis. *Journal of Family Violence,* (1), pp. 1–7. [Online] Available at: https://www.iassw-aiets.org/wp-content/uploads/2021/01/Covid-19-and-Domestic-Violence_an-Indirect-Path-to-Social-and-Economic-Crisis.pdf [Accessed 18th May 2022].

Solangaarachchi, D., Griffin, A.L. and Doherty, M.D. (2012). Social vulnerability in the context of bushfire risk at the urban-bush interface in Sydney: A case study of the Blue Mountains and Ku-ring-gai local council areas. *Natural Hazards, 64*(2), pp. 1873–1898.

Sommer, M., Likindikoki, S. and Kaaya, S. (2013). Boys' and young men's perspectives on violence in Northern Tanzania. *Culture, Health, and Sexuality, 15*(6), pp. 695–709.

Tarisayi, K.S. (2015). Some contemporary challenges faced by NGOs in disaster induced relocations at Chingwizi Transit Camp, Zimbabwe. *Journal for Studies in Management and Planning, 1*(9), pp. 316–320.

Tarisayi, K.S. (2018). Traditional leadership and the Tokwe-Mukosi induced displacements: Finding the missing link. *Jàmbá: Journal of Disaster Risk Studies, 10*(1), pp. a592. [Online] Available at: https://doi.org/10.4102/jamba.v10i1.592 [Accessed 8th May 2022].

Teater, B. (2010). *An introduction to applying social work: Theories and methods.* Berkshire: Open University Press.

Terre-Blanche, M. and Durrheim, K. (1999). *Research in practice: Applied methods for the social sciences.* Cape Town: University of Cape Town Press.

Tyupa, S. (2011). A theoretical framework for back-translation as a quality assessment tool. *New Voices in Translation Studies, 7*(1), pp. 35–46.

UN Women. (2020). *The shadow pandemic: Violence against women during COVID-19.* [Online] Available at: https://www.unwomen.org/en/news/in-focus/in-focus-gender -equality-incovid-19-response/violence-against-women-during-covid-19 [Accessed 8th May 2022].

UN Women. (2021). *COVID-19 and violence against women: The evidence behind the talk.* [Online] Available at: https://www.unwomen.org/en/what-we-do/ending-violence -against-women/facts-and-figures [Accessed 20th May 2022].

Van Raemdonck, L., Seedat-Khan, M. and Raeymackers, P. (2017). Assessing the capability approach as an evaluation tool for community networks on intimate partner violence in seven townships in KwaZulu Natal, South Africa. Social Work Review, *Revista de Asistenta Sociala, 15*(3), pp. 5–17.

Wisner, B. (1998). Marginality and vulnerability: Why the homeless in Tokyo don't count in disaster preparations. *Applied Geography, 18*(1), pp. 25–33.

Part II
Health

4 Autoethnography as a Lens to Understand Women and COVID-19 Care in South Africa

Kezia Lewins

Introducing the COVID-19 Context

From the outbreak of a seemingly localised epidemic in Wuhan, China, in December 2019 to the upcoming second anniversary of the global SARS-CoV-2 pandemic, with over 5.6 million deaths (Worldometer 2022), there has been contestation over if, what, who, how, and why the pandemic has had the effects it has. Recent data (2021) illustrates that the developing world accounts for 64% of globally reported COVID-19 deaths and 86% of estimated excess deaths (Schellekens 2022). Thereby signalling the aggregate health toll of the pandemic on the global South. In South Africa, Moultrie et al. (2021) estimate that 85–95% of natural excess deaths are attributable to COVID-19, with the remaining being 'collateral' cases resulting from an overwhelmed health system. These losses have been accompanied by the amplification of chronic unemployment rates, poverty, food insecurity, malnutrition, and gender-based violence (Onyeaka, et al. 2021; Dlamini 2021). From the first COVID-19 lockdowns (April–May 2020), half of those surveyed across sub-Saharan Africa actively 'reported mental health and emotional symptoms' (Langsi et al. 2021).

The continent's peri-urban majority, who live within vastly under-resourced communities, experience the pandemic as 'syndemic' (Bambara et al. 2020; Team and Manderson 2020; and Oppong et al. 2015). The compound and intersectional effects of structural and systemic vulnerability, socio-economic exploitation, and widespread deprivation render the poor, precarious, and those on the ever-increasing margins vulnerable, at risk, and exposed to COVID-19. Within this perspective, the extractive impact of colonial capitalism and its ongoing legacies holds specific significance for understanding the health disparities of the pandemic (Jolly 2022). As such, the widely acclaimed Public Health and Social Distancing (PHSD) measures that focus on limiting disease transmission make little to no pragmatic sense in a context and reality configured around exploitation and inequality (Wilkinson 2020).

The social determinants of disease demonstrate how, for those who develop moderate or severe COVID-19, access to hospital, COVID-19 treatment, care, the experience of hospitalisation itself, and the outcome correlate with social inequality. In South Africa, Phaswana-Mafuya et al. (2021) conclude that being black

DOI: 10.4324/9781003267133-6

African, marginalised, and of low socio-economic status within the Eastern Cape predicts poor COVID-19 outcomes. Their data shows that young black African women had the highest hospitalisation rates. Cevik and Baral's (2021) empirical findings on the networks of SARS-CoV-2 transmission demonstrate much of what Wilkinson (2020) argued concerning the epidemiological, health system, control measures, and systemic vulnerabilities that drive infectious disease transmission amongst the poor and marginalised.

Without appropriate interventions, the outcome of the first (and subsequent) waves in South Africa saw more patients admitted to hospitals. Whilst more patients were admitted to the private healthcare sector, a more significant proportion died within the public sector (NICD 2020). Whilst inequities in the global and local supply and distribution chain of medication, material stock, and health personnel are amongst the factors that shape the availability and quality of clinical COVID-19 care. These have been exacerbated by South Africa's long history of underfunding, maladministration, and 'crisis-upon-crises' within the public sector (Reynolds 2020). As such, we see Watts and Bohle's (1993) coordinates of vulnerability being affirmed with the poor and marginalised experiencing a triple burden: the risk of exposure, capacity risk due to a lack of resources to cope, and the risk of potentiality in facing the pandemic's most serious consequences (Delor and Hubert 2000, p. 1562).

Alongside competing mainstream narratives, policies, and approaches to care, the majority at the margins simultaneously live with COVID-19 in a context that adds another layer to their life stories of endurance, resilience, and resistance (Eyles et al. 2015). It is essential to recall this earlier work. It reminds us that people are not merely the victims of circumstances but actively respond, engage, shape, and resist context and circumstances.

The economic, psychosocial fallout and mounting health-related evidence of the pandemic and its concomitant lockdowns are compelling reasons for us, as sociologists, to engage our multiple audiences. We document, analyse, and explain why experiences such as 'the pandemic' are debilitating, devastating, and a catalyst for change for the individual, family, community, and society.

COVID-19 and Its Limitations and Potentiality

COVID-19 has challenged academics and conventional research, writing, and publication processes. The way and pace scientists have had to respond to SARS-CoV-2 has overwhelmed traditional methods. Scientists have responded by working rapidly, networking across the globe, publishing pre-prints and sharing results on social media, retracting work that has since become obsolete, etc. At the same time, social scientists appeared to be inert, particularly at the pandemic's start. Žižek (2020), quoted in Mathewman and Huppatz (2020, p. 679), asked: 'What is wrong with our system that we were caught unprepared by the catastrophe despite scientists warning us about it for years?' Whilst Connell (2020, p. 749) exclaimed, 'Sociology as we know it is not very good in handling a historical moment, unpacking a conjuncture, let alone grasping a radically new situation like this.'

Lockdown restrictions particularly impacted social scientists, isolating them from existing or potential research sites, and qualitative researchers were prevented from face-to-face interaction with participants (Ruppel 2020). Social scientists articulated the need to pause for deep thought, reflection, and critical introspection about the relevance of existing theorisation (Connell 2020; Will and Bendelow 2020). In a somewhat telling act of professional integrity and/or closure, blog sites were recommended as the preferred spaces for such individual and collective thought (Will and Bendelow 2020) and 'methodological cosmopolitanism' (Beck in Zinn 2021, p. 444). In mainstream journals, scholars drew from, amongst others, Beck's (1992) risk society, Klein's (2007) disaster capitalism, and Scambler's (2018) fractured society (Monaghan 2020; Ward 2020; Zinn 2021). Others revisited classic themes on inequality, invisibility, and vulnerability (Milan and Treré 2020; Will and Bendelow 2020). Whilst some envisaged new research agendas of 'cure' (Berghs 2021) and critiqued the very social construction of COVID-19 as an epidemic (Bhat and Dar 2020). The basic tenets of the sociological imagination became everyday vocabulary and a part of the lived reality during the pandemic. Hindsight will determine whether the academic approach within the social sciences has been beneficial, a shortcoming or a mix of context-specific complexities and contradictions.

Nonetheless, the pandemic can be thought of as an opportune time to engage and build public, critical, professional, and policy audiences (Burawoy 2005, p. 24) for social scientists. In 2005, Burawoy argued:

> the standpoint of sociology is civil society and the defense of the social. In the times of market tyranny and state despotism, sociology – and its public face – defends the interests of humanity.

In pandemic times, this is particularly vital, especially for both applied and clinical sociologists. In this chapter, I generally refer to clinical sociology as a type of applied sociology that specifically engages the health sector with practical and action-oriented interventions. Nonetheless, the history and trajectory of the sub-discipline are shaped by local and global contexts. For example, it has been widely documented, historically across the globe, that the delineation of clinical sociology has been retrospectively applied to those who have not necessarily used the term themselves, sometimes unaware of the field's existence, even though their practice fits squarely within the ambit of the field (Fritz 1991; Uys 2021). Another incongruity is that whilst not all medical or health sociologists have been identified or classified as clinical sociologists, neither have all clinical sociologists worked within healthcare (Fritz 1991; Uys 2021).

Friedman (1989, p. 54) states, 'Clinical sociology brings a sociological perspective to intervention and action for change. The clinical sociologist is essentially a change agent rather than a researcher or evaluator.' Bruhn and Rebach (1996) concur that whilst clinical sociology is concerned with problem-solving, its uniqueness lies in its explicit intention to lead to 'active intervention' (Hoppe 1998, p. 99). Fritz (1991, p. 18) stresses an endemic tension within the field when trying to 'meet both scientific and community needs.' Over time, practitioners have found ways to overcome these challenges. Fritz (1991, pp. 22–23) identifies six distinguishing factors as part of the clinical sociologists' toolbox: an excellent working theoretical base that can be practically applied, an ability to understand and intervene in the requisite social system, whilst being able to focus on a specific unit of analysis, using one's specialist subject knowledge, the discipline's methodology, and specialist intervention skills; as such, clinical sociology reflects all components of sociological knowledge identified by Burawoy (2005) whilst perhaps being mostly public and policy-oriented.

In South Africa, Uys (2021, pp. 111 and 118) notes the Carnegie Commission's influential role in profiling and establishing the field of (clinical) sociology in the 1930s and 1980s. Uys (2021) also documents how, given South Africa's racialisation, the field has experienced racialised tensions over whose interests have been served or pursued, the degree to which the 'state' has been supported or opposed, the extent of recognition of the field, and the focus (including whether healthcare has been prioritised) within clinical sociology in South Africa.

The Role of Clinical Sociologists in the Pandemic

During the COVID-19 pandemic, the unique positionality of clinical sociologists has necessitated revisiting these debates, including the purpose, role, engagement, and relationship between clinical sociologists and their diverse 'publics.' Metzl and colleagues (see Metzl and Hansen 2014; Metzl, Petty, and Olowojoba 2018, and Metzl, Maybank, and De Maio 2020) have long been writing about the importance of a structurally competent healthcare system in the United States, drawing attention to the need to 'reimagine and redesign the health care delivery and education systems through a lens of health equity and racial justice' (Metzl, Maybank, and De Maio 2020, p. 231). Their approach includes the:

> recognition of how social structures 'shape clinical interactions,' development of 'extra clinical language' of structure, rearticulating 'cultural presentations in structural terms,' planning 'structural interventions and development of 'structural humility.'
>
> (Metzl and Hensen in Metzl, Maybank, and De Maio 2020, p. 231)

These recommendations have extensive reach and speak specifically to the skill set of clinical sociologists, particularly those with an interest in medical and health sociology. By drawing on and from personal experience and observation of the impact of the COVID-19 pandemic on affected people and families, I aim to begin a reimagination of South African healthcare in which integrated patient-centred healthcare is provided by an array of stakeholders including clinical sociologists.

The COVID-19 pandemic presented a unique opportunity for clinical sociologists to solidify existing relationships by working within under-resourced clinical settings. Within the context in which we worked, the clinical care of COVID-19 patients had been the priority. During this time, I coordinated a team of social science gradu-ate women volunteers working with COVID-19 patients and families at a Gauteng Field Hospital in South Africa between June 2020 and August 2021. This group of volunteers worked alongside clinical staff, offering complementary psychosocial ser-vices, providing mainly telephonic family support, psychological first aid, targeted food packages, and referrals for further psychological, social, and medical services to patients determined at risk or in need by clinicians (see Lewins et al. 2020). This form of integrated care was deliberate and nuanced within this setting, at this time.

As per an application of Fritz's (1991) clinical sociology toolbox, our team aimed to intervene by contributing to racial, socio-economic, and linguistic justice, thereby reinforcing the overall Field Hospital's vision of health equity. We sought to do so through a targeted approach by focusing on patients and families most in need, as determined by those experiencing ill health (COVID-19, comorbidity, and long COVID), socio-economic, and geographic inequality (living in under-resourced areas and/or experiencing poverty, hunger, homelessness) and experiencing com-munication and linguistic marginalisation (limited or an absence of contact with the family upon hospitalisation and whose language preference was any language besides the dominant medical lingua franca of English, even if this was spoken). Our services were available in multiple South African languages, drew on insights from health sociology to reinforce the biopsychosocial approach, and utilised sociocultural communication skills to bridge the competence gap and minimise institutionalised systems of exclusion. Giustini (2020) reports that public service interpreters in the United Kingdom (UK) have been recognised as 'essential work-ers,' emphasising their centrality in broadening equity. Giustini emphasises, as was our experience, that this type of work largely remains 'invisibilised' in the broader COVID-19 and medical response. Given that women disproportionately use the healthcare system and comprise healthcare workers, further investigation is needed into this systematic marginalisation of women providing key components of care.

As per Friedman's earlier definition, our engagement with the Field Hospital was a classical clinical, sociological undertaking. Prior discussions with the clini-cal team revealed a need for psychosocial patient and healthcare practitioner (HCP) support. The former was a service we were able to provide. Several months into service provision, we reflected on the potential value the work held as 'reflections from practice' and the ways it could inform 'research.' We have written a collec-tive article about this (see Lewins et al., 2020). Here I further reflect on specific dimensions of this work from my own perspective and from what I was able to observe from those experiencing COVID-19 within the Field Hospital context.

Autoethnography as a Relevant Method

Adams and Manning (2015, p. 2) discuss how autoethnography as a qualitative research method can be used to deliver social justice. Researchers reflexively engage their positionality and experience and in so doing acknowledge, situ-ate, reflect, and critique the personal, cultural, social, and political dynamics and processes that make up the 'field' with 'intellectual and methodological rigour, emotion, and creativity' (Poulos 2021, p. 5). However, as most writers attest, tensions of interpretation, analysis, and ethics come to the fore when engaging in autoethnographic work (see Chang 2008). As such, the potential contribution of this exercise has been valued in principle but was morally, ethically, and pragmatically a challenge from start to finish – especially my own aims to fit it into professional parameters. Thus, it demonstrates the often-quoted tension between 'serving the public' and doing 'profession-worthy work.'

In this chapter, I provide deductions from my autoethnographic insights and reflections (written in personal diaries from the time and in retrospect) based on onsite encounters and engagements whilst providing person-centred care to patients in a Field Hospital to illustrate the potential contributions of clinical sociologists in a time of crisis. This material is complemented by the analysis of ten interviews with allied HCPs, in late 2021.

Autoethnography as a method, especially during the COVID-19 context, opened up many questions such as 'what is research'; 'what does it mean to be a sociologist in a pandemic'; 'can and should research be done during a pandemic'; 'what potential is there for sociologists to engage publics now and for the future'; 'what does it mean and feel to be a researcher with a voice on mute'; and 'how do we reclaim sociology and our right to be interlocutors and co-construct the stories of the pandemic with those most affected.' In short, COVID-19 raised questions about whether clinical sociologists (with their dual identities and roles) can act, research, produce, and know authentically, mainly whilst engaged primarily in service work. These are essential questions for clinical health sociologists whose existence and future sit at the intersection of medicine and sociology; and who potentially sit within 'no [person]' land doing under-appreciated care work of both disciplines.

These are questions without uniform or straightforward answers and whose situation and context-dependent solutions may be slippery and fluid even for the person (sociologist) themself. Nonetheless, as I hope the emergent discussion shows, there are valuable insights in sharing these stories. There is a distinct positionality and advantage of perspective that the clinical sociologist has and brings. There are unique conversations in 'the moment,' a specific intersection of time, space, and circumstance that cannot be recreated in shape or form. If not 'captured,' some insights may be lost, resulting in a more superficial understanding of the margins – and quite often the women who inhabit these. Furthermore, there are ways of recording broad macro brushstrokes of experience to guarantee individual anonymity, maintain confidence and privacy, ensure no harm is done, and maintain the trust and integrity of the clinical relationship. These enable marginal experiences to be shared as motivation for change, equity, and justice.

Insights from Autoethnographic Work during COVID-19

Patients' Clinical Experiences

Patients hospitalised at the Field Hospital had often been through a disease trajectory that included moderate or severe COVID-19. Whilst in designated COVID-19 (public) hospitals, patients were treated biomedically according to the specific hospital's protocol, the patient's presentation, and the risk profile. This commonly included medication, physiotherapy, and various supplementary oxygen treatments administered through intubation (mechanical ventilation), continuous positive airway pressure (CPAP) masks, and/or high-flow oxygen via nasal cannula. Patients had variously been treated in intensive care, high care, and/or general COVID-19 wards before being down-transferred to the Field Hospital. Patients' length of stay was variable, with some having been in the hospital for just a few days for up to a month before coming to the Field Hospital. Whilst in the Field Hospital, there was a distinct pattern to 'uncomplicated cases,' with the patient's condition determining the pace with which they moved through the processes of medication completion, supplementary oxygen downscaling, and completion of days in quarantine – sometimes taking just a few days, whilst in other cases, up to two weeks, and occasionally requiring a return to a tertiary hospital.

The in-ward and post-discharge recovery of those with comorbidities were often compounded by their physiological condition, especially for those with existing and newly diagnosed diabetes. Patients needing to be discharged with oxygen, particularly during the first and third waves, faced an uncertain future. Particularly in the latter case when provincial supplies reached a crisis point (SA News 2021). To varying extents, the COVID-19 illness was experienced by patients as a biographical disruption to an otherwise expected and known health trajectory (Bury 1982). The women's section of the Field Hospital was always fuller than the men's, with slightly more variation in the age range. Although as a non-clinician, it was difficult to make any decisive conclusions about the severity of patients' illness experience.

As non-clinicians, our team worked closely with the clinical team. Whilst HCPs handled the vital 'medical' aspects, we supported, facilitated, and reiterated explanations and the processes to the families and patients. Our presence and experience seemed to provide patients with some calm, reassurance, and simply the time for questions and answers as well as the retelling of patients' clinical experience – something that has historically been antithetical to patients' typical experience of a public hospital and traditional hospital cultures. This integrated and holistic approach allowed all members of the Field Hospital time to specialise in their tasks and time for reprieve in this tense environment where none of us could do our work without each other.

Experiences Affecting Patients' Mental and Emotional Well-Being

COVID-19 tested patients' physical, mental, and emotional health and well-being. Now in the Field Hospital, many patients were still afraid of, actively grappling with, or trying to blank out what they expected, perceived, saw, and heard in hospital COVID-19 wards. For example, patients may have witnessed the struggles and/or death of fellow patients, undergone intensive healthcare procedures, simply woken up to find their companion in the next bed gone (unsure whether they had been discharged or died) and battled to decipher their own experience and what components of it were real. Patients grappled with what this meant to and for them as COVID-19 patients (receiving care, in recovery, and post-recovery). Some explicitly asked for mental healthcare referrals, the clinical team referred others, some shared their struggles in conversations with support teams or family, whilst others sat privately in contemplation. Particularly at the start of the pandemic, approximately a third of patients had not had contact with their families whilst hospitalised. So, it was important for the Field Hospital to attend this role (see Lewins et al., 2020 for more).

Field Hospital patients either sought affirmation and connection by establishing small daily communication rituals, took each other's contact details before discharge, or waved ecstatically as they said goodbye to the ward. Others seemed to seek solace and quiet, with/from their bodily responses and own thoughts. Most had a positive rapport with members of the clinical team and clung each day to the hope of news of improved health stats and going home as round wards took place. At critical junctures, such as this, we explained several times why patients were staying longer, were now going home, and explained how to prepare for their discharge and how to acclimatise to being home. Each patient was unique, but patients +55 years tended to respond to verbal communication the most.

The second and third waves were accompanied by more personal and familial distress, loss, and grief. More patients grappled with their hospitalisation whilst simultaneously worrying about family members who were undergoing home-based COVID-19 care were hospitalised, or had died, and often could not attend funerals. For some patients, grief could just not be processed within the clinical space, at least not during the waking hours. At first, it seemed that women were more likely to be widowed, but we encountered both men and women in grief with time. Each responded to this in markedly different ways reflecting differentiation in their experience of vulnerability. The bureaucratic complexity involved in 'proving' their hospitalisation as a reason for delayed processing of spousal deaths or having to appoint a proxy to act on their behalf was particularly stressful for widows, whilst widowers were often more emotionally expressive at the loss of their 'lifelong friends.' Many patients expressed gratitude for 'time to talk,' indicative of how seldom it may have been the norm for them to be put first in their lives.

During the second wave, octogenarians (men, then women too) came to the Field Hospital with a history of intensive care psychosis or degenerative mental health conditions, an additional layer of complexity for patients and families. The experience of alienation was intense for the elderly and isolated patients – on occasion, home locations and families were untraceable, complicating the demands on the healthcare institutions. Silence and the apparent absence of social connection that hung over some patients were intractable concerns. It further emerged that some patients had been found or dropped at the hospital of origin without any contacts – some were homeless and were picked up by ambulances or passers-by, whilst callous employers had simply dropped a few staff off. Examples such as these revealed the pervasive fear and stigma in the early days of the pandemic and the gaps in the South African social welfare system.

Standard Patient Narratives

In conversations with patients, despite their diversity, a distinctly standard narrative emerged that included: firstly, questioning the source of infection and why 'they' were infected ('who brought it into the household?'; 'how did I get it?'; 'why did others not?'). This was often accompanied by a distinct deflection of blame away from the self, usually an elderly self who had been home sheltering ('I did everything I was supposed to, it was…'). During the third wave, some suspicion about the vaccine emerged, as elderly patients were admitted to the hospital shortly after receiving their first dose.

Secondly, patients reflected a degree of 'fear' of the virus. Thirdly, based on their hospital experiences, there was a unanimous agreement that 'this thing is real.' Throughout the three waves, varied public articulations to discredit the scientific explanation of the virus were circulating, and patients seemed to 'talk back to this.' Fourthly, many professed ahead of discharge, 'I am going to tell everyone about this,' signalling an intention to continue or commit more significant action to protect family, friends, and the community from the experience they had been through. This appears to be an emergent example of Frank's (1995) quest narrative whereby an illness experience provides special insight and may reshape one's perspective on life.

Fifthly, all were deeply grateful to the HCPs for treating them, readying them for discharge, and returning them to their families and their lives. Here, parallels could be seen with Frank's (1995) restitution narrative where people are glad to get well again and intend on staying well. Lastly, those who felt they had been to the brink 'thanked God!' for sparing them, bringing them back, and giving their life purpose. Some of these narratives were also viewed as 'prophetic' by those who experienced them.

This initial exploration of patients' COVID-19 narratives illustrates the ongoing relevance of Frank's (1995) *The Wounded Storyteller* and illustrates how patients very much experienced themselves as dyadic; how they struggled with the way tertiary hospitals had often reinforced separatism between themselves and their families, and fellow patients; and how the Field Hospital played a restorative role in facilitating the re-establishing of these connections.

Patients' Socio-economic Experiences

Our volunteer team's primary role was to support HCPs by attending to patients' psychosocial, emotional, and socio-economic challenges. Invariably these challenges varied and intensified with the pandemic. During the first wave, the need was most significant to establish initial communication between patients and families and provide primary COVID-19 health education, with only a few families requesting food support. Many patients were employed (with notable examples in the transportation, sanitation and hygiene, and the health sector) and requested proof of hospitalisation, for the return to work. From the second wave, a significant proportion of families needed food aid and cell phone data, while patients needed psychosocial and mental health interventions. During the third wave, the need for grief counselling was notably higher, and greater tension and difficulty were experienced in resolving social support needs within families because of prolonged economic hardships. Several older women and widows battled to find homes after experiencing pandemic-related losses. Whilst those who entered the Field Hospital already experiencing homelessness were more likely to be men. At this stage, family tensions (seeming absent or less significant earlier in the pandemic) meant the elderly were relegated to 'the state.' However, the burden of the pandemic itself meant rehoming such individuals was a lengthy and challenging process.

Families worried about patients' condition within the hospital context, and likewise, patients were concerned about their family's ability to manage without them. This was particularly articulated by grandmothers, mothers, and fathers – especially if the hospitalised person was the only family member in a 'parenting role' or was the primary economically active person in the household. The burden of knowing their families had reduced means of survival without their income-earning capacity or their cooking abilities caused great stress. Others whose familial context was characterised by strife that they (the patient) contained or managed were also concerned about the effects of their absence. In these families, the hospitalised patient often felt the difference that kept their family from poverty. Therefore, the provision of short-term resources was a stopgap for the family whilst their most vital link was unavailable.

Some patients ran small businesses and community-based organisations such as taxis, creches, women's empowerment groups or ran community food gardens – they worried greatly about how others were doing and whether these community interventions would survive. Daily motivation and prayers from 'their church groups' provided a way forward for the religious. However, regardless of context, patients sometimes needed to retreat from 'demands' and 'the goodwill' from the outside. However, the experience of hospitalisation for COVID-19 rarely, if ever, gave anyone the relief promised by 'the sick role.'

Whilst the psychosocial and food support interventions undoubtedly made a difference to the families, these had many shortcomings; they were on a small scale, were short term, and were an initiative at a single household level. That the pandemic affected whole communities, businesses, community projects, etc., was beyond our scope of intervention. These limitations demonstrate that whilst little has been done to cushion the vulnerability experienced; not much has been done to build lasting resilience strategies (Hufschmidt 2011). Such necessitates active and ongoing engagement with the personal and community networks already present within the communities. It was also hard not to feel overwhelmed by the systemic and bureaucratic challenges we faced when we did try to scale up and when we engaged broader structures, institutions, and departments. In the end, this has meant our intervention gathered a lot of insights but has struggled to transition into or inform sustainable and long-term interventions.

Allied Healthcare Professionals' Experience

Here broad-brush strokes from interviews with women HCPs (mostly working in psychosocial fields) complement the patient experience. Across the board, HCPs were acutely aware of the inaccessibility of psychosocial, emotional, and mental healthcare for patients and themselves. Some HCPs volunteered and used

HCP-support networks to sustain themselves through the pandemic. Allied HCPs (particularly psychologists, psychiatrists, physiotherapists, palliative care specialists, and social workers) experienced an increase in the demand for their services. Those in tertiary public hospitals continually found the demand more significant than the supply. As a result of being overwhelmed, HCPs often felt forced to care for the most severe cases. A few private HCPs felt compelled to provide pro-bono care, whilst HCPs in non-governmental organisations (NGOs) often took on COVID-19 project work to assist with pandemic gaps.

Depending on institutional protocol, select allied HCPs were allocated targeted responsibility to the following types of in-patients: those explicitly in COVID-19 and/or a person under investigation (PUI) wards or in other (non-COVID-19) hospitalised patients such as psychiatric patients, cancer patients, etc. Due to initial personal protection equipment (PPE) limitations, HCPs often felt directly at risk within and beyond the workplace, and several reported having contracted COVID-19 during the pandemic.

In some public hospitals, allied HCPs were given supplementary roles to screen and test fellow HCPs for COVID-19. Despite this 'essential task,' allied HCPs often felt their actual professional skills were not being put to best use for patients or fellow HCPs. This was echoed by some medical HCPs, who often reported a shortage of allied colleagues depending on whether located within specialised or general COVID-19 wards. Some allied HCPs (such as occupational therapists, physiotherapists, social workers) only began to see their regular out-patients after the first wave was declared over, an intervention that led to backlogs in service delivery. This affected the delivery of medical care and rehabilitation, but allied staff also noticed an increase in the socio-economic vulnerability of patients. Regardless of the role undertaken during the pandemic, allied HCPs (like their clinical counterparts) reported burnout, and many contemplated exiting the workplace and profession altogether.

This section adds important insight as it questions how 'essential' healthcare is determined and valued. As discussed in the patients' section, the services provided by allied HCPs were very much in need throughout the pandemic, both by COVID-19 and all patients, but were not uniformly available across the health sector. Hence, this role was taken up, in our example by volunteers and redeployed HCPs.

Personal Reflection

I think of myself as a creature of habit, who does not cope well with change and yet I was surprised how quickly I adapted and became accustomed to new things. During lockdown, I did not leave the house, even for groceries … However, when I learned of the opportunity to assist at the Field Hospital, I was right there! During the first few visits with the clinical team, we stayed in the 'green zone' … at the start of the second wave, it was deemed 'safe' for non-clinicians … so we went into the 'belly of the beast,' the actual hospital, all suited up like blue spacemen, the anxiety and heat my body generated set me on fire and all my senses were on hyper-alert … I asked myself, what did I expect ... Looking around, the patients were all 'normal,' not well, but not at death's door (if they had been, they were not now). I breathed a sigh of relief. They looked quiet and withdrawn ... Some looked up at the passing spectacle, in hope. The HCPs rushed about in busyness and in huddles, and then everything was still in the long, long corridors of repetition.

After that first visit, I assured myself the safety measures were in place, I could take responsibility for my safety, I could spend the necessary time finding out about the people (behind the label 'patient') and their needs, and I could be kind and caring (despite being a blue spaceman). I knew this is a job I could do and wanted to do.

In retrospect, over the next six months, the Field Hospital patients filled my heart and soul as much as I hoped I was able to help them, collectively. We refound our humanity in our COVID-19 ward. I still find myself wondering about the textured faces, abundant characters, and colourful lives that I had the privilege of glimpsing into for a short while.

Discussion and Conclusion

This material has implications for providing and accessing allied care, especially psychosocial and mental healthcare services. Allied HCPs work was often deemed secondary or 'non-essential' within the context of rising COVID-19 numbers. As a result, recognition of their contribution, services, and 'care' was often undervalued at the level of decision-making but greatly needed and missed in hospital wards by patients and fellow HCPs. The effort and adaptability required of all HCPs during the pandemic are acknowledged, particularly given the structural and process limitations. This further underscores the vital psychosocial role performed by colleagues within Field Hospitals as a down referral point for COVID-19 patients. Of course, additional gaps exist such as patients who needed care but who were not hospitalised (because of COVID-19 prioritisation protocols) and those who were hospitalised (but not for COVID-19) and who nonetheless required the range of psychosocial support services because of the pandemic and lockdown.

The overview of the patient experience has shown hospitalised patients' variable nodes of vulnerability in part due to their direct clinical state (due to viral, late presentation, and comorbidity effects); psychological experiences (clinical and social interactions); and as per the intersectionality of their political, social, economic, and geographic positionality (Wilkinson 2020; Delor and Hubert 2000). As has been shown, the patients met along this journey were both men and women, and both experienced vulnerability with different inflexions and to differing degrees. More detailed research is necessary and would further illuminate and quantify the patients' COVID-19 experience. Nonetheless, the observation that yielded this autoethnographic reflection demonstrates how and why patients, continued, endured, survived, and recovered. Their narratives tell us they do this for their family, community, and God, and not to be beaten by 'this tiny invisible thing.' There is far more about people's resilience, resistance, agency, and activism still to be learned, of which this account barely scratches the surface.

I would recommend much more active, deliberate, and considered autoethnography and participatory action research (PAR) to understand society's majority experience, often mislabelled the 'experience from the margins,' which should be given prominence front and centre to begin to do the essential work of equity, justice, and care. I argue this is of vital importance in the South African context. The Field Hospital example cited here demonstrates this can and has taken place, during the COVID-19 pandemic within the public health sector. Furthermore, clinical and applied sociologists can actively engage and participate in this process, moving toward a new form of socially just public health characterised by accountable and responsible professional relations and engagements with communities.

References

Adams, T. E. and Manning, J. (2015). 'Autoethnography and Family Research'. *Journal of Family Theory & Review*, 7 (4), pp. 350–366. https://doi.org/10.1111/jftr.12116.

Bambra, C., Riordan, R., Ford, J. and Matthews, F. (2020). 'The Covid-19 Pandemic and Health Inequalities'. *Journal of Epidemiological & Community Health*, 74, pp. 964–968.

Beck, U. (1992). *Risk Society: Towards a New Modernity*. London: SAGE.

Berghs, M. (2021). 'Who Gets Cured? COVID-19 and Developing a Critical Medical Sociology and Anthropology of Cure'. *Frontiers. Sociology*, 5, pp. 613548. https://doi.org/10.3389/fsoc.2020.613548.

Bhat, A. I. and Dar, F. A. (2020). Why Covid-19 Is a Pandemic: Seeking Answers from "Sociology of Knowledge and Social Construction". *IOSR Journal of Humanities and Social Science*, 25 (6), pp. 12–16.

Bruhn, J. G. and Rebach, H. M. (1996). *Clinical Sociology. An Agenda for Action*. New York: Plenum Press.

Burawoy, M. (2005). '2004 Presidential Address: For Public Sociology'. *American Sociological Review*, 70, pp. 4–28.

Bury, M. (1982). 'Chronic Illness as Biographical Disruption'. *Sociology of Health & Illness*, 4 (2), pp. 167–182.

Cevik, M. and Baral, S. D. (2021). 'Networks of SARS-CoV-2 Transmission'. *Science*, 373 (6551), pp. 162–163.

Chang, H. (2008). *Autoethnography as Method*. Walnut Creek, CA: Left Coast.

Connell, R. (2020). 'COVID-19/Sociology'. *Journal of Sociology*, 56 (4), pp. 745–751.

Delor, F. and Hubert, M. (2000). Revisiting the Concept of "Vulnerability" *Social Science & Medicine*, 50, pp. 1557–1570.

Dlamini, N. J. (2021). Gender-based Violence, Twin Pandemic to COVID-19. *Critical Sociology*, 47 (4–5), pp. 583–590.

Eyles, J., Harris, B., Fried, J., Govender, V. and Munyewende, P. (2015). Endurance, Resistance and Resilience in the South African Health Care System: Case Studies to Demonstrate Mechanisms of Coping within a Constrained System *BMC Health Services Research*, 15, pp. 432.

Frank, A. W. (1995). *The Wounded Storyteller: Body, Illness, and Ethics*. Chicago and London: University of Chicago Press.

Freedman, J. A. (1989). 'Defining Clinical Sociology'. *Sociological Practice*, 7 (1), pp. 7.

Fritz, J. M. (1991). 'The Contributions of Clinical Sociology in Health Care Settings'. *Sociological Practice*, 9 (1), pp. 4.

Giustini, D. (2020). 'Interpreting the COVID-19 Crisis'. The British Sociological Association. https://es.britsoc.co.uk/interpreting-the-covid-19-crisis/.

Hoppe, S. (1998). 'Clinical Sociology: An Agenda for Action'. *Clinical Sociology Review*, 16 (1), pp. 11.

Hufschmidt, G. (2011). 'A Comparative Analysis of Several Vulnerability Concepts'. *National Hazards*, 58, pp. 621–643. https://doi.org/10.1007/s11069-011-9823-7.

Jolly, R. J. (2022). 'Decolonising "Man", Resituating Pandemic: An Intervention in the Pathogenesis of Colonial Capitalism'. *Medical Humanities*, 48 (2), pp. 221-229

Klein, N. (2007). 'Disaster Capitalism'. *Harper's Magazine*, 315, pp. 47–58.

Langsi, R., Osuagwu, LU., Goson, PC., Abu, EK (2021). Prevalence and Factors Associated with Mental and Emotional Health Outcomes among Africans during the COVID-19 Lockdown Period—A Web-based Cross-Sectional Study. *International Journal of Environmental Research and Public Health*, 18 (3), pp. 899. http://dx.doi.org/10.3390/ijerph18030899.

Lewins, K., Seabi, T., Maphalela, K., Seotsanyana, L., Nyirenda, T. and Benvie, C. (2020). 'Reflections on First Wave COVID-19 Practice: Insights from Family-Patient-Liaisons'. *South African Review of Sociology, 51* (3-4), pp. 165–187

Mathewman, S. and Huppatz, K. (2020). 'A Sociology of Covid-19'. *Journal of Sociology*, 56 (4), pp. 675–683.

Metzl, J. M. and Hansen, H. (2014). 'Structural Competency: Theorizing a New Medical Engagement with Stigma and Inequality'. *Social Science & Medicine*, 103, pp. 126–133. https://doi.org/10.1016/j.socscimed.2013.06.032.

Metzl, J. M., Maybank, A. and De Maio, F. (2020). 'Responding to the COVID-19 Pandemic: The Need for a Structurally Competent Health Care System'. *JAMA*, 234 (4), pp. 231–232.

Metzl, J. M., Petty, J. and Olowojoba, O. V. (2018). 'Using a Structural Competency Framework to Teach Structural Racism in Pre-Health Education'. *Social Science & Medicine*, 199, pp. 189–201. https://doi.org/10.1016/j.socscimed.2017.06.029.

Milan, S. and Treré, E. (2020). 'The Rise of the Data Poor: The Covid-19 Pandemic Seen from the Margins'. *Social Media + Society*, September, pp. 1–5.

Monaghan, L. F. (2020). 'Coronavirus (COVID-19), Pandemic Psychology and the Fractured Society: A Sociological Case for Critique, Foresight and Action'. *Sociology of Health & Illness*, 42 (8), pp. 1982–1995.

Moultrie, T., Dorrington, R., Laubsher, R., Groenwald, P. and Bradshaw, D. (2021). *Correlation of Excess Natural Deaths with Other Measures of the COVID-19 Pandemic in South Africa*. Burden of Disease Research Unit, SAMRC, 23 February 2022.

National Institute for Communicable Diseases (NICD). (2020). 'Alerts'. https://www.nicd.ac.za/media/alerts.

Onyeaka, H., Anumudu, C. K., Al-Sharify, Z. T., Egele-Godswill, E. and Mbaegbu, P. (2021). 'Covid-19 Pandemic: A Review of the Global Lockdown and its Far-Reaching Effects'. *Science Progress*, 104 (2), pp. 1 –18.

Oppong, J. R., Mayer, J. and Oren, E. (2015). 'The Global Health Threat of African Urban Slums: The Example of Urban Tuberculosis'. *African Geographical Review*, 34 (2), pp. 182–195. https://doi.org/10.1080/19376812.2014.910815.

Phaswana-Mafuya, N., Shisana, O., Jassat, W., Baral, S. D., Makofane, K., Phalane, E., Zuma, K., Zungu, N. and Chadyiwa, M. (2021). 'Understanding the Differential Impacts of COVID-19 among Hospitalised Patients in South Africa for Equitable Response'. *SAMJ*, 111 (11), pp. 1084–1091.

Poulous, C. (2021). *Essentials of Autoethnography*. Washington DC: American Psychological Association.

Reynolds, L. (2020). 'The Coronavirus Crisis and the Struggle for Health'. *Amandla*, April 3, 2020. https://aidc.org.za/the-coronavirus-crisis-and-the-struggle-for-health/.

Ruppel, S. (2020). 'When Your Lab is the World but the World is Closed Down-Social Science Research in Times of Covid-19'. From: Elephant in the lab, 9 June 2020: https://elephantinthelab.org/when-your-lab-is-the-world-but-the-world-is-closed-down/

SA News. (2021). 'Gauteng Dealing with COVID-19 Third Wave Pressure'. *South African Government News Agency*, June 21, 2021. https://www.sanews.gov.za/south-africa/gauteng-dealing-covid-19-third-wave-pressure.

Scambler, G. (2018). *Sociology, Health and the Fractured Society: A Critical Realist Account*. Oxon, NY: Routledge.

Schellekens. (2022). 'The Global Picture of Excess Deaths is Disturbing'. https://pandem-ic.com/the-global-picture-of-excess-deaths-is-disturbing/.

Team, V. and Manderson, L. (2020). 'How COVID-19 Reveals Structures of Vulnerability'. *Medical Anthropology*. pp. 671–674.

Uys, T. (2021). 'The Emergence of Clinical Sociology in South Africa'. In Fritz, J.M (ed) *International Clinical Sociology*, Springer, Cham pp. 109–127.

Ward, P. R. (2020). 'A Sociology of the Covid-19'. *Journal of Sociology*, 56 (4), pp. 726–735.

Watts, M. and Bohle, H. G. (1993). 'The Space of Vulnerability: The Causal Structure of Hunger and Famine'. *Progress in Human Geography*, 17 (1), pp. 43–67.

Wilkinson, A. (2020). 'Local Response in Health Emergencies: Key Considerations for Addressing the COVID-19 Pandemic in Informal Urban Settlements'. *Environment and Urbanization*, 32 (2), pp. 503–522.

Will, C. M. and Bendelow, G. (2020). 'Processing the Pandemic'. *Sociology of Health & Illness*, 42 (8), pp. 1–3.

Worldometer. (2022). COVID-19 Coronavirus Pandemic. https://www.worldometers.info/coronavirus/.

Zinn, J. O. (2021). 'Introduction: Towards a Sociology of Pandemics'. *Current Sociology*, 69 (4), pp. 435–452.

Žižek, S. (2020). *Pandemic: COVID-19 Shakes the World*. New York: John Wiley & Sons.

5 Community Health Workers – COVID-19 Lived Experiences

The Case of Jharkhand, India

Ujjwala Gupta

Introduction

The World Health Organization (WHO, 2020a) International Human Rights (IHR) Emergency Committee on COVID-19 declared the 2020 outbreak a public health emergency of international concern. WHO (2020b) referenced the COVID-19 rate of infection triggered by SARS-CoV-2 as causing the severe acute respiratory syndrome. India's first reported SARS-CoV-2 case was documented in a 20-year-old woman in Kerala in January 2020. This case marked the beginning of India retaining its number 2 spot in the Worldometers (2022) live SARS-CoV-2 data.

India was unprepared for the magnitude of the pandemic, daily infections, deaths, and lack of hospital beds, personal protective gear, and treatment options (Singhal, 2020). The increasing number of SARS-CoV-2 cases intensified with unregulated safety screening, low testing protocol, and unreported cases. The absolute number of untreated and undocumented SARS-CoV-2 patients remained unclear, and current statistics offered only a rough estimate (WHOc, 2020).

The sudden appearance and upsurge of SARS-CoV-2 paralyzed the foundations of human lives across the globe. WHO (ND) reports claimed the COVID-19 pandemic is a more significant risk to frontline workers and women CHWs versus those infected with SARS-CoV-2. WHO (2020b; 2021) established that CHW activities adapted significantly to undertake various healthcare roles and patient responsibilities. CHWs faced increased occupational exposure risk of COVID-19, augmenting their social, physical, and mental vulnerability. WHO (2021) estimated that approximately 80,000 and 1,800,000 healthcare workers died from COVID-19 infections between January 2020 and June 2020 (*The Wire*, 2020).

The Charter of World Patient Safety Day (WHO, 2020g) called upon all governments to intensify the focus on vital lifesaving roles of frontliners and CHWs during the pandemic. The charter supported campaigns to highlight safety protocol efforts, personal protective gear, and hand washing to increase the health safety, and effective functioning of public health systems (WHO, 2020f). The charter was critical as India's public health system delivers varied quality in rural and urban areas with glaring differences between public and private healthcare systems. Expanding healthcare services across India presented a challenge where the population tipping 1.3 billion left the health sector in crisis (WHO, 2020j).

DOI: 10.4324/9781003267133-7

WHO's (2020d) report on Global Strategy on Human Resources for Health Workforce (2030) recognises the need for adequate investment in the healthcare workforce. The investment would deliver an overall upgrade in healthcare delivery to India's population. Low financial investment in public healthcare, state of education, and skill-oriented training failed to build an adequate workforce required for India. India's historical colonial past, the caste system, and systemic patriarchy entrench gross inequalities intersecting in the current state of its public health system. India's rural population accounts for 66% of its 1.3 billion people. Rural dwellers confront significant challenges accessing health services from registered medical practitioners, where a community population has 1:10,926 per healthcare professional, which stands against universal standards of WHO (2020b), recommending 1:1000 person–doctor ratio. WHO (2020e) reports that India has a shortage of 1.8 million doctors, impacting the workload of CHWs. The lack of healthcare professionals forced CHWs to serve a population of 10,000. Multiple instances documented indicate the ineffectiveness of the Indian rural health system in handling emergencies and the overloading of patients with their inadequate treatment in the urban health system (Kumar et al., 2020).

In 2005, the government of India, under the National Rural Health Mission (NRHM), introduced a cadre of capillary link workers between the health system and rural community by introducing women volunteers known as Accredited Social Health Activists (ASHAs). Voluntary CHWs constitute a significant number of women. A largely women-driven workforce was directly attached to India's pandemic health delivery system. CHWs served a pivotal role in communities amid COVID-19. CHWs confronted role overload, expected to fulfil pre-COVID-19 patient care in addition to COVID-19 patients. The burden imposed on CHWs acknowledged that CHWs have traditionally operated at peripheral levels independent of India's state healthcare system. CHW's distinguished competence and placement determined their undeniable status in the structured organisation of India's health system.

Nevertheless, CHWs have been under extreme pressure as the first line of defence, overstretched to continue routine activities and surveys, and responsible for managing potential COVID-19 education, safety, testing, and patient care. CHWs worked to dispel misinformation via health education advocacy and education in rural areas. CHWs function in indigent communities with limited personal protective equipment (PPE) increases their risk of infection, leaving them vulnerable to SARS-CoV-2 (Jha, 2020).

Santhosh et al. (2021) identify that despite the lack of structural integration, the independent CHW model has been instrumental in implementing 'culturally and linguistically' appropriate primary healthcare goals to respond to diverse community requirements. However, recurrent waves of the pandemic challenged their efficiency, overstretching the capacity of CHWs and bringing them to the forefront of discourse. There have been many instances of burnout and limited skills and abilities among healthcare workers, making things worse in the community, who eventually depended on them for health services (Loke and Fung, 2014). The focus on COVID-19 activities and tremendous work pressure substantially reduced other essential healthcare activities (Santra, 2021).

India's three-tier public health system has experienced an increasing trend of communicable and non-communicable diseases (epidemiological transition). The growing elderly population (demographic transition) and maternal and new-borne morbidity/mortality has been affected by immeasurable human resources shortages, financial inadequacy, failing infrastructure, skill limitations, and poor maintenance of healthcare facilities infrastructure. India looked forward to CHWs providing grassroots healthcare roles in communities. CHWs' relevance and role as India's largest voluntary group of women placed them at the forefront of the pandemic. The context of ASHA is examined and scrutinised for its invincible role in managing COVID-19 emergency services in India (Santra, 2021; Miyamoto, 2021). The political leadership and the central health system recognised CHW's proactive support in the fight against the COVID-19 crisis. Still, many of their challenges and difficulties remained unanswered in response to the rapidly evolving pandemic situation.

The lessons learned to date have helped not only to respond to public health emergencies but also to review the capacity, skills, and challenges of CHWs. It is, therefore, imperative to understand the supportive role of CHWs within the public health system and the challenges associated with their experiences and reflections. This chapter looks at the need for gender-based health policies and programmes in this context. This chapter relies on secondary data, reports, and documented responses supported by empirical data that capture the experiences of frontline workers in India. The author chose Jharkhand as one of the remote states of India to explore the scenario.

Profiling CHWs' Trajectories

ASHA-Linking Community and Public Health Systems

ASHAs are women volunteers from the same village, in the age group of 25–45 years. They are a cadre of CHWs with no permanent pay base. Their payments are on an honorarium basis based on the actual service delivery in the form of supporting Auxiliary Nurses and Midwives (ANMs) and simultaneously doing community awareness based on their rapport with the community through interpersonal communication. Thus, they connect the community to the primary healthcare system. ASHA bridged the human resource gaps given the ANM's inability to provide health services at the patient's doorstep. This initiative of the government of India, as part of the National Rural Health Mission, was seen as an innovative approach to achieving equity in healthcare, particularly maternal and child healthcare. Given the nature of the work, an ASHA per 1,000 population was promoted (Nayar et al., 2021).

ASHA COVID-19 Control

According to the Ministry of Health and Family Welfare, nearly nine lakh ASHAs were deployed in rural and urban areas for COVID-19 control activities. Even though their privileges are limited, and they have the lowest levels of education in the system, their role remains invincible. They were assigned to make door-to-door visits to trace COVID-19 symptoms, keep a vigilant track record of masses of migrant workers, and generate awareness by addressing myths and rumours in the community against the disease and vaccination (Behera et al., 2020). Awasthi (2020) and Ahmad et al. (2022) state that newer assignments added to their work-load and duty hours, leading to delays in other routine activities and causing falls in immunisation, antenatal check-ups, birth control measures, and other regular surveillance activities. Consequently, there were increasing cases of other diseases and maternal and child mortality/morbidity with an increase in the number of births.

With an increasing number of cases, very high mortality, and highly risk-laden prevention coverage without health insurance or adequate PPE, the vulnerability of ASHAs further increased. Beyond these, they remained the first-hand witness to the plight of COVID-19 victims in hospitals fighting the disease with their families pleading for beds in hospitals, oxygen cylinders, and medicines with the apathy of the hospital staff towards patients and pricey treatment that added to their psycho-logical trauma (Bhowmick, 2021). Above all, ASHA workers dying of COVID-19 because contracting the disease during their field duties without adequate personal protective cover created insecurity among them, raising several ethical questions about the health system (Chandra, 2022). *Indian Express* (2022) reported the dis-bursement of a small honorarium for CHWs to reach rural communities and expand healthcare to a larger area. Despite the insignificant payment, poor medical sup-plies, limited training access, no PPE, employment benefits, health insurance, sick leave, and travel allowances, women CHWs responded to the call for help. Women CHWs experienced elevated stress levels impacting their familial and domestic responsibilities. Countering perceptions of people towards COVID-19 (Gupta and Nayar, 2021) and mobilising the community against misinformation regarding the infection was a significant problem faced by ASHAs that negatively influenced their preventive work, including vaccination.

Methodology

This fieldwork was conducted from April to May 2021 in the Gumla district of Jharkhand, India, and occurred in a post-COVID-19 context phase between 2020 and 2021. Given the conceptual context and the current role of frontline CHWs (ASHA called *Sahiyaa* in Jharkhand) in the pandemic response, especially in identifying patients with COVID-19, by liaising with the primary healthcare system and monitoring confirmed cases, this study explores CHWs' narratives in the context of their experiences. Following the mandated pandemic protocol of social distancing, hand washing, and use of masks, researchers conducted in-depth interviews with CHWs from different communities in rural areas. The field-work followed a data saturation approach and included ten respondents of various social and geographical criteria from Jharkhand, one of India's economically marginalised states. Since the research involved mapping lived experiences and insights of CHWs and COVID-19, face-to-face and telephone interviews, using open-ended questions in the local language (*Hindi and Saadri*), with verbal con-sent from respondents, were conducted. The responses were transcribed, coded, and analysed thematically to extract lived experiences and pandemic insights.

Findings

ASHAs Undertaking COVID-19 Care

Catchment Area

Jharkhand has poor socio-economic and development conditions, with a 26% tribal population. Unlike the rest of India, COVID-19 intensified the poor living conditions in Jharkhand. Jharkhand state was the first to experience the fatal second wave of COVID-19 during the first quarter of 2021, exposing additional pressure on previously ill-equipped healthcare infrastructure. The lack of essential healthcare equipment and services worsened to the extent that it failed to give medical care even to critical patients. The reliance on ASHA facilitated access to women in rural communities to monitor active COVID-19 cases and track migrant movement.

> In the first phase of Corona, my area had no active, positive cases but later, several people in one family were affected with no noticeable symptoms. There were no quarantine centers, and people were home-quarantined, which affected many people. It increased the number of families screened and surveyed in the community. My work area is an urban ward of 1,000 in population, but my catchment area was increased to nearly 2,500 during the COVID-19 pandemic, overloading me.

Trust

Many workers revealed that people usually did not respond to them due to fear of stigma/anxiety associated with COVID-19 or mistrust in the public health system. Especially during the first phase of COVID-19, social isolation, lack of trust, and ostracism were the critical phenomena felt by most workers as they were not allowed to enter many houses due to the pervasive practice of casteism (differences based on caste classification). COVID-19 protocols, guidelines, and instructions increased the challenges and frustrations of CHWs, which were intensified by a series of imposed lockdowns and curfews. ASHA workers shared their lived experiences:

> Before COVID-19, people contacted me, but when COVID-19 hit, people did not trust us, and they refused to cooperate with us, saying- we are all Ok here! They interacted with us differently and talked to us from a distance.
>
> People escaped and passed comments saying – Corona wali aa gae! (Corona woman has come). They covered their faces and closed their eyes, seeing us coming or passing the road.

However, lately, the central government's response to the multifaceted approach to COVID-19 with the integration of various institutions has supported ASHAs in community engagement and mobilisation for vaccination. Panchayats, NGOs, youth, farm groups, and self-help groups helped ASHAs address misconceptions and challenges and gain community trust.

Panchayat and Mahila Mandal actively volunteered to mobilise people in our village to conduct door-to-door investigations, organise quarantine facilities, maintain the list of migrants, and in COVID-19 vaccination.

ASHA's COVID-19 Knowledge

Besides their personal beliefs, ASHA workers demonstrated a broad understanding of COVID-19 because of the brief formal instructions they received from their medical supervisors. Participants considered this a deadly viral infection spread due to killing wild animals for eating. They knew no specific medicine was available for its treatment, and it spread even by touch, with a runny nose, sneezes, and fever as its common symptoms. Many also knew that it affected the liver and so on. The first phase of the pandemic went a lot less prepared, with no time for training. In the subsequent step, training sessions aimed to improve knowledge of COVID-19 and deliver appropriate scientific preventive measures, such as using PPE kits, and masks, caring for COVID-19 patients, social distancing, and isolating, giving ASHAs a lot more confidence.

This was the first time we heard of such a disease which took each person into fear and doubt for one another. My grandmother, who is 90, says that we have the experiences of 'Mahamari' epidemics like cholera, diarrhea, and plague repeating year after year when the entire community was affected but never of such a disease called 'COVID-19.' However, getting it will not survive, and there is no medical treatment. People are wearing plastic!

My experience with the first round was very tragic. In the second phase, after familiarity with the nature of the disease and the use of the PPE kit despite the fear, I was very confident.

Role Overload

The pressure to perform existing and additional tasks due to the pandemic was a severe issue that affected women workers. It involved many people mentally and physically, and some of them found it hard to do domestic work and care for their children, sick and elderly at home. CHWs had to play a dual role in terms of increased work pressure and requests from the family that significantly impacted their work.

We needed to complete the everyday targets and do the paperwork work after the day's schedule until midnight.

Our catchment area increased by twice its size, and we had to work overtime at a stretch with no leaves in between, which exhausted us.

Stigma

The fieldwork of healthcare workers is an essential dimension of pandemic response efforts. The other healthcare personnel expressed that ASHA workers gave their full potential to detect COVID-19-positive people and provide all necessary assistance during this period. Simultaneously, they had to face much opposition to home visits.

> People often expressed discontent when we visited them regularly; we found out about their health. Home visits were the most labour-intensive tasks. Though the patients families remained supportive of their duties, difficulties in the community emerged with the stigma and fallacies attached to a 'corona carrier' and expressions witnessed.

Tackling people's perceptions was ASHA workers' most severe and threatening task. People from different backgrounds had different beliefs and often reacted with hostility making it harder for them to encourage government guidelines. Many people attributed the situation as a punishment due to sins and harms perpetrated by humans against nature.

> Corona is a form of curse of God of this Janma (Lifetime), and it will keep circling, no matter how many vaccines and precautions we take to prevent it; Nature is taking a turn, and our air is poisoned.

There were views from people that considered the pandemic as an International Political agenda,

> It is an international politics where each wants to overpower the other. It is a well-planned and managed intervention to distract the attention of ordinary people and governments of all nations of the world and to evolve as a superpower.

Pre-COVID-19

Jharkhand being prone to vector-borne and water-borne diseases like dengue, malaria, and typhoid made the matter worse for the healthcare system, in addition to the high number of COVID-19 cases.

> Last time, we were involved in surveys, testing, and community mobilisation. In this phase, we are engaged in the COVID-19 vaccination drive and simultaneously other duties related to dengue and malaria, which are also rising.

Occupational Health and Safety

During the second wave, the situation in rural Jharkhand remained even more debilitating, with no definite estimate of the upsurge in cases and mortality rate. ASHAs underwent constant fear of contracting SARS-CoV-2 due to limited or low-grade

PPE kits provided predominantly to them. Their needs are largely ignored due to enormous pressure on the health system to tackle the increasing number of cases.

> We were given masks and gloves during the first phase, which got old and torn off. In the second phase, most of us were either buying our own or using thin clothes like our stole or dupatta *(veil)* as masks which were neither safe for ourselves nor anyone else. We feel left out and inferior in the system where most privileges are given to doctors and nurses in regular employment. The health system does not compensate for any damage to our health. My family pressures me to quit my job and stay home like other women in the village.

Concealing Evidence

Intersecting pandemic contexts included transmission, misinformation, and *infodemic*. Families and migrant workers refused to provide travel information, occupational roles, demographic details, and medical histories for fear of isolation and stigmatisation. Missing data compromised the tracing of contacts. SARS-CoV-2 conditions created daily challenges for ASHA workers' accurate collection of COVID-19 data.

> Many families hide their fever and cold symptoms, fearing being taken away by the health services for having Corona. We did our duties of convincing such families because we did not have the option to leave this job.

Payment Delays

Paying honoraria remains a contentious issue across the state of Jharkhand. COVID-19 government incentives included Rs. 1,000 per month and post-COVID-19 incentives escalated to Rs. 1,00,000 per annum (*New Indian Express*, 2022). Incentive payments were disbursed as awards for pandemic responses. Costs were problematic, and instances of payment divergence were reported across the state of Jharkhand, leaving healthcare workers to need more time to receive payments. Unregulated employment and work records compounded the costs for the delivery of routine healthcare. The pandemic context delayed overpayments, while they have suffered extreme neglect from the health system. Declining income forced women CHWs to extend and increase their debts and mortgages. The state's irregular payments to the *Sahiyaa*/ASHA in tribal and nontribal areas were commonly reported. *Sahiyaa*/ASHA workers blamed officials for payment delays, and government administrators demanded bribes from *Sahiyaa*/ASHA to receive payments for work.

> Due to COVID-19, even our previous payments are held up. Your duty records are still pending to be signed by ANM due to COVID-19 work pressure. In the main office, getting the sanction to get the payment is possible by bribing the babu. I also participated in the ASHA demonstration

for offsetting our COVID-19 premiums. All ANMs and healthcare workers received compensation on time, and we worked like slaves and still struggled for our payments!

Response to Healthcare

Towards COVID-19 Care

ASHA workers expressed dissatisfaction and extreme negativity towards their care role during COVID-19. They complained about the need for more remuneration for their activities, the inconsistent work schedule, and the lack of status in the structured organisation of the healthcare system. ASHA workers witnessed the proliferation of COVID-19, unprecedented hospitalisations, and expenses first-hand. They still dared to take up their duties in COVID-19. During the second wave, the situation remained even more debilitating, with no definite estimate of the cases and mortality rate increase.

> I work as a Sahiyaa simply because we need some money, and the small stipend I get by working here is also a significant support for us.
> We do not have any specific time of duty. We could be called anytime in 24 hours, and for that, my family does not support me.
> My family members do not allow me to meet and talk to outside male members.
> I was compelled to continue my duty despite testing positive for COVID-19. I was forced to continue because I feared losing my job and the stipend.
> Several Sahiyaa workers tested positive at work, and some even died, but our loss in this disaster neither counted nor mattered to anyone. Last time, we had masks, sanitiser, and gloves, but nothing this time.

COVID-19 Healthcare

ASHAs, despite all challenges, still demonstrated a sense of accountability towards the role assigned to them. As the second phase of the disease wholly devastated life, they continued offering their best services to distressed families. They showed a willingness to work but were waiting for additional training, safety measures, and appropriate compensation for other tasks. Although they were underpaid, overloaded with work, surrounded by many negative experiences, and come from backward socio-economic backgrounds, most ASHAs find their wages a hope and continue contributing to COVID-19 activities. Women in the community were also highly dependent on them.

> My family tested for COVID-19, so I requested time off, but my supervisor declined. However, our duty and interaction with people were in no way compromised, even though we had minor protective covers.

I work as a Sahiyaa because I have a large family to feed, and the little allowance I get from working here also supports us.

The Future of Universal Health Care and CHWs in India

The study highlights the experiences of CHWs, who demonstrate that they are ready to work in difficult situations despite enduring challenges. They have remained the primary choice for any population health claim due to their reach and proximity to the community. This study demonstrates some of the critical factors that have impacted their ability and willingness to take on the COVID-19 services that, if appropriately addressed, could strengthen the disease response in Jharkhand. Primarily, there is a lack of compensation for their work in conjunction with workload and inappropriate scheduling during the COVID-19 phases. The destructive COVID-19 virus and its subsequent variants undoubtedly broke the spine of India's health system, especially regarding the limited provisions for managing public health emergencies, the lack of staff, the quality of infrastructure support, and the unequal gender hierarchy. Most women workers face gender inequalities and expectations in their work within the healthcare system. Secondly, there was a common ground between the urban and rural CHW (ASHA/*Sahiyaa*) concerning pressures on healthcare workers and additional efforts to counter misinformation. Supporting frontline healthcare workers in primary emergency healthcare spaces is essential to counter unpleasant human interactions, maintain security, and counter misinformation that hinders positive health actions. It is vital to revive the preventive protocols in health programmes to strengthen the health service system at the grassroots level, significantly enhancing the trust between workers and people. The COVID-19 pandemic presents an opportunity to recognise, improve primary care workers' roles, and develop effective and gender-sensitive control strategies. India experiences frequent epidemics and natural disasters, so understanding the needs and functions of CHWs are critical. They were motivated by the need for safety and protection from occupational health risks by providing PPE kits, training, disinfectants, vaccines, etc., in addition to their convenience in terms of transportation, work schedules, free time at work, and subsequently, to make their job less taxing. Existing literature facilitated new knowledge with the findings that indicate the need for collaborative efforts between government and non-profit agencies, NGOs, and the private sector to establish the political will for transformation.

References

Ahmad, S.S.A., Karimi, A., Mojdeganlou, H., et al. (2022). "Impact of COVID-19 pandemic on routine vaccination coverage of children and adolescents: A systematic review". *Health Science Report*, 18,5(2), pp. 1–12.

Awasthi, P. (2020). *The Life of ASHA Workers in the Time of COVID-19*. Available at: https://www.theweek.in/news/india/2020/04/10/the-life-of-asha-workers-in-the-time-of-covid-19 (Accessed: 3 May 2021).

Behera, D., Praveen, D. and Behera, M.R. (2020). "Protecting Indian Health Workforce during the COVID-19 pandemic". *Journal of Family Medicine and Primary Care*, 9, pp. 4541–4546.

Bhowmick, N. (2021). "Our lives do not matter. India's female community health workers say the government is failing to protect them from COVID-19". *Time*. Available at: https://time.com/6045836/india-covid-19-healthcare-workers-asha/ (Accessed: 4 May 2021).

Chandra, J. (2022). *Honours the Role of ASHA Workers for their Crucial Role in Linking the Community during the COVID-19 Pandemic.* Available at: https://www.thehindu.com/news/national/who-honours-asha-workers-for-their-crucial-role-linking-community-during-covid-19-pandemic (Accessed: 3 August 2022).

Gupta, U. and Nayar, K.R. (2021). "COVID-19 and popular discourses in Jharkhand: A qualitative study". *Journal of Anthropological Survey of India*, 70(2), pp. 1–10.

Jha, N. (2020). *India's First Line of Defense against the Coronavirus is an Army of 900,000 Women without Masks or Hand Sanitiser.* Available at: https://www.buzzfeednews.com/article/nishitajha/india-coronavirus-cases-ashas (Accessed: 24 June 2021).

Kumar, A., Nayar, K.R. and Koya, S.F. (2020). "COVID-19: Challenges and its consequences for rural health care in India". *Public Health in Practice*, 1 (100009), pp. 1–3.

Loke, A.Y. and Fung, O.W.M. (2014). "Nurses' competencies in disaster nursing: Implications for curriculum development and public health". *International Journal of Environmental Research and Public Health*, 1, pp. 3289–3303.

Miyamoto, I. (2021). "COVID-19 healthcare workers: 70% are women". *Asia-Pacific Center for Security Studies*, pp. 1–3. Available at: Security-nexus-COVID-19-Healthcare-Workers-miyamoto.pdf (dkiapcss.edu) (Accessed: 5 May 2023)

Nayar, K.R., Vijayan, B., Sunitha, S.B., Sivanand, S., Kapila, V.S. and Gupta, U. (2021). "The role of Community Level Workers in COVID-19 control activities: A Case Study from India". The Independent Panel for Pandemic Preparedness and Response. Entering communities in pandemic preparedness and response, Background paper 10, WHO.

New Indian Express. (2022). "ASHA workers get kudos but need good pay". *The New Indian Express*. Available at: https://www.newindianexpress.com/cities/bengaluru/2 (Accessed: 3 August 2022).

Santhosh, J., Durbach, A. and Joshi, R. (2021). "Charting the rights of community health workers in India: The next Frontiers of universal health coverage". *Health and Human Rights Journal*, 3(2), pp. 225–238. Available at: https://www.hhrjournal.org/2021/08/charting-the-rights-of-community-health-workers-in-india-the-next-frontier-of-universal-health-coverage/ (Accessed: 24 June 2021).

Santra, S. (2021). *Maternal and Child Health Sidelined Amidst COVID-19 Emergencies.* Available at: https://www.villagesquare.in/maternal-and-child-health-sidelined-amidst-covid-19-emergencies/ (Accessed: 24 June 2021).

Singhal, T. (2020). "A review of coronavirus disease-2019 (COVID-19)". *Indian Journal of Pediatrics*, 87 (4), pp. 281–286.

The Wire. (2020). *More than 2000 Healthcare Workers have Tested Positive for COVID-19.* Available at: https://thewire.in/health/delhi-healthcare-workers-covid-19-positive (Accessed: 15 June 2022).

WHO, World Health Organization. (2020a). *COVID-19 IHR Emergency Committee.* Available at: https://www.who.int/groups/covid-19-ihr-emergency-committee (Accessed: 22 July 2022).

WHO, World Health Organization. (2020b). *Here is a Current Outbreak of Coronavirus (COVID-19).* Available at: https://www.who.int/health-topics/coronavirus (Accessed: 18 June 2022).

WHO, World Health Organization. (2020c). *India Situation Report 2020*. Available at: India-situation-report (Accessed: 18 June 2022).

WHO, World Health Organization. (2020d). *Health Workforce Policy and Management in the Context of the COVID-19 Pandemic Response: Interim Guidance*. Available at: https://apps.who.int/iris/bitstream/handle/10665/337333/WHO-2019-nCoVhealth_workforce-2020.1-eng.pdf (Accessed: 10 July 2022).

WHO, World Health Organization. (2020e). *COVID-19: Occupational Health and Safety for Health Workers: Interim Guidance*. Geneva: World Health Organization. Available at: https://apps.who.int/iris/handle/10665/339151 (Accessed: 7 July 2021).

WHO, World Health Organization. (2020f). *Keep Health Workers Safe to Keep Patients Safe*. Available at: https://www.who.int/news/item/17-09-2020-keep-health-workers-safe-to-keep-patients-safe-who (Accessed: 10 July 2022).

WHO, World Health Organization. (2020g). *Patient Safety*. Available at: https://www.who.int/docs/default-source/world-patient-safety-day/health-worker-safety-charter-wpsd-17-september-2020-3-1.pdf (Accessed: 22 July 2022).

WHO, World Health Organization. (2021). *Health-and-Care-Worker-Deaths-during-COVID-19*. Available at: https://www.who.int/news/item/20-10-2021-health-and-care-worker-deaths-during-covid-19. (Accessed: 7 July 2021).

WHO, World Health Organization. (no date). *Decade for Health Workforce Strengthening in SEAR 2015–2024, the Mid-term Review of Progress*. Available at: https://apps.Ho.Nt/iris/handle/10665/333611 (Accessed: 22 July 2022).

Worldometers. (2022). *Coronavirus Updates*. Available at: https://www.worldometers.info/ (Accessed: 22 July 2022).

6 The Association of People with Sickle Cell Disease (APEDFI) and Associated Black Women in Ilhéus-BA (Brazil) during the COVID-19 Pandemic

A Sociological Analysis

Flávia Alessandra de Souza and
Maria Noemia das Neves Conceição

Translated from Portuguese to English by Iraiza de Souza Pereira.

Sickle Cell Disease (SCD) and the Health Issue of the Black Population in Brazil

According to Silvia Lúcia Ferreira, Ana Luiza de Oliveira Carvalho, and Enilda Rosendo do Nascimento,

> The term sickle cell disease is used to define hemoglobinopathies in which at least one of the abnormal haemoglobins is HbS. It is the genetic alteration more common in our population, characterised by a type of mutant haemoglobin called haemoglobin S (or HbS) that causes the erythrocytes to distort, making them take the shape of a 'sickle' or 'half-moon' (Pnud et al., 2001; Carvalho, 2010).
>
> (Apud Carvalho, Ferreira, and Nascimento, 2013, p. 16)

> The most frequent sickle cell diseases are sickle cell anaemia (or Hb SS), S thalassemia or micro drepanocytes and double heterozygosity. HbSC and HbSD (PNUD, 2001).
>
> (Apud Carvalho, Ferreira, and Nascimento, 2013, p. 17)

> Sickle cell anaemia is one of the most common inherited haematological diseases worldwide. It appears approximately 50 to 100 thousand years ago, between the Palaeolithic and Mesolithic periods, in the countries of Central-West Africa, India and East Asia (Galiza-Neto; Pitombeira, 2003).
>
> (Apud Carvalho, Ferreira, and Nascimento, 2013, p. 17).

SCD has a prominent occurrence in the Brazilian population, which is marked by African ancestry. Bahia is the State with the highest known incidence of SCD in Brazil. In Bahia, for every 650 children that are born, one has SCD, and, for every

DOI: 10.4324/9781003267133-8

17 children that are born, one has the sickle cell trait (Brasil, Ministério da Saúde, 2013, p. 18).

It is of great importance to highlight that the Health of the Black Population (Saúde da População Negra) constitutes, at the same time, a category of analysis and a political category, which was built by the historical struggle of black women and men in Brazil. Jurema Werneck rightly points out that the black Brazilian political mobilisation present in the Marcha Nacional Zumbi dos Palmares (National March Zumbi dos Palmares), in 1995, in Brazil, and in the III World Conference against Racism, Racial Discrimination, Xenophobia, and Related Intolerance, in 2001, in South Africa, were fundamental milestones for the institutional design and implementation of public health policies for the black population in Brazil – including here specific policies for the treatment of people with sickle cell diseases. At the same time, Jurema Werneck draws attention to the systemic limitations informed by structural racism, which prevent the full implementation of these policies in the Brazilian context, and to the fact that we still do not have the issue of black women's health as a conceptual and political field in the Brazilian context within health research and in the Brazilian health system (Werneck, 2016).

In Brazil, in 2005, due to the black struggle, the National Programme for Comprehensive Care for People with Sickle Cell Disease and other hemoglobinopathies was structured, as well as the National Policy for the Comprehensive Health of the Black Population, in 2009 – both linked to the Unified Brazilian Health System – SUS. However, the Brazilian black movement has been struggling with enormous difficulty for the maintenance and implementation of these devices, which have lost a significant portion of their financial and human resources, especially since the establishment of a Brazilian federal government openly racist, misogynistic, denialist, genocidal, and warmonger. In its lethal orientation, according to official data, we have lost approximately 700,000 lives due to COVID-19 in Brazil. The majority killed by COVID-19 in Brazil are black and impoverished.

The APEDFI and Black Women with Sickle Cell Disease in Ilhéus during the COVID-19 Pandemic

Ilhéus is a Brazilian city located in the south of the State of Bahia, approximately 460 km from Salvador, the capital of Bahia. Worldwide, the region of Ilhéus became known through the novels of the writer Jorge Amado, for its social history intensely linked to the production of cocoa (its symbol fruit), for the extraordinary biodiversity of its Atlantic forest, and for its outstanding coastline – the largest of the State of Bahia. In Ilhéus is located the Universidade Estadual de Santa Cruz – UESC (State University of Santa Cruz), an institution of great impact in the South Coast Identity Territory, which is classified as the best state university in Bahia at the Times Higher Education ranking.

According to the last census carried out in Brazil in 2010, the total population of Ilhéus was estimated at 184,236 inhabitants. Of this total, 155,281 lived in urban areas while 28,955 lived in rural areas; 94,796 were women and 89,440 men; by self-declaration, 58.6 were *pardos*, 18.7 were black, 2.1 were indigenous, 19.5

were white, and 0.9 were yellow (IBGE, 2010). In Brazil, the total *negro* population is computed by adding the contingents of *pretos* (blacks) and *pardos* (browns),
given the predominance of people of African descent in the *pardos* group – a fact
highlighted by the Brazilian black movement for decades, in its historic struggle
against racism and against the myth of racial democracy in the country. From this
perspective, *negro* (black) in Brazil is a political, sociological racial category, not
a biological category (see Nascimento, 1978; Gonzalez and Hasenbalg, 1982;
Munanga, [1999] 2020). Therefore, Ilhéus had 77.3% of its population self-identi-
fied as black in 2010, configuring itself as a majority black city. At the same time,
it is important to emphasise the strong indigenous presence in Ilhéus and in the
region, which contrasts greatly with the small number of indigenous people identified in the mentioned census (see Santos (Casé Angatu), 2021; Santos (Tupinambá)
and Mello, 2021; Mello, 2021; Santos (Ayra Tupinambá), 2021).

Historically, in Ilhéus and its surroundings, racism and patriarchy underlie a
radical and persistent social inequality, which incisively affects black and indigenous people in the region. Here we mention some important historical events
involving terrible social disadvantages and pains for non-white peoples in Ilhéus
and its region, as follows: the Cururupe Massacre (euphemistically called the
'Battle of the Swimmers'), a large slaughter of indigenous people promoted by
Mem de Sá in Olivença, around 1560 (Santos (Casé Angatu), 2021, pp. 58–59);
the repression of white masters against the revolts of black people enslaved in
Engenho de Santana, in the 18th and 19th centuries (Marcis, 2000; Pinto, 2020);
the 'coronelista' persecution against Índio Caboclo Marcelino de Olivença, in the
first half of the 20th century (Santos (Casé Angatu), 2021, pp. 58–61); the profound social impoverishment linked to the great crisis of the 'vassoura de bruxa'
(witch's broom) (*Moniliophthora perniciosa fungus*) in cocoa plantations in southern Bahia, from 1989 onwards (Guimarães, 2014).

It is in this context that the Association of People with Sickle Cell Disease of
Ilhéus (APEDFI) is situated, as the first entity of its kind in the State of Bahia. Its
existence based on mobilisation is directly associated with the social history of
Ilhéus and its region. In accordance with the official document of the institution,
APEDFI was created in 1997, initially as the Association of Anaemic Sickle Cells
of Ilhéus – AAFI (Minutes of the constitution meeting of the AAFI, made official by the Special Registry of Titles and Documents and Civil Registry of Legal
Entities of Ilhéus-BA. Physical cadastral database of APEDFI). In 1998, people
with SCD in Ilhéus started to be treated in an outpatient clinic by a haematologist.
Years later, on 10 April 2014, AAFI established a new board and was renamed
APEDFI. The name change happened as a request of the entity's new presidency,
to combat the stigmatising idea that a person is synonymous with disease and that
sickle cell anaemia is the only possibility of sickle cell disease.

After a period of relative retraction (as AAFI), APEDFI streamlined its activities and helped to achieve, for people with SCD in Ilhéus and region: the hiring of
a multiprofessional team composed of 'haematologist, psychologist, nurse, social
worker, nutritionist and nursing technician'; the normalisation of the 'dispensing
of drugs for continuous use'; and the guarantee of 'participation in events related to
SCD inside and outside the city' ('Association of People with Sickle Cell Diseases

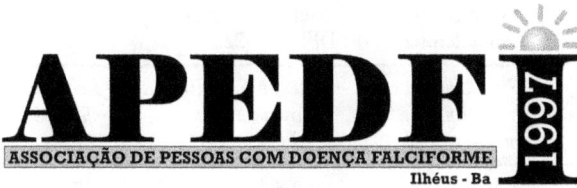

Figure 6.1 Graphic art symbol of APEDFI. Source: APEDFI digital collection.

of Ilhéus is advancing every day,' 2018). It is important to stress that both the World Day for Awareness of Sickle Cell Disease, celebrated on June 19th, and the National Day of Struggle for the Rights of People with Sickle Cell Disease, celebrated on October 27th, are fundamental dates for APEDFI, since they provide more visibility to people with SCD and an opportunity to expand society's awareness of the fight against SCD. Below we fully reproduce an essential statement made in 2018, by the coordination of APEDFI (Figure 6.1).

> With struggle and resistance, we will overcome institutional racism so that we have the care we need. 'Pain' is a force that moves us and keeps us firm, … we are a family in solidarity with the pain of the other, because the pain of one is the pain of all and if you don't feel pain, don't underestimate ours.
>
> ('Associação de pessoas com doença falciforme de Ilhéus
> vem avançando a cada dia,' 2018)

The APEDFI works in partnership with the Care Program for Sickle Cell Disease of Ilhéus – PRODOFI, a multidisciplinary and multiprofessional health local staff, and is a public utility entity, autonomous, itinerant, which configures a social movement and carries out social control in the State, in defence of comprehensive care for people with SCD (according to Municipal Law n.3788 of March 11th, 2016 – APEDFI physical cadastral database). APEDFI is the oldest association of people with SCD in the State of Bahia, has a seat on the Municipal Health Council of Ilhéus, and is part of the board of the National Federation of Associations of People with Sickle Cell Disease in Brazil – FENAFAL, as a northeast coordinator. Currently, APEDFI has a total of 157 patients registered as associates in its database and, of this total, 37.6% are women, 23.6% are men, and 38.8% are children – 21% are girls and 17.8% are boys. Among women 83.1% are black, among men 81% are black, and among children 90.1% are black. Most of the entity associates are low-income people (APEDFI physical cadastral database and post 'Dados estatísticos mostram falta de oportunidade das pessoas que vivem com doença falciforme,' 2022).

As a rights-claiming agency, APEDFI works systematically to seek quality of life for its associates, since, in general, SCD has unfavourable consequences, especially for its patients, such as hardships in achieving higher levels of education and employment. Many patients with SCD must live on the Continuous Payment

Table 6.1 Data on occupational status, profession, and sources of income of the total number of women and men associated with APEDFI in 2022

	Unemployed (%)	Public service or commerce professionals (%)	Receive continuing payment benefit – BPC (%)	Receive sickness allowance
Women	32.2	3.4	52.5	1.7
Men	16.2	8.1	51.6	5.4

Source: Authors' elaboration based on the physical cadastral database of APEDFI and the post 'Statistical data shows lack of opportunity for people living with sickle cell disease' on Facebook from APEDFI, January 30, 2022, accessible at https: //m.facebook.com/story.php? story_fbid=2982224712029232&id= 100007251972972 – accessed on January 30, 2022, at 9:35 pm.

Benefit (BPC), a monthly financial resource in the amount of only one minimum wage provided by the Organic Law of Social Assistance (LOAS) of Brazil for low-income elderly people or people with disabilities (APEDFI physical cadastral database and post 'Dados estatísticos mostram falta de oportunidade das pessoas que vivem com doença falciforme,' 2022). Below we present APEDFI percentage data that allow us to establish some comparisons between associated women and men (Table 6.1).

The data in Table 6.1 shows that more than half of the women and men associated with APEDFI depend on BPC for a living, which means that these groups have health limitations caused by sickle cell disease and low purchasing power. Comparatively, the data also shows that female associates have an unemployment rate twice as high as that of male associates; that they have less access to more profitable professions than male associates do; and that they receive less sickness allowance than males do. To explain the position of intersectional disadvantage projected against black women in Brazil, historically, it is essential to turn to Lélia Gonzalez (2020), Beatriz Nascimento (2007), Luiza Bairros (1995, 2002, 2008), and Sueli Carneiro (2019), black feminists avant-garde Brazilians in the Social Sciences and Humanities. Lélia Gonzalez – one of the black Brazilian feminists often referenced by the also black feminist Angela Davis – draws our attention to the sociological fact that:

> The process of exclusion of black women is patented, in terms of Brazilian society, by the two social roles assigned to them: 'domestic' or 'mulatto'. The term 'domestic' encompasses a series of activities that mark her 'natural place': housekeeper, school lunch lady, servant in supermarkets, in the hospital network, etc. The term 'mulata' implies the most sophisticated form of reification: it is called an 'export product', that is, an object to be consumed by tourists and the national bourgeoisie. Here we have the misleading offer of a pseudo job market that works like a funnel and that, ultimately, determines a high degree of alienation.
>
> (Gonzalez, 2020, p. 50)

In Ilhéus and in the surrounding areas, many women with sickle cell disease experience a very hostile and adverse social reality: a considerable part of them raises their children alone, as they are abandoned by their partners who, given the limitations that SCD imposes on the family, are absent from the responsibility of offering paternal support within the home. There are cases in which these mothers with SCD have children with SCD and take on various jobs to support themselves and their needs at home. In several cases, even mothers of children with SCD who the disease does not have find themselves unable to work outside the home or to seek professional qualifications, because they need to be with the children with SCD in medical consultations, exams, and hospitalisations due to the children's pain crises, resulting from SCD. This problem has a significant and generational impact on the lives of the families involved. These mothers, in general, start to realise that their own trajectory, marked by the lack of access to education and desired professions, tends to be repeated in the lives of their children with SCD, who have a great chance of not being able to achieve success in their educational and professional goals (APEDFI physical cadastral database and post 'Dados estatísticos mostram falta de oportunidade das pessoas que vivem com doença falciforme,' 2022).

We still do not have research on the lives of black women with SCD during the COVID-19 pandemic in Ilhéus – not only in Ilhéus, but considering cities all around the world, we believe. It is in this context of the lack of studies that we pioneered the clinical sociological research that made this chapter possible. Our objective is to sociologically study APEDFI and its associated black women, through avant-garde intellectuals of Brazilian black feminism, to share with the association, in conversation circles, the knowledge collectively built in our analysis. Knowing in depth their own collective history is essential to strengthening the group and its struggle for rights in society, remembering that clinical sociologists can do a very positive job in this process, helping groups to achieve their goals through interventions based on social justice (Fritz and Rhéaume, 2014).

Before March 2020, our interactions with APEDFI women took place in person, in spaces of the city occupied by them, in favour of the rights of people with SCD. From March 2020 – when the COVID-19 pandemic became both known and a close and scary reality for us – APEDFI monthly face-to-face meetings were interrupted. In Ilhéus, patients with SCD began to face great difficulty in performing imaging and laboratory tests, since they were suspended via SUS. As all the attention of the health system was focused on COVID-19, the great concern of people with SCD was to die from a chronic disease, isolated at home, but because of hardships imposed by the respective pandemic, not from SCD itself. On the other hand, there was also the fear of getting infected by COVID-19 when leaving home, already having SCD as a prevalent disease. In Ilhéus, the use of *hydroxyurea* by patients with SCD was not discontinued in the COVID-19 pandemic only because haematological consultations, which used to be in person, quickly became remote – that reality was possible due to the struggle of APEDFI in partnership with the PRODOFI.

From the beginning of the social isolation imposed by the COVID-19 pandemic, we focused our research on the analysis of physical documents from the

APEDFI database and on the analysis of the entity's Facebook, simultaneously. The most complete archive of APEDFI is Facebook since the main activities of the association are registered there. Through these two archives, we were able to access references on the life dynamics of black women with SCD from APEDFI, with attention to the pandemic moment. Considering the decrease in face-to-face human contact in this period, APEDFI's Facebook has established itself as the possible path of encounter, mutual support, affective, and collaborative interactions for people affected by SCD. As Mariam Seedat-Khan points in her autoethnography, participating in online mutual support networks formed by people facing common diseases is vital in times of the COVID-19 protocol (Seedat-Khan, 2022).

On APEDFI Facebook, the first post alluding to the COVID-19 pandemic was made on 14 May 2020. It is a photo without text, portraying alcohol gel in the hands of a black woman. Still on APEDFI Facebook, the second post regarding the pandemic was made on 16 March 2020, with the sentence 'Em tempo de pandemia' (in time of a pandemic), showing the card of the IX Brazilian Symposium on Sickle Cell Disease in Belo Horizonte-MG, June 2020, event cancelled due to the COVID-19 pandemic.

It is relevant to draw attention to the imagery presence of black women in the first posts about the COVID-19 pandemic that APEDFI published on its Facebook. The hands of black women are pictured sanitising, and, in the second one, there is a stylised black woman, in a prominent position next to the stylised map of Brazil. These representations are linked to the 'protagonism of black women in the struggle for the rights of people with sickle cell disease, which is not a coincidence. According to data from Dreminas, 92% of the families of these people are led by single mothers' (solo mothers, in fact) ('Mulheres negras lideram a luta das pessoas com doença falciforme,' 2019).

Based on APEDFI records, most women with SCD at the entity have low schooling levels and work informally as cleaners, laundresses, babysitters, bar maids, peanut sellers on the beach, and caregivers for the elderly. These are professions historically performed by black women, very poorly paid in Brazil in particular. During the COVID-19 pandemic, most of them lost their jobs and had to stay at home, generally taking care of their children, who stopped going to school because classes were suspended. In a context of scarcity or lack of resources at home, many of them experienced violence from their partners, marital divorce, and tensions of different orders in the family, in addition to various mental health problems. In the pandemic, hunger became a problem for many families linked to APEDFI, a reality that had not happened before, and the association was no longer able to raise and distribute food parcels to all of them. The emergency aid instituted in Brazil during the pandemic – paid by the federal government to vulnerable people, due to the struggle of social movements and left parties and against the will of the Brazilian presidency and its government team – was insufficient in the face of such a social crisis (APEDFI physical cadastral database).

It is worth noting that, in a 2010 survey on the quality of life of black women with sickle cell anaemia, carried out in Salvador-BA, Ana Luiza de Carvalho Oliveira reached the following conclusions – which we consider to be also applicable to most women with SCD from Ilhéus:

No statistically significant differences were identified between women and men [with SCD in the State of Bahia] in the analysis of global quality of life. **When classifying the quality of life into levels, it was found that women had a lower quality of life than men. There was a statistically significant difference for variables related to specific aspects: energy and fatigue, personal relationships and sexual activity, financial resources, physical environment, and transportation**. It is concluded that the use of a gender focus in health research is necessary, as a transversal axis, as it allows the visualisation of inequalities between women and men, ... [*which makes it possible*] to impact public policies to reduce such inequalities.

(Carvalho, 2010, p. 6. Emphasis added)

Even with all the adversities faced during the COVID-19 pandemic, APEDFI managed to build paths and strategies to continue with its mobilisation for the lives of people with SCD. In this process of struggle, a group of black women from APEDFI stands out – remembering that the presidency of this institution is exercised by a black woman with SCD, a long-term mobiliser in the struggle for people with SCD in Ilhéus and the region. Here, we present two APEDFI events, held in 2020, which are emblematic and symptomatic of the mobilising existence of black women with SCD in the association.

In 2020, APEDFI celebrated the World Day of Awareness on Sickle Cell Disease, on June 19th, publishing on its Facebook a series of videos of people with SCD and supporters of the cause, which were filmed at home mainly by associates, respecting social isolation as a measure to combat the spread of COVID-19. We analysed seven videos, in which are starring black girls and black women from APEDFI. In these videos, while each narrative keeps its own specificity, they all reveal a lot of knowledge and practical awareness of SCD, as well as a sense of belonging to an association that, in the presence of intense pain, can support and foster self-love and collective love, paradoxically. Seeking to favour the understanding of the narratives in question, in the following, we present seven thematic categories that we built from the subjects that black girls and black women mentioned in the videos:

When emphasising the World Sickle Cell Disease Awareness Day, APEDFI presidency made a very significant post on the Facebook of the association in 2020:

Today, June 19th, is an allusive date to remind those who know and to show to those who don't know that sickle cell disease exists and that it affects a large part of the Afro-descendant population. And that these people with sickle cell disease, in addition to suffering from physical pain, also suffer

Table 6.2 Narratives of black girls and women with SCD from APEDFI due to World Sickle Cell Disease Awareness Day – 2020

Thematic category	Narrative description
Disease qualification	Sickle cell disease is a serious, dangerous, degenerative, and deadly disease.
Affirmative	I am (name). I am a person with sickle cell disease.
Surgical and therapeutic procedures performed	Surgery to remove the spleen. Surgery to remove the gall bladder. Lung drainage. Blood transfusion.
Sensitive body experience	Lots of pains. Pain crises. Pains experienced during winter.
SCD-derived health problems	Leg necrosis. Infections.
Specific challenges	Having a life marked by hospitalisations. Waiting for stem cell transplantation. Transfusions in times of a pandemic.
Social appeal	Donate blood. Save lives. Help us. Become aware. Join your city's association. Understand that SCD is not a rare disease. Meet the motto 'assume, know and care.'
Wishes	Quality of life. Living free from discrimination in society.

Source: Authors' elaboration based on videos posted on APEDFI Facebook on June 17 and 18, 2020.

from pain in the soul, but many will not understand what I am talking about. The pain in the soul exists when we are discriminated, when we are naturally ignored because we are black and poor, because we experience a disease that represents a social bother, which requires extra attention from the family, from the health professional, from managers, because sickle cell disease is degenerative, and the risk of death is imminent. That's why we need to come out and not give up, to fight against all kinds of prejudice is our goal, we need to empower ourselves and occupy spaces to gain visibility. We need to sleep and wake up dressed in the shirt that represents us. #doençafalci-formeélutaouluto #doençafalciformenadadenóssemnós.

(APEDFI Facebook post, June 19th, 2020)

On November 20th – established by the Brazilian black movement as the National Day of Black Consciousness in Brazil, following the death of the black leader Zumbi dos Palmares in 1695 – APEDFI held, in 2020, an event starring young black women linked to the entity. The activity extraordinarily took place in person, outdoors, and with a few participants, in the northern part of the city of Ilhéus. At this event, surrounded by banners with the messages 'We are all APEDFI,' 'Racism kills – Black lives matter,' 'Sickle cell disease – the most common hereditary disease in Brazil,' 'Sickle cell disease is not a rare disease,' and 'Raising awareness to better treat,' they performed the recitation of the poem 'Gritaram-me Negra,' by Victoria Santa Cruz, and a dance choreography with Afro-Brazilian and African steps to the rhythm of the song 'Jerusalema,' performed by Nomcebo Zikode[1]. These presentations would be performed at the IX Brazilian Symposium on Sickle Cell Disease in Belo Horizonte-MG, in June 2020, if it were not for the cancellation of the meeting due to the COVID-19 pandemic.

As Flávia Alessandra de Souza and Valquiria Pereira Tenório accentuate, 'celebrating the life and crowning the beauty of Black women constitutes a challenging, pedagogical, and political manifest that definitely matters' (Souza and Pereira, 2021, p. 331). In this sense, the performance of the young black women in the APEDFI 2020 Black November favoured and still favours the self-esteem and the positive mirroring of black women. This sort of expression transforms bodies into 'live sickles' against racism, sexism, classism, and against the pain of SCD itself – particularly in times of COVID-19, when social injustices against destitute people deeply increased in Brazil. These are insistent, insurgent, and resistant bodies which fight the most varied battles to stay on their feet, earning respect. Via declamation and dance, every word, and every step, counts as a bonus to exist beautifully and gladly. The sentence 'Black lives matter' is embodied with love and energy in the fierce struggle to maintain the lives of people with SCD.

Unfortunately, until February 2022, APEDFI lost a total of three associated members with SCD due to COVID-19. They were two black women and a black man who died without receiving vaccination in Brazil. Three deaths may seem like a small number in the cold letter of statistics – according to official data, until the end of February 2022, Brazil lost approximately 650,000 lives and Ilhéus lost 630 lives to COVID-19, but taking into account that these are preventable deaths, they represent a high number, considering that each life really matters, and that each death is particularly felt when it happens within a group that struggles all the time to maintain life.

APEDFI fought hard, in 2020, for people with SCD to access the COVID-19 vaccine as a priority. According to an initial determination by the Ministry of Health, a ministry led by a denialist government, people with SCD would not have priority in vaccination. But each Brazilian state had the autonomy to intervene in the national vaccination schedule for itself. When the Bipartite Inter-management Commission (CIB) of the State of Bahia established the priority groups for vaccination against COVID-19 in Bahia, it placed the immunosuppressed group in the fourth position, leaving people with sickle cell disease in the 24th position, the last of the positions. Faced with this occurrence, APEDFI began to categorically challenge CIB Bahia, as well as the Health Department of Ilhéus, questioning whether the exclusion of people with SCD from the immunosuppressed group for vaccination meant invisibility due to institutional racism or ignorance. As a result of this APEDFI protest, Ilhéus was the first city in Brazil to offer the first dose of the COVID-19 vaccine to people over 18 years old with SCD on 4 May 2021 – a historical fact that served as jurisprudence for the vaccination of this public in other Brazilian cities. This achievement was held due to the persistent mobilisation of the coordination of APEDFI during the pandemic, an entity whose board is composed mostly of black women (physical cadastral database of APEDFI).

Final Considerations

APEDFI is located in Ilhéus, a place known worldwide due to the former cocoa colonels, the beaches, and the *grapiúna* literature, but not due to the resistance, protagonism, and achievements of black women. Furthermore, the associations of people with SCD which have greater visibility are in the country's capitals, in large urban centres, while the struggles and conquests of their counterparts in country-side cities tend to be relatively disregarded.

Aware of this disproportionality, we focused on the countryside and, in our research, we found that: APEDFI is the oldest association of people with SCD in the State of Bahia – the state with the highest incidence of SCD in Brazil; people with SCD from Ilhéus were the first to receive the first dose of the COVID-19 vaccine in Brazil, mainly as a result of protest by APEDFI; through the National Federation of Associations of People with Sickle Cell Disease in Brazil – FENAFAL (see Lira and Queiroz, 2013, p. 135), APEDFI works in partnership with similar associations throughout the country, playing the role of northeast coordination within this entity.

Under the leadership of black women with SCD, the APEDFI audience knows that fighting collectively along the entity is much more fruitful than fighting alone, as they know how powerful the act of association is. Altair dos Santos Lira and Maria Cândida Alencar de Queiroz rightly highlight how fundamental is the protagonist of the struggle of people with SCD, family members, and associations of people with SCD in the promotion of health for the public with SCD (Lira and Queiroz, 2013).

But our study points up a very worrying matter: during the COVID-19 pandemic, most black women linked to APEDFI are carrying on themselves, in a much more deepened way, the weights of mourning, unemployment, loss of purchasing power and autonomy, famine, domestic tensions or loneliness at home, shattered self-esteem, deteriorated mental health, among others. Jurema Werneck was right when she proposed, in a hearing held on June 24th, 2021, at the Parliamentary Commission of Inquiry (CPI) of the pandemic, the creation of a memorial to the victims of COVID-19 and a plan of state accountability and national reparation to the individuals, families, and the community affected by the government's lack of control over the pandemic (Brasil, Senado Federal, 2021).

Because of the overload they have been managing in this pandemic, black women with SCD from APEDFI are part of a sociological sample to which the State owes great constitutional reparations. We will not have a better society if black women are not recipients of love, affection, well-being, care, zeal, respect, and rights assurance, on the part of all individuals, social groups, and institutions.

Note

1   See: https://www.youtube.com/watch?v=us67dfmFngw for APEDFI Black November 2020 performances by black young ladies; https://www.youtube.com/watch?v =RljSb7AyPc0&t=19s for "Gritaram-me negra", by Victoria Santa Cruz; https://www .youtube.com/watch?v=fCZVL_8D048 for Jerusalema song. Access on February 10th, 2022, 9 pm.

Bibliography

APEDFI Facebook post published on March 14th, 2020, picture portraying alcohol gel in the hands of a black woman, accessible at https://www.facebook.com/photo/?fbid =2486239294961112&set=a.1388891481362571 – accessed on February 10, 2022 at 1:59 pm.

APEDFI Facebook post published on March 16th, 2020, picture portraying the IX Brazilian Symposium on Sickle Cell Disease in Belo Horizonte-MG, June 2020, canceled due to the COVID-19 pandemic, accessible at https://www.facebook.com/anemiafalciforme .ilheus/posts/2488130728105302 – accessed on February 10, 2022 at 2:20 pm.

APEDFI Facebook videos posted on June 17th and 18th, 2020, about the Mobilization of APEDFI on the World Sickle Cell Disease Awareness Day – 2020, accessible at https://www .facebook.com/anemiafalciforme.ilheus/videos – accessed on February 10, 2022 at 7:05 pm.

APEDFI Facebook post on June 19th, 2020, about the World Sickle Cell Disease Awareness Day related by the APEDFI presidency, accessible at https://www.facebook.com/ anemiafalciforme.ilheus/posts/2561023677482673 – accessed on February 10, 2022 at 9:33 pm.

APEDFI Facebook post on November 21st, 2020, about the APEDFI event in celebration of Black Consciousness Day in 2020, accessible at https://www.facebook.com/photo?fbid =2688015154783524&set=a.1384905888427797 – accessed on February 10, 2022 at 8:15 pm.

APEDFI Ilhéus. Vidas negras importam. Youtube video accessible at https://www.youtube .com/watch?v=us67dfmFngw – accessed on February 10, 2022, 9 pm.

'Associação de pessoas com doença falciforme de Ilhéus vem avançando a cada dia', August 31, 2018, posted at https://cabrest.blogspot.com/2018/08/associacao-de-pessoas -com-doencas.html – accessed on January 3, 2022 at 8:05pm.

Bairros, L. (1995). Nossos feminismos revisitados. *Estudos Feministas*, v.3, n.2. Florianópolis, Universidade de Santa Catarina.

Bairros, L. (2002). Lembrando Lélia Gonzalez. Afro-Ásia, n.23. Salvador, Centro de Estudos Afro-Orientais da UFBA 2000. In Werneck, J., Mendonça, M., and White, E. (orgs.) *O Livro da Saúde das Mulheres Negras: nossos passos vêm de longe*. Rio de Janeiro: Pallas/Criola.

Bairros, L. (2008). A mulher negra e o feminismo. In Costa, Ana Alice Alcantara e Sardenberg, Cecilia Maria B. (orgs). *Relatório do Seminário Nacional: O feminismo no Brasil – reflexões teóricas e perspectivas*. Salvador: NEIM / UFBA, 1990. / O feminismo do Brasil: reflexões teóricas e perspectivas. 2ª ed. Salvador: NEIM / UFBA.

Brasil. Ministério da Saúde. (2013). Secretaria de Atenção à Saúde. Departamento de Atenção Especializada. *Doença falciforme: saiba o que é e onde encontrar tratamento / Ministério da Saúde, Secretaria de Atenção à Saúde, Departamento de Atenção Especializada*. 1. ed., reimpr. Brasília: Ministério da Saúde.

Brasil. Senado Federal. (2021). 'Médica Jurema Werneck defende responsabilização pelas mortes e danos da pandemia', post published on June 24, 2021 at https://www12.senado .leg.br/noticias/videos/2021/06/medica-jurema-werneck-defende- responsabilizacao-pe las-mortes-e-danos-da-pandemia – accessed on January 5, 2022 at 16:10am.

Carneiro, S. (2019). *Escritos de uma vida / Sueli Carneiro. Prefácio de Conceição Evaristo e apresentação de Djamila Ribeiro*. São Paulo: Pólen Livros.

Carvalho, A. (2010). *Qualidade de vida de mulheres negras com anemia falciforme: implicações de gênero*. Dissertação (Mestrado em Enfermagem) – Escola de Enfermagem, Universidade Federal da Bahia, Salvador.

Carvalho, A., Ferreira, L., and Nascimento, E. (2013). Qualidade de vida e saúde de pessoas com doença falciforme: aspectos conceituais. In Cordeiro, R., and Silvia, L. (orgs.). Salvador: EDUFBA.

'Dados estatísticos mostram falta de oportunidade das pessoas que vivem com doença falciforme', APEDFI Facebook post published on January 30, 2022 accessible at https://m .facebook.com/story.php?story_fbid=2982224712029232&id=100007251972972   – accessed on January 30, 2022 at 9:35 pm.

Daltro, G., et al. (2008). Tratamento da osteonecrose da cabeça femoral com células progenitoras autólogas em anemia falciforme. *Acta Ortop. Bras*, v.16, n.1, p.23–27.

Fanon, F. (1968). *Os Condenados da Terra*. Rio de Janeiro-RJ: Editora Civilização Brasileira.

Fritz, J. M., and Rhéaume, J. (2014). *Community Intervention: Clinical Sociology Perspectives*. Dordrecht: Springer.

de Galiza, Neto, G. C., and Pitombeira, M. (2003). Aspectos moleculares da anemia falciforme. *Jor. Bras. de Pat. e Med. Lab., Rio de Janeiro*, v.39, n.1, p. 51–56.

Gonzalez, L. (2020). *Por um Feminismo Afro-Latino-Americano: Ensaios, Intervenções e Diálogos. Organizadoras: Flávia Rios e Márcia Lima*. Rio de Janeiro: Zahar.

Gonzalez, L., and Hasenbalg, C. (1982). *Lugar de negro*. Rio de Janeiro: Marco Zero.

Gritaram-me negra. Youtube video accessible at https://www.youtube.com/watch?v =RljSb7AyPc0&t=19s – accessed on February 10, 2022, 9 pm.

Guimarães, E. (2014). Ciência, técnica e tecnologia: Vassoura de Bruxa, Cacau Cabruca e a ideia de progresso no Sul da Bahia. Anais Eletrônicos do 14º Seminário Nacional de História da Ciência e da Tecnologia – 14º SNHCT.

IBGE. Censo 2010 accessible at https://cidades.ibge.gov.br/brasil/ba/ilheus/panorama – accessed on January 4, 2022.

Jerusalema song. Youtube video accessible at https://www.youtube.com/watch?v=fCZVL _8D048 – accessed on February 10, 2022, 9 pm.

Kikuchi, B. (2007). A. Assistência de enfermagem na doença falciforme nos serviços de atenção básica. *Rev. Bras. Hematol. Hemoter.*, v.29, n.3, p.331–338.

Lira, A., and Queiroz, M. (2013). O protagonismo das pessoas e seus familiares na implantação do Programa de Atenção Integral às Pessoas com Doença Falciforme. In Cordeiro, R. e Ferreira, S. (orgs.) *Qualidade de vida e cuidados às pessoas com doença falciforme*. Salvador: EDUFBA.

Marcis, T. (2000). *Viagem ao Engenho de Santana*. Ilhéus: Editus.

Mello, F. (2021). Fronteiras internas do Brasil: demarcações de terras indígenas e ações afirmativas. In Souza, F. (org.) *Ações afirmativas no Brasil contemporâneo: dinâmicas e perspectivas* [online]. Ilhéus-BA: Editus.

Mulheres negras lideram a luta das pessoas com doença falciforme, NUPAD Medicina UFMG post published on July 23, 2019 accessible at https://www.nupad.medicina.ufmg .br/mulheres-negras-lideram-a-luta-das-pessoas-com-doenca-falciforme / – accessed on January 12, 2022 at 1:02 pm.

Munanga, K. (1999, 2020). *Red013iscutindo a mestiçagem no Brasil: Identidade nacional versus identidade negra*. 5 ed. Belo Horizonte: Autêntica. Coleção Cultura Negra e Identidades.

Nascimento, A. (1978). *O genocídio do negro brasileiro*. 1 ed. Rio de Janeiro: Paz e Terra.

Oliveira, F. (2003). *Saúde da população negra: Brasil ano 2001*. Brasília: Organização Pan-Americana da Saúde.

Panepinto, J. A., Brandow, A., Mucaloena, L., et al. (2020). Coronavirus disease among persons with sickle cell disease. United States, March 20–May 21, 2020.

Pena, S. (2007). *Anemia falciforme: uma doença molecular. Coluna Deriva Genética – Instituto Ciência Hoje*.

Pinto, A. (2020). *Revolta, negociação e autoridade: o levante dos escravos do Engenho Santana, Ilhéus (1789)*. 2020. 184 f. Dissertação (Mestrado em História) – Universidade de Brasília, Brasília.

Pnud et al. (2001). *Política nacional de saúde da população negra: uma questão de eqüidade*. Brasília: Sistema Nações Unidas.

Ratts, A. (2007). *Eu sou Atlântica: Sobre a Trajetória de Vida de Beatriz Nascimento*. 1. ed. São Paulo: Imprensa Oficial/Instituto Kuanza.

Santos (Ayra Tupinambá), Vanessa Rodrigues dos. (2021). Território e resistência: Os Tupinambá de Olivença no período da globalização. In Souza, F. (org.) *Ações afirmativas no Brasil contemporâneo: dinâmicas e perspectivas* [online]. Ilhéus-BA: Editus.

Santos (Casé Angatu), C. (2021). Lutas indígenas e ações afirmativas no Brasil contemporâneo. In Souza, F. (org.) *Ações afirmativas no Brasil contemporâneo: dinâmicas e perspectivas* [online]. Ilhéus-BA: Editus.

Santos (Tupinambá), M., and Mello, F. (2021). A educação escolar indígena como ação afirmativa e instrumento de luta para valorização e revitalização da cultura indígena – O exemplo Tupinambá de Olivença. In Souza, Flávia Alessandra (org.) *Ações afirmativas no Brasil contemporâneo: dinâmicas e perspectivas* [online]. Ilhéus-BA: Editus.

Santos (Tupinambá), M., and Mello, F. (2021). A escola indígena como instrumento de luta para valorização e revitalização das culturas e identidades indígenas – O exemplo Tupinambá de Olivença. In Souza, Flávia Alessandra (org.) *Ações afirmativas no Brasil contemporâneo: dinâmicas e perspectivas* [online]. Ilhéus-BA: Editus, 2021.

Seedat-Khan, M. (2022). A clinical account of breast cancer amid COVID-19. In Heath, M., Darkwah, A., Beoku-Betts, J., and Purkayastha, B. (eds.). *Global Feminist Autoethnographies during COVID-19: Displacements and Disruptions*, 1st Edition. Routledge.

Souza, F. (org.). (2021). *Ações afirmativas no Brasil contemporâneo: dinâmicas e perspectivas* [online]. Ilhéus-BA: Editus.

Souza, F., and Tenório, V. (2021). Sites of resistance: Black woman and beauty in Black Brazilian communities of São Paulo and Bahia (chapter). In Hobson, J. (org.) *The Routledge Companion to Black Women's Cultural Histories* (book). Routledge.

Souza, N. *Tornar-se negro ou As vicissitudes da identidade do negro brasileiro.*

Werneck, J. (2016). Racismo institucional e saúde da população negra. *Saúde Soc. São Paulo*, v.25, n.3, p.535–549.

Zago, M. (2000). Anemia falciforme e doenças falciformes. In Hamann, E., and Tauil, P. (orgs.) *Manual de doenças mais Importantes, por razões étnicas, na população brasileira afrodescendente*. Brasília: UnB.

7 Filipina Caregivers and Mental Health under COVID-19

Impacts of Transnational Obligations and Precarious Work on Migrant Care Workers in the United States of America

Valerie Francisco-Menchavez, Elaika Janin Celemen, Edwin Carlos, and Chloe Janelle Punsalan

Introduction

Filipinos in the United States (US) have suffered disproportionately from deaths during the COVID-19 pandemic because of their over-representation in frontline care industries, such as nursing and formal caregiving (Wang et al., 2020; Chan and Litam, 2021). As an increasing number of 'baby boomers' (i.e., those born between 1946 and 1964) have moved into long-term care facilities, there has been a corresponding increased demand for caregivers. Consequently, many Filipino/a migrants have answered the call to become 'formal care workers' in the US partly because of a historic immigrant labour stream of care workers to the US (Choy, 2003). Unlike 'informal' caregivers, who are unpaid for the care they provide to their family members or friends, formal care workers or caregivers are in fact paid for the work that they provide to their clients. This sector of home care workers in the US is not required to fulfil the 160 minimum hours of medical training required for positions like Certified Nursing Assistants (CNAs) or Home Health Aides (HHAs). Instead, the lowest tier of care workers which are caregivers assist clients with daily living activities such as moving from one place to another, toileting, cooking, and cleaning. Despite these differences, Filipino caregivers in our study admitted that they are asked to provide care for medical issues (e.g., managing and administering medications, and changing bandages) even if they are not compensated in line with other classified care workers. In sum, caregivers are typically the least paid group of home care workers in the eldercare and long-term care industry. While Filipino caregivers were not equally compensated, they were working with the most vulnerable to COVID-19, those 65 and older with pre-existing health conditions. Thus, given their elevated exposure in COVID-19 hot spots, such as assisted living and long-term care facilities, there were high incidence rates of COVID-19 seen in Filipino caregivers.

DOI: 10.4324/9781003267133-9

Filipino migrants to the US, especially in the port cities of California like San Francisco and Los Angeles, have long occupied these positions due to a confluence of neoliberal state abandonment of funding to long-term care (Tung, 2000), as well as a history of domestic and medical labour migration from the Philippines to the US (Choy, 2003). Scholars and researchers have established that the eldercare and long-term care industries have largely relied on low-wage, disposable labour to care for the country's ageing and ill populations (Shah, 2017). Filipino caregivers in the US have been at the centre of the so-called 'crisis of care,' as they constitute one of the biggest ethnic migrant groups that have answered the call for care work, and disproportionately experience wage theft, substandard live-in work conditions, non-compensated overtime work, etc. The authors of this chapter have previously argued that Filipino caregivers have normalised their exploitation and workplace-related abuse due to their transnational obligations to financially support their families in the Philippines (Francisco-Menchavez, Celemen and Osorio, 2021). The COVID-19 pandemic became an added layer of crisis on the work conditions for Filipino caregivers, exacerbating the existing gaping wounds in the labour practises in eldercare (Nasol and Francisco-Menchavez, 2021). The coupled crisis of a broken long-term care industry in the US and the global health pandemic rendered caregivers and their work an invisible frontline and invisible frontline workers.

While we understand that Filipino caregivers' work conditions were quite arduous before the pandemic, and then exacerbated under the pandemic, we aim to explore the gendered processes that inform caregivers' decisions to continue with paid caregiving under such difficult work conditions, especially during the COVID-19 pandemic. How do gendered narratives of obligation to family and, even to the clients they cared for, shape their mental health outcomes, especially as invisible frontliners? With evidence from surveys and qualitative data, we explore the gendered narratives of filial piety that kept Filipina caregivers working in their precarious and, at times, unsafe work environments, to provide for their families in the Philippines. Their filial duty stems from Filipino gendered norms tethering Filipinos to various grades of exploitation in the caregiving industry. Although our study includes both men and women, we focus on the data from Filipina migrants for our findings, given that they are disproportionately represented in this care work occupation and in our study.

Literature Review

Scholars have established that Filipino migrant workers, especially in health and care industries, have high rates of mental health issues related to their occupation, specifically burnout (Maglalang et al., 2021, Chan and Litam, 2021). Due to the challenging tempo of the work in caregiving, and the chronic understaffing in long-term care facilities, caregivers experience various workplace stressors that can in turn negatively affect their mental health (Shah, 2017). Often caregivers in the US normalise the exploitative conditions in their workplace that can affect their mental health because they feel a strong responsibility for the clients they care for (Francisco, Celemen and Osorio, 2021). Caregivers liken their relationships with their elderly clients to mimicking how they would treat their own elderly relatives (Tung, 2000). The tension between local and transnational obligations of care, both paid (for their clients and employers in the US) and unpaid (for their biological and fictive kin in the Philippines), can produce stressors that impact mental health outcomes, especially exacerbated by the COVID-19 pandemic (Sabar, Babis and Sabar Ben-Yehoshua, 2022). In our study, Filipina care workers attest to their excellence in providing care to their clients while continuing to support their families abroad through the pandemic as actualising 'good' womanhood and daughterhood. In this way, their gendered understanding of their paid work as caregivers is linked to the ways they understand their duty to their transnational families. As scholars have argued, transnational filial obligations have and continue to influence the decisions and behaviour of Filipino migrants, more so for women than men (Parreñas, 2001; Asis, Huang and Yeoh, 2004).

Even before they leave the Philippines, patriarchal ideologies of domesticity have long shaped the lives of Filipino women in the Philippines and in the diaspora (Cruz, 2012). The Philippines, a site for overlapping empires of Spanish, American, and Japanese colonialism, has developed multiple gendered narratives constructing Filipino femininity as mobile (in terms of labour migration), yet subservient, docile, and domesticated (Rodriguez, 2005). For Filipinas, both when they are in the Philippines or when they are working abroad, the gendered expectations are to care for their families (Guevarra, 2014). In short, many Filipinas consider their decision and tenure as labour migrants as a part of their filial duty and gendered responsibility to the Filipino family (Francisco-Menchavez, 2018). The obligation to financially support families in the Philippines is a thick social bond that informs how Filipina migrants navigate the various work environments and conditions in the diaspora. The remittance-oriented nature of contemporary Filipino labour migration requires that migrants conceptualise their transnational financial responsibilities first and above their own local well-being, often creating internal conflicts about maintaining jobs that might be exploitative or hazardous (Francisco-Menchavez, 2020). This follows from the scholarship that remittance behaviours are a gendered process, producing different sending patterns and internalisation of financial responsibilities (Rahman and Fee, 2012). For Filipino women, gendered roles of caretaking are conflated with their breadwinning obligations as labour migrants abroad.

As the lives of Filipina caregivers straddle their local and transnational obligations, we examine the health outcomes and behaviours of Filipino migrants working as caregivers by contextualising these individuals in their social and cultural contexts. Scholars in sociology and social work have used 'critical feminist narrative inquiry' to centre the lives and knowledge of research participants while exposing the structural conditions that produce the hardships of their lives (Pitre et al., 2013). In this chapter, we use narrative inquiry to understand how systems of emigration and immigration in both sending and receiving contexts, the Philippines and the US, respectively, impact the lives and decisions of Filipino migrants in their workplace. We look at the narratives of Filipina care workers to assess participants' adherence to social and cultural gendered norms around care obligations. This line of inquiry frames the stories of Filipina migrants in the social and structural systems that produce them as docile and submissive workers for a global gendered market of domestic work. Scholars of critical feminist narrative inquiry

> contend that it would be useful to analyse the content (what) of the stories that were told with a view to understand the forces and conditions that shape particular experiences and delineate the boundaries of individual or collective agency, voice, identity, and reflexivity.
>
> (Pitre et al., 2013, p. 119)

By what is told in the stories of Filipina migrants, we can pull out the larger social forces that produce psychosocial outcomes on their mental health, such as emotional dissonance, stress, and anxiety (Perkins, Palmer, and García-Ramírez, 2011). Moreover, we will also highlight their ability to be resilient in the face of these social forces.

Studies in Social Work and Sociology of Labor and Work (Roberts, 1993) define that 'psychosocial' hazards on workers include 'aspects of work organization, design and management that have the potential to cause harm on individual health and safety' (Bretones, Jain, Leka, and García-López, 2020, p. 1). In this chapter, we juxtapose the effects of local work conditions to the transnational obligations as told in the narratives of Filipina migrants to bring a psychosocial assessment of their mental health outcomes. Building on the few scholars that centre Filipino migrant worker experiences and the psychosocial impacts of precarious work, especially in healthcare (Maglalang et al., 2021; Kaur-Gill, 2020), we hope to highlight how their work stressors as care workers are amplified by the transnational factors in migrant workers' lives.

Methods

The findings for this chapter are based on a mixed-methods study called 'The CARE Project' study, led by Dr Valerie Francisco-Menchavez, part of the data we use comes from the 'Filipinx Count!' survey administered by the Carlos Bulosan Centre for Filipinx American Studies at the University of California, Davis. The survey instrument measured for mental and physical health outcomes in the Filipino American community, specifically targeting Filipino/a care workers' health under COVID-19, which included items such as access to basic needs such as food, healthcare, COVID-19 testing, internet, and financial assistance. This chapter also draws qualitative data collected by a researcher on the team, which included the authors of this chapter, utilising a data collection method, '*kuwentuhan*,' a Filipino word that refers to a Filipino cultural practice of talk-story (Francisco-Menchavez, 2021). Kuwentuhan, is like a focus group, where two or more people participate in a semi-structured interview led by a researcher. The distinction of kuwentuhan from a traditional focus group is that the researcher allows for participants to build on themes or questions that one another may bring up during the session. While the open-ended prompts in the interview guide allow for later comparable data analysis, participants can explore important aspects of their experiences based on what the group builds on.

We collected 56 surveys through Filipinx Count. Separately, we recruited 32 caregivers to participate in virtual kuwentuhan since the beginning of the COVID-19 pandemic. Our recruitment strategy was two-pronged. The first: we worked with Filipino migrant organisations in the San Francisco/Bay Area that provided political education and collective action for Filipino caregivers, specifically Pilipino Association of Workers and Immigrants (PAWIS) in the Silicon Valley and the Filipino Community Centre in San Francisco. The second approach was a snowball sampling approach wherein we tapped our team's families and networks to recruit for our study since many of us had relatives that worked in the home care industry. This community-centric recruitment strategy allowed us to tap into our epistemological knowledge as members of the Filipino community, which has a formidable population working as caregivers and home care workers. The caregivers in our study came from a variety of backgrounds but trends emerged in looking at some of the descriptive statistics. The mean age of participants in our study is 53 years old, indicating that our participants are likely to be parents and/or have parents in the Philippines who may need financial support. Only 9% of our participants identified as male, the rest were female, which emphasises the gendered nature of care work. Half of the sample reported they were immigrants and 23% reported they were US citizens. The mean household income for four people ranged from $25,000 to $34,999, indicating that many of the workers hover a bit over the US poverty line, thus informing the decisions they make about working in precarious but easy-to-obtain jobs like caregiving. Over a third of participants reported they had some college education. This sample reflects the demographics of Filipino migrants to the US in the past two decades characterised by middle to late life course migration, educated, English-speaking, and majority female (dela Cruz et al., 2002).

For this chapter, we used descriptive analysis of the survey data to summarise Filipino/a care workers' access to basic needs and the mental and health outcomes they self-reported. We used both grounded theory analysis and narrative analysis with the qualitative data collected. While the grounded theory is often conceptualised as methodology, many qualitative sociologists use it as a data analysis method by adjusting qualitative interview guides during concurrent data collection and analysis (Charmaz, 2008; Walker and Myrick, 2006). For example, emergent themes in the kuwentuhan sessions pointed to transnational and gendered constraints, for both male and female caregivers; therefore, we ensured that we included time for caregivers to explore this issue. Grounded theory as a data analysis strategy helped us identify important categories in our data that organised the ideas and themes 'grounded' in the stories of the participants. After all the kuwentuhan sessions were collected, we used narrative analysis, wherein we identified core narratives in the kuwentuhan sessions and analysed the structures of caregivers' self-narratives (Burck, 2005). For example, we analysed how the women in our study constructed the narratives of their filial obligations based on the changing and ascribed gender roles placed on Filipino and Filipina migrants.

In what follows, we present the narratives of Filipina migrants and aim to discuss the structural forces that influenced their mental health as frontline workers in the COVID-19 pandemic.

Gendered Work: For the Family, from Abroad

Although some scholars have suggested that migration disrupts patriarchal gender roles in the family for migrant women, where women are caretakers and men are breadwinners, the ideologies of gendered obligations remain, especially when women migrate (Dreby, 2010; Hondagneu-Sotelo, 1994). Transnational obligations to one's family through economic sustenance and emotional labour shape how Filipina migrants approach their interactions with families abroad. In turn, these transnational concerns inform their behaviours and decisions to work in the US. Richelle, a 52-year-old caregiver in the US and mother whose children remain in the Philippines stated:

> Like, you go to the US to earn big bucks, but then the result of what happens to your family back home, sometimes it's good. It is good. But sometimes it's bad, like the children would, you know, do things that they're not supposed to do. They would lack direction. They would lack supervision, and everything goes, you know, really crazy while you're here trying to give them a good life. And then they're not having a good life because some stuff happens.

Richelle structures her narrative based on an 'immigrant bargain' (Smith, 2005) wherein her labour migration was based on the intention of giving her children a better life in the Philippines, and therefore they might repay her sacrifice with good behaviour and gratitude. However, in this quote, she demonstrates that her decision to be the breadwinner for the family can induce emotions of guilt and regret with Filipina migrants as she reflects on her inability to give her children direction so that they do not 'do things they're not supposed to.' When the gendered work of nurturing and giving 'direction' continues to remain in Filipina migrants' psyche as a part of their role as a mother, their inability to attend to that emotional labour and guidance brings feelings of ambivalence for migrant women. While Filipinas are grappling with these complex emotional schemas, they are confronted with daily decisions to work so they can indeed provide the financial assistance their families need.

Richelle's original contract to work as a caregiver in the US had almost expired, but she was granted an extension for her labour visa by her employers. Rather than going back to the Philippines, Richelle recounts:

> The boss here, help me get an extension from the immigration so I was granted another six months. But then I thought, I have no more work there and a lot of still bills to pay, because my eldest daughter's going to go to college and then my second daughter is eventually going to go to college as

well. So, I just decided to stay so I didn't prepare my kids that I'm not coming back, you know, for a long time. I didn't prepare them for that.

In this quote, we argue that the gendered transnational family obligations that Richelle carries have shaped her interactions with her daughters in the Philippines, and it also informed her decision to stay in the US to work despite her own and her family's emotional health. Richelle's decision of whether the income she is providing to her family is worth not taking her immigration extension to go back home to be with her children is filled with emotional dissonance. Richelle is communicating her guilt about not fulfilling the patriarchal gendered definition of motherhood which is staying in proximity and caring for her own children. Rather, she is migrating abroad to work – a seemingly masculinised decision – to be the breadwinner for her family. Her inability to tell her children about her decision of not returning in her story demonstrates that the contradiction in the definition of gendered familial obligation is difficult for her. Based on her story, she lists her financial responsibilities first and then discusses acting on a decision that belied her desire to return to the family. We read this structure in her narrative as a contradiction in the gender roles for Richelle that stretch her idea of 'good' motherhood as a breadwinner and caretaker in her family. Richelle's narrative is representative of the transnational scaling that influences the work conditions and lives of Filipino/a migrants working in the care industry. We lay this as the foreground to the decisions that were made by Filipino/a caregivers before and during the pandemic.

This provides the essential transnational context as to why the risks for COVID-19 contraction were higher for Filipino/a caregivers. Their risk-taking behaviour to work on the frontlines as precarious care workers was undergirded by the gendered responsibilities in supporting their families. Opting to not work as caregivers under the COVID-19 pandemic was not an option given the financial obligations they had in the Philippines. However, compounded by mental health stressors of supporting families in the Philippines, Richelle's narrative structure shows us that care workers' decisions to continue to work with the most vulnerable population to the virus, those 65 and older with pre-existing conditions in COVID-19 hot spots, is shaped by their transnational contexts. In what follows, we explore the nature of care work in the US for Filipina migrants as their occupations are not folded into the American health infrastructures that informed and protected other frontline healthcare workers through the most difficult time of the pandemic.

Caregiving through COVID-19

Among the caregivers we interviewed during the COVID-19 pandemic, 25% reported issues of anxiety and isolation. Early in the pandemic, information on the way the virus was transmitted or cared for by those ill with the virus was unclear. The lack of information trickling down to for-profit and privatised care facilities for the elderly demonstrated the fact that long-term care for the elderly was not considered a part of the larger American healthcare system. Therefore, we find the lack of clear communication and information about the COVID-19 virus produced feelings of anxiety for Filipina caregivers. Belle, a 48-year-old caregiver, reflected on adjusting to new protocols with her client:

> And I was doing a lot more than I felt qualified for. And because no one's trained me on that. And then she had IV antibiotics um that she was given through a pump, and I've never [done that]. They [quickly] trained me at the hospital, but I was so nervous about it. And I had to do that every day for six weeks. So that was, I felt like someone should have been paying me somehow, but, because I wasn't doing something I was comfortable with, and it was something I've worried about all the time. So, yeah, I wish maybe there was also a medical training or something for caregivers or something in addition to compensation just to relieve anxiety.

In Belle's narrative, we can see that the failure in including caregivers in the formal healthcare system did not provide them with training and lessened their confidence to take care of their clients. In this narrative structure, Belle's quick-paced response to our question about the changes in her workplace post-COVID-19 signalled that the stressors at work took a toll on how she performed as an effective caregiver, especially as new information about COVID-19 added to her workload. Still, with or without ample training, Belle still attended to the needs of her clients. However, we point to her narrative to highlight the psychosocial impact of her workplace environment, resulting in her feeling undervalued, undertrained, and undercompensated.

Such sentiments and feelings can still be seen even if caregivers work in facilities that provide proper training and safety measures (e.g., personal protective equipment (PPE)). For example, Linda, a 52-year-old caregiver, lamented the experiences that were affecting her mental state. Though many of her interactions with other clients were positive, there were numerous instances where, in her words, clients could be quite 'verbally abusive' during her workdays. When asked how this made her feel, Linda stated through tears:

> I get like upset sometimes. So, it's like I just wanted to just quit or something. I give up one client, because I just couldn't take it anymore. They, you know, they abuse [us]. You know what they do it to us ... the way they treated their caregivers as like they're paying a lot of money and therefore that they wanted to get their money's worth ... It makes me feel so low. They make you feel like you're nothing.

In contrast to Belle's reflection on the institutional issues she was facing, Linda's account reveals how interactions with clients lead to mental strife. She shared that her clients and their families used the fact that she was being paid to justify verbal abuse and mistreatment. In her narrative, Linda had many pauses (represented by the ellipses above) as she demonstrated in real time the difficulty and stress these types of employer relationships present for care workers like her. To further illustrate this point, Linda detailed a particular interaction with a client and her daughter:

The family too. It's like they don't understand. They say that 'You guys are not doing good enough. You guys – It's your fault that my mom's … bedsore is not getting better.' It's like 'we're paying a lot of money you know' … The patient [too], yes, she's very mean to us. She's just like 'Oh, I don't have anybody that helped me. They are nothing. They're not doing enough.' It's just like, instead of being thankful of what you know the caregivers are doing [for] them, they are belittling us. They are kind of mean to us.

To make matters worse, Linda largely had to deal with these emotions on her own, as her position as a one-on-one caregiver under COVID-19 policy (i.e., one caregiver to one client) meant that she was usually isolated from co-workers or the administration that could mediate the situation. While she was caring for a client on her own, with multiple demands such as lifting, bathing, feeding, changing bedding, and administering a schedule for medicines, Linda's efforts were cast aside as worthless, explicitly by both her client and the client's family. These experiences produce a low sense of self-worth, even pushing some to quit entirely, which in turn may be part of the reason why there is such a high turnover rate amongst caregivers. Building on scholarship that identifies burnout because of 'work overload, lack of job control, insufficient reward or recognition, poor work collegiality, inequity in decision making, and conflict between worker and organisational values' (Maslach and Leiter, 2016), we present the narratives of Filipina migrant care workers to concur that care workers, especially under the pandemic, suffered negative outcomes to their mental health. These testimonies from Belle and Linda demonstrate how continuous exposure to stressful and/or negative life or environmental events can contribute to feelings of anxiety and fear, and even exploitation (National Institute of Mental Health, 2018).

Caregivers' feelings of fear and uncertainty were exacerbated as the pandemic set in. 39% of the caregivers in our sample believed that their increasing feelings of anxiety could be attributed specifically to issues regarding COVID-19. Given that the COVID-19 virus transmissibility did not have a definitive answer in the early part of the pandemic, caregivers often discussed how anxiety induces working as an essential worker on an invisible frontline in long-term care. Ian, a 43-year-old, caregiver stated:

It's a lot more difficult now, first because there's that fear of uncertainty. You don't know what the case will be or what the set up will look like. Not just for me but in general, caregivers today are careful with the patient that they work with. As much as possible, [caregivers] stay away from [multi-bed] facilities because there will be a lot of people. Second, if the patient has had COVID in the past, of course that's scary because I wouldn't want to catch COVID and spread it to other people. Third, how much is the rate today, if it's okay or if it's the same. There's a lot to consider today because of the situation.

Ian gives an account of the multiple factors that caregivers had to juggle and the decisions they had to make in terms of maintaining their positions as care workers.

In the throes of the pandemic, this quote shows the cost and benefit analysis caregivers implement when choosing to continue with various work commitments, and we found that many caregivers suffered from job insecurity under COVID-19. Overall, 40% of the participants in our initial study on caregiver's pre-pandemic confirmed that one caregiver can have multiple jobs in full-time and part-time care work at any given time (Francisco-Menchavez, Celemen, and Osorio, 2021). Among those who worked multiple jobs, 26% worked two jobs and 9% worked three jobs which demonstrated that one caregiving job is not enough for a formidable population of caregivers to sustain a livelihood. On the other hand, while some caregivers lost their part-time jobs, those who were full time and live-in, found themselves in intensified workload, which is an indicator of burnout. Rita, a 55-year-old caregiver with family in the Philippines, said:

> I gave up two days of work. But at the same time, another co-worker said that she wasn't gonna come into work because her spouse was sick, maybe COVID. So, I had to cover for her. And I just worked full time, covering her duty and mine. So, it was like I just quarantined myself, but before I go to sleep, I'm always thinking, 'Oh my god, what will happen if I get COVID? What if I got sick? What will I do? What will my family [in the Philippines] do?'.

Even in the face of possible contraction of COVID-19, caregivers like Rita and most of the caregivers in our study did not consider stopping their work as caregivers because they had their responsibilities to their families abroad. Even when the issues about the pandemic, transmission and ill-prepared work conditions were at the forefront, caregivers did not have the privilege to step down from their positions for their own health and safety. Whether their workload increased, or they lost their part-time jobs, caregiver concerns were heavily tied into migrants' transnational obligations.

Chief in caring for their transnational responsibilities is demonstrated by financial remittances. We have provided evidence that through the pandemic, the pattern of remitting money to their families in the Philippines stayed consistent, regardless of the job insecurity caregivers faced. In our study, 30% of caregivers reported that they still sent remittances back to the Philippines despite the conditions of job insecurity and lower monthly wages. Sonny, a 39-year-old caregiver and father of two who is in the Philippines, responded to a question about what percent of his monthly pay cheque is remitted, 'Maybe, seventy or eighty. In dollars? Four thousand. Under COVID, I am sending the same.' While many caregivers reported that their work hours decreased during the pandemic, remittances continued which demonstrates that caregivers continued to find work, however dangerous the conditions were. In the present study, among caregivers who sent remittances, 47% reported that the value of dollars they sent had decreased, acknowledging their ability to provide for their family decreased during the pandemic. This may have led to a higher likelihood of risk-taking behaviours like working more jobs to continue sending the necessary money back.

Tess, a worker leader in a Filipino/a migrant workers' organisation and caregiver, reflected on the transnational obligation that caregivers shoulder through their remittances. She starts by talking about how earning in dollars a critical lifeline for Filipino/a migrants and their families in the Philippines is, she asserts:

> So that's a big money if they send [dollars] to the Philippines, to their families. So, their focus is not really about rights. It's more of the money that they – especially, now the what the [COVID] condition in the Philippines that they're there you know its life is so hard. They lost jobs, a lot of people are not employed, so they need support, more than anything. So, if we could work here, why not? We could work doubly to support them! So that's what's happening with most of the caregivers since they're mostly breadwinners.

In this quote, we learn that many caregivers' approaches to working under the COVID-19 pandemic, in an already underfunded eldercare industry, are foremost motivated by their obligations to the families they left behind in the Philippines. In Tess' quote, she mentions that caregivers often dismiss their 'rights,' which include their health and well-being, because their paycheque in US dollars goes a long way for their families back home. Based on the data, caregivers indicated that over $200 to $1,000 dollars of their monthly personal income were spent on remittances alone. This money can go toward their own well-being and care in the US, but it is often prioritised on family rather than themselves.

Still, scholars have argued that patterns of remittances are codified by gendered roles in their families. Cynthia, a 48-year-old caregiver who left one child and ageing parents in the Philippines, reflected on how she thinks about working non-stop during the pandemic:

> We all have a lot of different reasons why we leave the Philippines. Some, because it's hard to earn a livelihood there, parents need to go abroad, so that all family members can be sustained. But that's my point, why we came here, because we earn in dollar. When we send it back to the Philippines, the value is higher. But for mothers, we will persevere through it all, just so that we can send something home to them.

Cynthia lays bare what we discussed in the prior section of this chapter. Much of the gendered ideas on good motherhood follows Filipina migrants in their migration. It shapes how they think of their role as breadwinners, thus informing how they make decisions about working in a low-wage, precarious job as a caregiver. Under the COVID-19 pandemic, both Ian and Cynthia, two migrant parents, demonstrate that the pressures of remitting as a practice of care work have gendered consequences. For Ian, the amount of his remittances echoes the expectations for breadwinning, while Cynthia's comments around self-sacrifice and perseverance shore up ideas around nurturance and caretaking as women's ascribed labour in the family. Still, in all the evidence presented here, we argue that migrants' vulnerability to workplace violations, especially under COVID-19, is mitigated by their transnational obligations and compounded by the different gendered ideas about their roles in the family.

Conclusion

In this chapter, we presented evidence that the gendered and transnational obligations of Filipina migrants impact their decisions to overwork and endure difficult working conditions as caregivers to the elderly in the US. The narrative analysis we provided is key to understanding how the transnational family demands of Filipina migrants are stressors that add to the psychosocial impacts of working in a caregiver position that is often underpaid and undervalued. In the COVID-19 pandemic, the privatised eldercare industry and the lack of structural funding for long-term care in the US further intensified the care workers' risks of contracting the virus or suffering from various psychosocial outcomes such as stress and anxiety. Care workers did not have the privilege of refusing work because of their transnational responsibilities. We hope that the scaling we have done geographically, and through psycho and social aspects of the lives of Filipino/a migrants, demonstrate that the mental health of migrants must consider the transnational lives they live, and how that bears upon their local daily decisions.

Scholars have urged a multi-method approach and action-oriented approach to studying the mental health impacts of migratory cultures and transitions so that meso-level interventions and social policies might be able to mitigate the systemic ills that can arise for immigrants (Perkins, Palmer, and García-Ramírez, 2011). Our chapter's findings lead us to recommend that interventions for Filipino migrant workers in the home care industry include increased social support from culturally relevant, community-based organisations that not only address the labour rights infringement on Filipino migrants, but also consider their holistic concerns as migrant parents and transnational family members.

References

Asis, M. M. B., Huang, S., and Yeoh, B. S. (2004). 'When the light of the home is abroad: Unskilled female migration and the Filipino family', *Singapore Journal of Tropical Geography*, 25(2), pp. 198–215.

Bretones, F. D., Jain, A., Leka, S., and García-López, P. A. (2020). 'Psychosocial working conditions and well-being of migrant workers in Spain', *International Journal of Environmental Research and Public Health*, 17(7), p. 2547. doi:10.3390/ijerph17072547.

Burck, C. (2005). 'Comparing qualitative research methodologies for systemic research: The use of grounded theory, discourse analysis and narrative analysis', *Journal of Family Therapy*, 27(3), pp. 237–262. https://doi-org.jpllnet.sfsu.edu/10.1111/j.1467-6427.2005 .00314.

Chan, C. D., and Litam, S. D. A. (2021). 'Mental health equity of Filipino communities in COVID-19: A framework for practice and advocacy', *Professional Counselor*, 11(1), pp. 73–85.

Charmaz, K. (2008). 'Grounded theory as an emergent method', in Hesse-Biber, S. N., and Leavy, P. (eds.), *Handbook of Emergent Methods*. New York: The Guilford Press, pp. 155–170.

Choy, C. C. (2003). *Empire of Care*. Durham: Duke University Press.

Cruz, D. (2012). *Transpacific Femininities: The Making of the Modern Filipina*. Durham: Duke University Press.

dela Cruz, F. A., McBride, M. R., Compas, L. B., Calixto, P., and Van Derveer, C. (2002). 'White paper on the health status of Filipino Americans and recommendations for research', *Nursing Outlook*, 50(1), pp. 7–15.

Dreby, J. (2010). *Divided by Borders*. Berkeley: University of California Press.

Francisco-Menchavez, V.(2018). *The Labor of Care: Filipina Migrants and Transnational Families in the Digital Age.*University of Illinois Press.

Francisco-Menchavez, V. (2020). 'Researching Queenila and living in-between: Multisited ethnography, migrant epistemology and transnational families', *Migration and Development*, 9(1), pp. 56–73.

Francisco-Menchavez, V. (2021). 'Kuwentuhan as a method', in Liamputtong, P. (ed.), *Handbook of Social Inclusion*. Cham: Springer International Publishing, pp. 1–23. doi:10.1007/978-3-030-48277-0_83-1.

Francisco-Menchavez, V., Celemen, E., and Osorio, K. (2021). 'Filipino formal caregivers to the elderly and normalized exploitation in the workplace', *Alon: Journal for Filipinx American and Diasporic Studies*, 1(1), pp. 51–67. doi:10.5070/LN41149607.

Guevarra, A. R. (2014). 'Supermaids: The racial branding of global Filipino care labour', in Anderson, B., and Shutes, I. (eds.), *Migration and Care Labour. Migration, Diasporas and Citizenship Series*. London: Palgrave Macmillan, pp. 130–150. doi:10.1057/9781137319708_8.

Hondagneu-Sotelo, P. (1994). 'Regulating the unregulated?: Domestic workers' social networks', *Social Problems*, 41(1), pp. 50–64. doi:10.1525/sp.1994.41.1.03x0424h.

Kaur-Gill, S. (2020). 'The COVID-19 pandemic and outbreak inequality: Mainstream reporting of Singapore's migrant workers in the margins', *Frontiers in Communication*, 5.

Maglalang, D. D., Sorensen, G., Hopcia, K., Hashimoto, D. M., Katigbak, C., Pandey, S., ... Sabbath, E. L. (2021). 'Job and family demands and burnout among healthcare workers: The moderating role of workplace flexibility', *SSM-Population Health*, 14, 100802.

Maslach, C., and Leiter, M. P. (2016). 'Understanding the burnout experience: Recent research and its implications for psychiatry', *World Psychiatry*, 15(2), pp. 103–111.

Nasol, K., and Francisco-Menchavez, V. (2021). 'Filipino home care workers: Invisible frontline workers in the COVID-19 crisis in the United States', *The American Behavioral Scientist*, 65(10), pp. 1365–1383. doi:10.1177/00027642211000410.

National Institute of Mental Health. (July). *Anxiety Disorders*. U.S. Department of Health and Human Services, National Institutes of Health. Available at: https://www.nimh.nih .gov/health/topics/anxiety-disorders (Accessed: 11 December 2021).

Parreñas, R. S. (2001). 'Mothering from a distance: Emotions, gender, and intergenerational relations in Filipino transnational families', *Feminist Studies*, 27(2), pp. 361–390.

Perkins, D., Palmer, N. A., and García-Ramírez, M. (2011). 'Psychosocial studies of migration and community: Introduction to the special issue', *Psychosocial Intervention*, 20(3), pp. 237–242. doi:10.5093/in2011v20n3a1.

Pitre, N. Y., Kushner, K. E., Raine, K. D., and Hegadoren, K. M. (2013). 'Critical feminist narrative inquiry: Advancing knowledge through double-hermeneutic narrative analysis', *Advances in Nursing Science*, 36(2), 118–132.

Rahman, M. M., and Fee, L. K. (2012). 'Towards a sociology of migrant remittances in Asia: Conceptual and methodological challenges', *Journal of Ethnic and Migration Studies*, 38(4), pp. 689–706.

Roberts, J. T. (1993). 'Psychosocial effects of workplace hazardous exposures: Theoretical synthesis and preliminary findings', *Social Problems*, 40(1), pp. 74–89. doi:10.1525/sp.1993.40.1.03x0073u.

Rodriguez, R. M. (2005). *Domestic Insecurities: Female Migration from the Philippines, Development and National Subject-Status*. Working Paper. UC San Diego: Center for Comparative Immigration Studies. Available at: https://escholarship.org/uc/item/7q75k44h (Accessed: 5 November 2021).

Sabar, G., Babis, D., and Sabar Ben-Yehoshua, N. (2022). 'From fragility to empowerment through philanthropy: The Filipino labor migrant community in Israel during COVID-19', *Journal of Immigrant & Refugee Studies*, 20(1), pp. 49–64.

Shah, H. B. (2017). 'Understaffed and overworked: Poor working conditions and quality of care in residential care facilities for the elderly', *Publications*, p. 788. Available at: https://digitalcommons.law.ggu.edu/pubs/788 (Accessed: 5 November 2021).

Smith, R.C.(2005). 'Mexican New York', in *Mexican New York*. University of California Press.

Tung, C. (2000). 'The cost of caring: The social reproductive labor of Filipina live-in home health caregivers', *Frontiers: A Journal of Women Studies*, 21(1/2), pp. 61–82. doi:10.2307/3347032.

Walker, D., and Myrick, F. (2006). 'Grounded theory: An exploration of process and procedure', *Qualitative Health Research*, 16(4), pp. 547–559. doi:10.1177/1049732305285972.

Wang, D., Gee, G. C., Bahiru, E., Yang, E. H., and Hsu, J. J. (2020). 'Asian-Americans and Pacific Islanders in COVID-19: Emerging disparities amid discrimination', *Journal of General Internal Medicine*, 35(12), pp. 3685–3688. doi:10.1007/s11606-020-06264-5q.

Part III
Work

Part III

Work

8 Supermarket Women Cashiers Closing Social Distancing Gaps

The Artificial World of Affective Labour?

Amber Blake, Khayaat Fakier, and Marjorie L. Naidoo

Introduction

Purpose of the Research

This chapter considers the emotional and affective labour performed by women cashiers during the Covid-19 pandemic in a coastal town in the Eastern Province of South Africa. Media coverage of frontline workers did not mention the role that cashiers had to play, although their work and contribution deserve recognition. Firstly, we looked at how cashiers' practice of emotional and affective labour increased during Covid-19. Attention shifted to how these forms of labour contributed towards bridging 'social distancing' gaps through the form they lent to enriched social encounters with certain customers. Secondly, the theory of 'sociability' aptly described the interactive service work between cashiers and pensioners, which allowed for momentary relief from the otherwise inhuman circumstances imposed by a global pandemic.

The Town

Yellow Bay[1] is a 'holiday town,' accommodating seasonal influxes of visitors, for its beaches and for water sports. Many residents of retirement age have settled in the town and have lived there for many years. The town has welcomed young families and has become increasingly diverse in terms of racial and age demographics, but most middle-class suburbs are habited by white locals, interspersed with holiday homes, empty for most of the year.

Grocery Shopping during Covid-19

From March 2020, the state restricted the sale of non-essential goods and services. Most shops were closed for nearly 8 months, except grocery stores and pharmacies which were considered 'essential' and remained open, during which time the research was conducted. In this period, everyone was confined to their homes for 'home isolation.' When in public, a 1.5 m 'social distance' gap between persons

DOI: 10.4324/9781003267133-11

and wearing face masks became mandatory. The state banned social gatherings and access to public spaces, such as beaches, parks, and sit-down restaurants, as one of the primary methods to limit contagion (Turner, Grange & Nkgadima 2021).

The supermarket of this research is in the town's one shopping mall. Prior to the outbreak of the virus, it had hosted regular social activity. Its location is a distance from the suburbs and requires transport to reach, influencing the race and class demographics of patrons who can shop there. The manager of Yellow Bay supermarket[2] for more than 20 years observed that their customer base is a mix of race, working people, families, and young people, but predominantly white and the elderly.

As essential service workers, cashiers and grocery packers were positioned on the frontline. They were provided with personal protection equipment (PPE) and seated behind a Perspex screen to protect themselves and the customer against cross-contamination throughout the Covid-19 outbreak.

Methodology

While the shopping mall had always been 'enlivened' by families with children, single people, and working people, of different racial groups – after the outbreak the numbers dwindled drastically. But many elderly shoppers, we noticed, continued to come. This intrigued us, as they were categorised as a group highly susceptible to contagion – and therefore in a fragile situation. We also noticed how 'social distancing' affected the behaviour of shoppers during the lockdown – towards each other in the isles and towards the cashiers, seated behind their Perspex partitions. From these informal observations, the idea of the research was borne.

We contacted various supermarkets in town via their public email address or by telephone; however, none were interested in the proposed research, until September 2020 when we contacted Yellow Bay supermarket via email and presented our research request to the store manager. She responded tentatively and referred us to the store owner. In a virtual meeting with the owner, one of us discussed the formalities of the research, our interest in cashiers' experiences of their work during Covid-19 and the ethical conditions of anonymity and privacy to which cashiers taking part would be entitled. The owner was sensitive to our request and the research was conducted in November 2020.

Limitation

Face-to-face research at the time of this study was prohibited. Therefore, we were unable to make any direct contact with the cashiers of Yellow Bay supermarket, all of whom were women. The inability to directly observe their interactions with customers as part of the research is a limitation of the study.

Introductory Video

We navigated this by making a short video to introduce one of us as a researcher and our interest in their work with customers during Covid-19. Further, the video explained that the research was not affiliated with their workplace, that their employment position would remain secure, that participation was voluntary and anonymous, and that their identity, privacy, and the confidentiality of their information would be protected, should they choose to take part.

One of our telephone numbers was made available on the notice board in the staff locker room. The first attempt to secure participants for the study was disappointing, but not surprising. In the second week, after the video was shown, a group of seven women contacted us and agreed to be interviewed; Black[3] Xhosa-speaking women and coloured Afrikaan-speaking women, whose age varied from 29 to 42 years.

My Positionality

It is reasonable to suggest that our interest in cashier–customer interactions, amid a global pandemic with new legally authorised safety protocols, would arouse suspicion from any supermarket.

The supermarket owner's willingness to allow us to contact the cashiers and the video presented to cashiers by their manager could have influenced how the research was received by participants and their willingness to take part in the research. In addition, it is not clear how they perceived me, whether this was a barrier or an invitation. It is unclear why participants came to contact me, whether there was influence from management, a hope of improving their situation or position as staff members, or simply because they wanted to share their experiences with another person.

Interviews

The participants were interviewed individually during November 2020 through semi-structured telephone interviews of approximately 45 minutes, which is determined by the availability of the cashiers. Consent to record the interviews was given in all instances. These were transcribed with careful attention to voice modulation and hesitations – as facial expressions and body language could not be observed for analysis.

In our analysis of participant interviews, we aimed to understand the quality of their labour beyond what they directly said. Clear themes emerged from participant interviews regarding their experiences between themselves and certain customers. Distinctions of the class and race of customers could not be accurately deduced in every instance. The findings of this chapter are, therefore, not generalisable, but novel in its consideration of a small group of women cashiers' experience of the dynamics with customers, particularly pensioners, in a coastal town, during the Covid-19 pandemic.

Literature Review

This study made use of three theories: emotional labour (Hochschild 1983), affective labour (Hardt & Negri 2001), and sociability (Simmel 1949). Firstly, some brief definitions are provided, followed by applied studies of the theories in the retail space.

Emotional Labour

In her 1983 book, *The Managed Heart*, Hochschild proposed her theory of emotional labour. Her seminal study of flight attendants' encounters with mainly white, middle-, and upper-class men showed how flight attendants had to school their outward emotional displays to present the corporate 'feeling rules' of caring and being catered for in the service recipient. In later studies, emotional labour emerged as an expected form of labour and was considered a key qualifier for employment in contemporary service jobs (Dahiya 2017). The application of emotional labour has been applied in many ways for different purposes. Various typologies of emotional labour have been proposed (Kang 2003; Bolton 2009). The concept remains useful to our understanding of service-based labour processes.

Interviewed mid-Covid-19 in September 2020, Arlie Hochschild applied her theory of emotional labour to emergency and frontline workers. She noted three types of responses: 'bracketing,' the need to temporarily detach oneself from one's own concerns or feelings that arise from interaction with patients or customers; 'bridging,' the need to empathise with patients or customers and identify with their fears or frustrations; and 'balancing,' the need to be in touch with one's own emotions to avoid inner fragmentation (Stix 2020).

For this chapter, emotional labour, as described by Stix (2020), is applied to cashiers' interactions with customers during Covid-19.

Affective Labour

Affective labour differs from emotional labour by going beyond emotional responses, to the creation and maintenance of organisationally determined relationships based on the deliberate production of affects (outcomes). First theorised by Hardt and Negri (2001), affective labour is used to describe the 'invisible' labour involved in the production of human relationships through 'immaterial' outputs. Most contemporary forms of employment involve a degree of affective labour which 'produces' communication, information, and knowledge exchange in human interactions (Oksala 2016).

Affective labour is fundamental to service work, through capitalising on human capacities for sociability, it has been used to illustrate the exploitation of contemporary workers (Weeks 2011; Waters-Lynch & Duff 2021). It employs the emotional and social skills of employees in organisational as well as social relationships and is regarded as essential in our advanced form of capitalism. The question of how to compensate for this form of labour remains unanswered. Furthermore, it has been applied in the analysis of gendered forms of work in its paid and unpaid variants which has shown that jobs with the highest affective labour requirements are positions predominantly held by women workers (Oksala 2016; Veldstra 2020). Oksala (2016) raises the importance of understanding how different forms of affective labour contribute to the production of various forms of life within and beyond the workplace, which this chapter aims to address with its findings.

Sociability

Simmel's (1949) relational perspective is premised on the fact that 'society' and its formal institutions are created by the micro-interactions between people. For the creation of any 'society,' Simmel identifies reciprocity as fundamental to the creation of any social realm (Pyyhtinen 2009). Two types of social interactions, first and second orders, are identified as the forms which impact the way human interactions are shaped.

First-order social forms are those human relations that are determined by inter-actions between superior and subordinated subjects and encompass the division of labour (Ruggeri 2017: 54). Applied to a workplace setting such as a supermarket, this is where different people come together, interacting under specific conditions, to work for money required for their continued existence. In this material environment, the nature of the social interactions between cashiers and customers is facilitated by company display rules, which are taught by management and learnt by members in secondary staff positions.

Second-order social forms may be articulated concurrently to first-order forms and derive from our innate human impulse to be sociable, to derive satisfaction from the mere being together with others (Simmel & Hughes 1949: 255). This is sociability, a sociological ideal type, in which social interactions are for the mere purpose of being with others, where conversations are without an explicit end or content. Sociability relies on each member being treated as symbolically equal.

Kaplan (2018) applied Simmel's theory of sociability to the interactions between members who belonged to the same social clubs and argued that out of the necessary tact required of previously unaffiliated people, feelings of familiarity, exclusivity, and loyalty were created, an ode to the frequency of contact regarding a common interest. Furthermore, it is suggested that within institutional and non-institutional collectives, such as schools and social networking sites, the form of interactions – sociability – is taken for granted in studies of national attachments. While the supermarket cannot be considered a 'social club' in a conventional sense, the interactions between cashiers and pensioners took on a similar form in Covid-19. As McNair (2012) illustrates, sociability can occur simply because of how one associates with another, despite personal differences, but through 'good form' the encounter enables mutual satisfaction, although momentary and fleeting.

The Theories Applied to the Retail Sector

The application of these three theories to the retail space is obvious, given that this is one of the key areas of interaction in a sophisticated market system. The supermarket serves as an important linkage between people who otherwise may have had no encounter with each other at all (Houssay-Holzschuch & Teppo 2009).

In the retail setting, customers are placed at the apex of service interactions, which automatically places the cashier in a position of deference. Deference is to place oneself on a 'lower' standing vis-à-vis another, a condition demanded of all people in structurally disadvantaged positions (Wharton 2009: 149). This type of labour is a part of most jobs where interactions with the public are required and where workers are positioned at the interface between the organisation and the customer. The employee is therefore held responsible for maintaining the reputation of the organisation, which mandates the regulation of employee's emotional displays in service encounters. Both emotional and affective labour are 'required' from and delivered by retail cashiers – in managing their own emotions in preference to a positive attitude and in 'managing' the customer experience through the projection of company behavioural rules which garner positive brand association.

The service encounter at the checkout station is essentially constructed around the frontal contact between cashiers and customers, sometimes with a packer who packs the customer's groceries in bags or boxes, while the customer completes the transaction with the cashier. The interactive service by cashiers was well articulated by Rafaeli (1989), who illustrated, in Israeli supermarkets, the range of influences on cashier's behaviour while the transaction at the checkout station was being completed. While limited in the consideration of race and class, it was argued that customers exert immediate influence on cashier behaviours for several reasons: their physical proximity, time spent together, the opportunity to exchange information, and the customers being, for the cashier, a direct source of communication, verbally and non-verbally (Rafaeli 1989: 253). Lawless's (2014) study of cashiers in the United States found that cashiers were likely to accept mistreatment from customers as an accepted part of their work and attributed this to the notion of customers' superiority over the service worker. This often manifested as verbal mistreatment because of negative stereotyping associated with cashiers' race. The differential treatment of people according to race, ethnicity, gender, and class is intertwined with the development of the division of work and labour in South Africa historically (Kenny 2016). The workplace was the battle terrain for the political inclusion of black South Africans during and after apartheid (Kenny 2015, 2016). Kenny (2016) argued that in their struggle for equal treatment in the workplace, black workers were represented as disruptive and deserving of low-status, low-skilled, and low-wage employment; stigma which has downstream consequences to how black retail workers are perceived and treated by others. When interactions between cashiers and customers escalate, cashiers must mediate and resolve any (affective) tension caused by the interaction. The creation of the service hierarchy imposes undue responsibility of customer satisfaction onto the cashiers, especially during the pandemic.

The literature also suggests that the size of a store, its location within a geography that is stratified by class, and racial demographics impact the priority placed on customer service (Kang 2003; Agius & Lee 2006). The implication is that the 'better-class' customers are to be treated with more sensitivity. Interestingly, research done in various countries on different continents shows the same challenges faced by frontline workers, e.g., Italy (Carls 2007), the United States (Ikeler 2015), and

India (Dahiya 2017). Furthermore, it has been found that work stress linked to emotional labour can cause mental harm and negatively affect workers and therefore the retail bottom line (Grandey, Rupp & Brice. (2015) ; Cho et al. 2013).

During the pandemic, the same principles of 'good service' were required of the cashiers, but the execution thereof was met with heightened emotional challenges when customers showed negative attitudes towards cashiers. Hochschild describes it as 'the emotional balancing act required to juggle fear for one's personal safety with a professional steadiness in the face of a circulating pathogen that can sicken and kill' (Stix 2020).

This chapter attempts to highlight the overlapping nature of emotional and affective labour and first- and second-order social interactions in the retail setting. While still a labour, the functioning of sociability operates simultaneously to emotional and affective labour but to a different end. Simmel's second-order social form has a particularly intriguing manifestation in South Africa, depending on customers' attitudes when entering the service encounter with cashiers in Covid-19. Sociability allows us to consider how certain interactions in the retail space contribute to moments of democratic exchange. The concepts that have been introduced in the literature review will be used to analyse the social interactions that had taken place between cashiers and customers, in Yellow Bay supermarket, during Covid-19.

Findings

Applying the lens of the theory to the interviews, the following revealed itself:

Emotional Labour in the Retail Setting

When we asked cashiers about their interactions with customers during the pandemic – after conversations about adhering to Covid-19 mitigation protocols, e.g., sanitising hands and checkout stations – they stated that customers had changed the way they behaved since the pandemic. The cashier and packer remain in the closest proximity to customers in the service encounter and experienced firsthand how the dynamic changed because of the pandemic. Rafaeli (1989) found that cashiers ignored customers' bad behaviour and resisted attempts to control the checkout process to safeguard their sense of autonomy. This remained relevant in the Covid-19 situation; however, cashiers' ability to control the checkout process was diminished due to the institution of state-enforced precautionary measures that enabled customers to behave in ways that were experienced as negative by the cashiers. During the pandemic, the cashiers set apart their own emotions to continue performing their work through bracketing (Stix 2020) in the face of customer responses. This is illustrated in the following quotation where that cashier women remained silent, despite feeling emotions in the situation, during the interaction with a patron:

I greeted the customer. It was an old guy. I did greet him, he didn't respond. Then I sanitise everything ... When I was helping him to pack in his own plastic bag, he grabbed those bags, just like that out of my hand … I just looked at him and didn't say anything. So that was really hard … But I do understand that he is scared of Corona but that was very rude of him.

(Black cashier)

In addition, the cashiers used the emotional labour of balancing (Stix 2020) their emotions by recognising how certain encounters with customers were unpleasant to them. They navigated their negative experiences with customers by bridging (Stix 2020) their emotions, through empathising with customers' fear of Covid-19. They attributed most of the customers' hostile reactions to the circumstance of the pandemic, rather than to themselves as a strategy for managing their emotions during and after their interactions with customers.

The 'social' distance, intentionally created through wearing masks and Covid-19 protocols, functioned as one barrier between cashiers and customers, but it extended into the ways customers treated cashiers, through surveillance and recrimination. The interactions below illustrate:

We were busy at the till, there was one lady by me, a customer. Then there was a customer standing there shaking his head – I don't know if he was in a hurry or what – so I said, 'Sir, you can come' and he was, 'No! You don't know the rules. You must social distance yourself!'

(Coloured cashier)

There was one day…I think I sneezed – I have a problem with my sinus – then she asked, 'Are you sick? You can't sit here!' and I said, 'No ma'am,[4] I am not sick.' Do you know what she did? She pissed off to another cashier… that was humiliating. Now everyone is going to think there is something wrong with me.

(Coloured cashier)

Cashiers classify customers' behaviours as negative when they intercept when cashiers tried to assist them with card payments and packing their groceries, questioned their competency, raised their voice during conflicts, ignored them and, during Covid-19, were suspicious of them, accused them, re-sanitised, and grabbed items from their hands as they performed the tasks that are required of them for their work. Emotional labour forms part of service work generally but heightened customer negativity resulted in emotion management strategies in excess by cashiers during the pandemic. When 'the customer is always right' in service encounters, it means that cashiers have limited recourse against rude customers, apart from the assistance of the superior and particularly in Covid-19. The service encounters from behind the checkout stations took on a new level of intensity because of customer responses which did not allow for fair and reciprocal exchanges to take place.

Affective Labour in the Retail Setting

Yellow Bay supermarket is branded on its website, newspaper inserts, and social media platforms as a much-loved store with 'strong and unique family values,' 'catering to customers' evolving needs.' Yellow Bay supermarket places high priority on customer service. The following statement made by the supermarket manager points towards what is expected of the cashiers:

> We give our cashiers and our packers quite extensive customer service training, not just, 'Hi Ma'am, plastic bag? Loyalty card?' **We tend to give a little bit more than that**.
>
> (White store manager, emphasis added)

Cashiers at Yellow Bay are trained to communicate with customers, greet them, respond to their questions, and write the customer's name in a book to 'rain check' items that are sold out so that they can be contacted when it is back in stock. It is expected and communicated to them by management that they should leave a lasting impression on customers that reflect their willingness to help them to create customer loyalty because of the quality of their service. Affective labour relies on the cashiers' capacity to show genuine interest in others and directs it towards the creation of relationships with customers through the additional interest taken in customer requests. The affective labour relationships with customers during the pandemic became increasingly demanding of the cashiers when other options to be sociable were severely limited.

To be employed as a cashier in Yellow Bay supermarket is demanding in terms of affective labour because of the frequency of contact with 'regular' customers and especially with pensioners; in fact, cashiers refer to many elderly customers by their surnames or names. In many instances, the familiarity that cashiers' affective relationships created with certain customers enhanced the service encounter and provided cashiers with the skills to mediate the service encounter with 'regular' customers, some of whom were described as 'difficult.' Despite the difference in power enabled by conditions of domination and subordination in the service encounter, the affective labour of cashiers was met with reciprocal exchanges with certain customers that brought some relief to the cashiers during the pandemic. Certain customers, described as 'supportive and motivating,' shared stories with cashiers, encouraged them, and purchased items from the store to give to them as gifts to thank them. It is dependent on the customer that some retail encounters can become two-way relationships, rather than one-sided productions of affective outputs from the cashiers. A cashier provides an example of a reciprocal affective exchange:

> They're asking us, 'Are you still coping? You must be safe' and they would also say, 'You must be safe, look after yourself.' We have nice customers. Yeah, our regular ones that we know.
>
> (Black cashier)

Affective labour, being the human capacity for the creation of relationships, can be reciprocated by customers and it does impact the cashier's ability to perform their work, as well as the demands of their emotional labour. When I asked the cashiers how they would like to be treated by customers they simply requested that their labour throughout the pandemic be acknowledged and that the customers recognise them as people, not only as workers, as described by one cashier:

> All they can do is just be thankful and appreciate us that we are always at the frontline. We are just helping them to get food to their houses... I think the customers must just respect us as we do them. They must know that I am a person just like them when it comes to shopping and to treat me like he is treating his family.
>
> (Black cashier)

It is not to say this form affective labour is not exploitative nor draining for the worker, but affective labour during the pandemic became a necessary constituent in the smooth accomplishment of sociability in the workplace setting. This will be further illustrated through cashiers' sociability with elderly customers during Covid-19.

Sociability with Pensioners

For many, being socially separated from others for the duration of the pandemic increased the rate of negative health outcomes (Xiong et al. 2020). Cashiers understood this need in certain elderly customers and entertained pensioners that would ask them questions unrelated to their work, e.g., regarding cashiers' families, or whether they watched the previous evening's television drama. The manager confirmed this:

> There are pensioners who come into the shop to buy a milk and a loaf of bread, but they stay in the shop for an hour ... They don't want to come to the till and just hear, 'Plastic bag? Loyalty card? Thank you, enjoy your day.' They actually want to talk about the weather and something that they saw on the news.
>
> (White store manager)

Covid-19 protective regulations created physical barriers between cashiers and customers, but it did not prevent cashiers from closing social distancing gaps to interact with pensioners. The cashiers hesitantly shared that they moved physically closer to elderly customers, behind the Perspex partitions, to engage them in conversation. The cashiers at Yellow Bay supermarket performed emotional labour of bracketing and bridging their own emotions to engage in affective relationships with elderly customers, to set aside their fear of contagion, and to empathise with the elderly customers and perform affective labour to communicate and connect with them:

> The old ones, they don't get to talk to people. They are nice old people and I like talking to them because they are stuck in their old age homes and there's

no one to talk to and when they come to the shops, I make their day. I talk to them, I make jokes, all that kind of things and I like it. When I am with them, I talk to them, even if there is someone waiting.

(Coloured cashier)

The older people ... They would make me laugh and we would laugh and it's nice.

(Black cashier)

All the cashiers remarked on their encounters with elderly customers with a light-hearted tone when the encounters took on the character of sociability – the form of an interaction in which the content of the conversation is drawn from the conditions of reality but is not affected by reality's seriousness (Simmel & Hughes 1949: 261). As this quote illustrates:

At that time [high Covid-19 infection period] when the old people still want to come shopping ... we [cashiers] would normally ask, 'Why did they send you Mama? Mama[5] knows it's Covid, but Mama still comes herself to the shop?' Like that and then we just laugh.

(Coloured cashier)

The example illustrates one of many interactions with pensioners described by the cashiers. We see that the risks associated with public interactions during the pandemic turned into a shared experience of risk for the customers and the cashiers and that mutual recognition elicited positive outcomes.

Discussion

The findings illustrated that emotional and affective labour is performed by the cashiers in their interactions with customers. When customers entered service encounters without recognising the service worker's position as being equally valuable to their own, the domineering logic of the first order shaped the outcome of the social encounter and created negative feelings that cashiers had to endure. This manifested itself in the strenuous performance of emotional and affective labour by cashiers with certain patrons.

In South Africa, the historical difference in the treatment of people according to their race and further by their class, at the level of the state, economy and interpersonally, has been acknowledged as the barrier to the creation of a democratic society. However, the 'artificially constructed' world of service relationships, mediated by emotional and affective labour, became an example of how, within the existing social and economic structures, sociability created momentary feelings of equality, from the bottom up, between people who were positioned differently within society. As Kaplan (2018) argued, these moments of 'public intimacy' between unaffiliated persons should not be disregarded as insignificant. For moments of sociability demand that members of the 'better-class' disregard their superior position to cashiers to gain satisfaction from the encounter – in those encounters, cashiers were subordinate only because of the service relationship, but valued as socially equal. The findings illustrated how the form of the interaction determined the nature of the outcome, which had the potential to place people of different races and class positions into encounters where the mutual recognition of value became possible, however fleeting. This should not be overstated, the research was limited in its scope and further research is required to evaluate whether moments like those articulated in the study impacted social relationships on the ground, beyond the pandemic.

By applying Simmel's seminal theory of sociability to interactive service work, we can understand the value of face-to-face customer service relationships in a new way. The findings produced here are not generalisable; however, as a theoretical endeavour, the potential for using sociability to better understand workplace interactions in South Africa was brought to the forefront by its application to the retail encounter in Covid-19.

Conclusion

The experiences articulated in this chapter illustrate the three theories in action. It is evident that 'social' distance revealed its layered formation as a physical and emotional phenomenon that expressed itself uniquely in affect-laden social interactions in the retail space. While physical distance was necessary to protect the health of both cashier and customer in retail encounters, the desire of customers to be sociable fostered interactions whereby the cashiers' affects were reciprocated in unexpected ways by (mostly) elderly patrons.

While it is the purchase of groceries that keep places like Yellow Bay supermarket open, the longevity of any functioning 'society' relies so heavily on this kind of association which maintains equality, if only on a moment-to-moment basis. For the pensioners of Yellow Bay, we suggest that cashiers had played a role in the creation of symbolic equality between pensioners who depended on them, through their affective labour and sociability. In South Africa, where people are socially separated by material differences, interactions like these which are artificially created – fleeting but valuable – could point towards moments of nation-building during the pandemic.

Notes

1 The original name of the town has been changed to a fake name.
2 The supermarket and the cashiers have been referred to by fake names.
3 This chapter makes use of superficial race categories, reminiscent of apartheid, because it is still a way many South Africans classify themselves and people with whom they interact.
4 In South Africa, white customers are most frequently referred to as "Ma'am" in service encounters as a sign of respect.
5 When cashiers refer to customers as 'Mama,' instead of 'you,' it is meant as a sign of respect.

References

Agius, J.A. and Lee, J. (2006). Raising the status of the cashier: Latina–White interactions in an ethnic market. *Sociological Forum*, Springer US, 21(2), pp. 197–218.

Bolton, S.C. (2009). The lady vanishes: Women's work and affective labour. *International Journal of Work Organisation and Emotion*, 3(1), pp. 72–80.

Carls, K. (2007). Affective labour in Milanese large scale retailing: Labour control and employees' coping strategies. *Ephemera Theory and Politics in Organization*, 7(1), pp. 46–59.

Cho, Y., Rutherford, B.N., and Park, J. (2013). The impact of emotional labour in a retail environment. *Journal of Business Research*, 66, pp. 670–677.

Dahiya, A. (2017). Extroversion and emotional labour: A study on organized retail sector. *International Journal of Research in Commerce & Management*, 8(4), pp. 50–54.

Grandey, A.A., Rupp, D., and Brice, W.N. (2015). Emotional labour threatens decent work: A proposal to eradicate emotional display rules. *Journal of Organizational Behaviour*, 36(6), pp. 770–785.

Hardt, M. and Negri, A. (2001). *Empire*. Cambridge, MA: Harvard University Press.

Hochschild, A.R. (1983). *The Managed Heart: Commercialization of Human Feeling*. California: University of California Press.

Houssay-Holzschuch, M. and Teppo, A. (2009). A mall for all? Race and public space in post-apartheid Cape Town. *Cultural Geographies*, 16(3), pp. 351–379.

Ikeler, P. (2015). Deskilling emotional labour: Evidence from department store retail. *Work Employment and Society*, 30(6), pp. 966–983.

Kang, M. (2003). The managed hand: The commercialization of bodies and emotions in Korean immigrant–owned nail salons. *Gender & Society*, 17(6), pp. 820–839.

Kaplan, D. (2018). Social club sociability as a model for national solidarity. *American Journal of Cultural Sociology*, 6, pp.1–36.

Kenny, B. (2015). Retail, the service worker and the polity: Attaching labour and consumption. *Critical Arts*, 29(2), pp. 199–217.

Kenny, B. (2016). The regime of contract in South African retailing: A history of race, gender, and skill in precarious labour. *International Labour and Working-Class History*, 89, pp. 20–33.

Lawless, M.E. (2014). Checking out: A qualitative study of supermarket cashiers' emotional response to customer mistreatment. *USF Tampa Graduate Theses and Dissertations*. [2022, May 25] https://digitalcommons.usf.edu/etd/5058

McNair, P.A. (2012). Your comfortable shopping. *Critical Arts*, 26(3), pp. 442–446.

Oksala, J. (2016). Affective labour and feminist politics. *Signs: Journal of Women in Culture and Society*, 41(2), pp. 281–303.

Pyyhtinen, O. (2009). Being-with: Georg Simmel's sociology of association. *Theory, Culture & Society*, 26(5), pp. 108–128.

Rafaeli, A. (1989). When cashiers meet customers: An analysis of the role of supermarket cashiers. *Academy of Management Journal*, 32(2), pp. 245–273.

Ruggieri, D. (2017). Georg Simmel and the "Relational Turn". Contributions to the foundation of the Lebenssoziologie since Simmel. *Simmel Studies*, 21(1), pp. 43–71.

Simmel, G. and Hughes, E.C. (1949). The sociology of sociability. *American Journal of Sociology*, 55(3), pp. 254–261.

Stix, G. (September 2020). Emotional labour is a store clerk confronting a maskless customer [2022, April 13]. www.scientificamerican.com/article/emotional-labor-is-a-store-clerk -confronting-a-maskless-customer/.

Turner, K.J., Le Grange, K., and Nkgadima, R. (2021). Timeline: 10 months of Covid-19 in SA. [Online]. TIMELINE: 10 months of Covid-19 in SA (iol.co.za) [2022, 11 April].

Veldstra, C. (2020). Bad feeling at work: Emotional labour, precarity, and the affective economy. *Cultural Studies*, 34(1), pp. 1–24.

Waters-Lynch, J. and Duff, C. (2021). The affective commons of Coworking. *Human Relations*, 74(3), pp. 383–404.

Weeks, K. (2011). *The Problem with Work: Feminism, Marxism, Antiwork Politics, and Postwork Imaginaries*.Durham, NC Duke University Press.

Wharton, A.S. (2009). The sociology of emotional labour. *Annual Review of Sociology*, 35(1), pp. 147–165.

Xiong, J., Lipsitz, O., Nasri, F., Lui, L.M., Gill, H., Phan, L., Chen-Li, D., Iacobacci, M., Ho, R., Majeed, A., and McIntyre, R.S. (2020). Impact of COVID-19 pandemic on mental health in the general population: A systematic review. *Journal of Affective Disorders*, 277, pp. 55–64.

9 Lest We Forget the Individual behind the Successful Woman

Chronicles of Indonesian Domestic Workers in Malaysian Households

Kalai Vaani Rajandram

Introduction: The Urban Malaysian Woman

Urbanisation has broken down some traditional barriers that hold women back from pursuing their share of economic opportunities. Lifestyles have changed whilst gender, identity, and culture have become more negotiable amidst a landscape that celebrates the pride of the working woman. Women account for 39% of all employed workers in Malaysia (Department of Statistics Malaysia, 2020). The healthy upward trajectory promises to create more productive employment and labour force participation in Malaysia. Considering this development, these ambitious women have grown to leverage on the support provided not only from family but also from domestic workers who eventually become 'family members' and are seen as 'helpers' in many households. This study will therefore proceed to use the term 'helper(s)' to refer to these women to acknowledge their significance beyond the clinical sphere.

As multi-faceted women with multiple roles to play, the duties of the urban Malaysian woman extend beyond the home, traversing into the workplace that demands societal and community needs be met in this hustle and bustle nation nested in modern Asia. The dawn of the pandemic saw an exacerbation in the stranglehold their careers had on them. As schools stayed closed since the movement control order, many women had to bear additional domestic work on top of their professional responsibilities. According to the Department of Statistics Malaysia, the first quarter of 2020 witnessed a noteworthy number of persons leaving the workforce. They justified 'housework and family' as the primary root cause. Hence, their dependence on domestic help has increased twofold since despite the freeze on foreign maids during the pandemic.

The Indonesian Community: Context, Culture, and Communication

There are an estimated 2.7 million Indonesian migrant workers in Malaysia although firm figures are difficult to come by as only about one-third of workers are believed to be documented (Aljazeera, 2021).The migrants take up jobs ranging

DOI: 10.4324/9781003267133-12

from domestic helpers to construction and plantation workers. While Malaysia plays host to approximately 92,481 foreign maids in the country, 58,438 are Indonesian domestic helpers, as of April 2022 (FMT Reporters, 2022). Statistics and figures do little to illustrate the disruptive nature of the pandemic on many of these individuals who facilitate their employers to make ends meet. As if their pre-pandemic situation was not enough to drive them to foreign soils, the current situation at hand plagues them in a way that they struggle to find the right words to even describe how their predicaments have worsened.

Research in the area has often focused on the plight of migrant workers. Similarly, with domestic workers, stories about their abuse and exploitation have been central to studies attempting to offer solutions and reform initiatives (Tandos, Rhu & Krever, 2022; Cheah, 2022; Flambonita, Novianti & Febriansyah, 2022). Hierofani (2021)'s work is particularly interesting because it talks about power play in the light of performativity and observes these domestic workers as social actors. The study discusses practices at the micro-level (home) and links it to racialisation of occupation, occupational identities, and the marginalisation of these women as aliens which completely desexualises them in the process.

With the pandemic in play, the trend has been one that highlights domestic workers' vulnerabilities related to Covid-19 such as the implementation and practice of health protocols, ignorance, and indifference to the dangers of transmission of the virus, and of the vaccination programme (Anaf, Ibnu, Romdiati & Noveria, 2022; Anam, Warsito, Al-Fadhat, Pribadi & Sugito, 2021). These have been studied in relation to the prolonged migration processes that they have to endure during the period of the pandemic. While these are without a doubt, pertinent issues that deserve attention, there is a lack of work that brings to the fore the dynamism that these migrant domestic workers embody despite their tragic tales.

The maid community featured in this collection is a close-knit one that subsists on solidarity and camaraderie. Although they live separately in various households, the inevitable bond that they share is one that has been carefully woven over the years in the heart of their homeland. They have a hub, a headquarter belonging to an *Ibu Sumi*. A domestic helper, just like the rest, cleverly engineered the meetups that have over the years drawn the other four to her backyard. In the absence of her employer who works abroad, she is left to tend to the empty home that she is more than delighted to do. Hence, by default, she assumed the role of Head Honcho. Weekend get-togethers were the pivotal moments of their week. Some have their partners in tow, while others would have cooked up a storm to celebrate their Sundanese heritage of *tempeh, nasi timbel*, and an assortment of *ulam* interlaced with a concoction of *sambal tumis* (fermented soybeans, rice, leafy vegetables, and chilli paste). The men were in it for the food, drinks, and chain-smoking. The banter was incomprehensible, but they were falling off their chairs!

The women always seemed to have an agenda of their own. Clad in their so-called party outfits that nicely tied-in with their psychedelic headscarves, their whispering and eye-rolling antics paralleled that of the typical women we have grown accustomed to seeing. Their conversations were intellectual to them; their gestures were animated. They were not merely making merry. They were making calculated moves, developing strategies, and plotting their next story. The serious-ness with which they discussed their children and family that they left behind was a poignant one. The men faded in the background, insignificant to the transpiring findings that *Irum, Yati, Siti, Ike,* and *Ibu Sumi* brought to the table. They brought to light their dreams, their hopes, and their ambitions as aspiring role models in their community of domestic helpers.

Their hearts were in the right place. It was not accidental that they were bestowed the role of chosen breadwinners of their families or so it appeared. The men who tagged along, all construction site workers, were reduced to uncouth, rough around the edges type of men who did little to alleviate the damnation the women felt that they were condemned to. The patriarchal structure that is firmly grounded back home was seen to erode just a little bit gnawing at the men at the back of their heads. The displeasure was evident as their ammo was observed in their loud voices and slightly larger stature to the women within their grasp. The women humoured them, giving them the respect they needed to keep the peace. Family is key. The women know this.

Empirical Data: The Wrath of the Pandemic

Ibu Sumi's Story

She made it. She secured a Malaysian-bred husband. They even referred to her dif-ferently out of respect or seniority, one cannot tell. She enjoyed the perks of being Malaysian as she gradually moved away from staying full-time with her employers to owning a modest home in the rural parts of Kuala Lumpur city. She still tended to the needs of her employers commuting back and forth daily. In her new home she not only nurtured a son, but it also became the headquarters of this group of women before lockdowns became the new normal.

The pandemic was a game-changer for *Ibu Sumi.* Her husband lost his job and had a tighter leash around her neck. Her employer's businesses abroad downsized making them homebound most of the time. Her movements became restricted and expectations of her increased. In other words, she finally experienced a full-fledged life as a domestic helper. She went from hostess to guest quite quickly. She was still privy to the privileges of marrying a Malaysian; hence, the other women did not empathise with her situation. Perhaps, she was only now feeling some of the brunt; she was only now in their shoes, or so to speak. *Irum* recollects how *Ibu Sumi* had grown distant since, although they try to maintain their circle of trust.

Irum's Story

The sudden distance from *Ibu Sumi* forced *Irum* to be content with her own com-pany. She had been working for the same employer for 17 years now. Once plump with heavy locks of deep-black hair that she would neatly pile into a high bun, *Irum* was now a frail and gaunt-looking 48-year-old who ambled her way through the chores. Make no mistake as looks can be deceiving. Her grip is of iron; her strength is of ore; and her heart is pure gold. She has three teen girls and a mother who looked after them in her absence. Her husband left her for another woman, and with this woman, another son. Poverty drove *Irum* to Malaysia, *'saya orang susah, orang miskin'* (she reminds us several times about how difficult it is being poor). She recollects how she was the chosen one. She was the one chosen among several siblings to save this family from further ruins.

The pandemic brought with it a divorce, a marriage, and a new baby. Alongside this, the death of *Irum*'s mother. She bawled like a baby for days. The worst had yet to come. The series of events that followed suit was like a dark cloud that would not leave her. Her daughter was facing a divorce and had a baby at the same time. *Irum*'s ex-husband returned with his son and began setting up camp in whatever was left of a shattered home. With zero income at hand, he was planning a wedding for the youngest daughter. All eyes were on *Irum* to beg, borrow, or steal, and all she wanted was to provide '*makan*' for her family, which loosely translates to food. The monetary demands and expectations have taken a physical toll on her. She spends hours confiding in *Yati*, who lives next door. From milk to court expenses, from more mouths to feed to holding on to whatever little shelter they have left in Indonesia – who would pay for these?

Yati's Story

Yati, being the younger woman in her early thirties, has always been like a little sister to *Irum*, and that sisterhood has only strengthened over the years. She would tippy-toe into the backyard, pull up a rickety chair, and peer into the house from over-the-wall searching for *Irum* from one end to the other. She always had her long raven black hair in a tousle. Standing at not more than 4 ft 5 in., she was a feisty one that always had to have the last say. Her employer is a 90-year-old grand lady who takes pride in keeping house and keeping herself youthful. Much of this has rubbed off on *Yati*. She once fancied a young Indonesian lad from a nearby construction site; he took her as his wife here in Malaysia, only to later find out that he had a wife and two children back home. She chuckled re-living the episode without a care in the world.

Yati became a dispatch-cum-runner girl for *Irum* during the pandemic. With all households tightening belts, none of these women were allowed to leave their workplace except for *Yati*. Employers were concerned about them contracting Covid-19, since these domestic helpers can have a rather lackadaisical attitude towards following standard operating procedures (SOPs) during the pandemic. She scurried to withdraw cash for *Irum* and would lend her money at times so that she can *'bayar hutang'*, or pay up debts. *Yati* would purchase items that *Irum* needed ranging from vegetables to bath products. Their over-the-wall activities, updates on court proceedings, and ploys on how to get things across to Indonesia. While on these heroic rescue missions, *Yati*'s pleas, and cries, as she hangs on to her Samsung in the wee hours of the morning, revealed another story – one that her eyes attempt to hide but that is betrayed by her tears. There was no wall to climb over for this one. *Ike* revealed what she heard through the grapevine.

Ike's Story

Ike bridges gaps. She is that one person who knew who's who and made it a point to get the group together via WhatsApp's video call feature. Her private conversations with the other women kept her abreast of their current situations. She learnt that *Yati*'s spouse is an illegal immigrant. He was hunted down by the authorities in their *kongsi*, a squatter-like living arrangement, and now faced deportation. The conditions at detention centres cannot be defined. One can only imagine hundreds of sweaty-bodied men reeking of *Gudang Garam*, a low-range cigarette brand, being shuttled like a herd of cattle into cooped-up cage-like cells far from the city centre. Malaysia does not take illegal immigrants lightly, and that is an understatement. The pandemic has only made the authorities more aggressive. We knew too much already about *Yati*.

Ike's reveal ironically sheds light on her own predicament. As she shoved her brittle-looking hair behind her ears, she lamented the quandary that she was in as she rubbed her tummy. She is with a child and her partner is in hiding. Unlike the rest, she only worked part time on an ad-hoc basis. Her travels here are undocumented. She narrates the day-to-day hunt for food and living off other *kongsi* members who can no longer accommodate her as it will not be long before their fate is sealed. One thing was certain, they cheated their way here and got away with it for the longest time. The pandemic unleashed the truth; it was a bomb waiting to go off. Her check-ins with the rest of the women have not ceased. What lies beneath those layers of uncomfortable and awkward socialising is her key to putting down roots that she severed the night she and her husband got on the boat and travelled eastwards to Malaysia. She is thriving, holding on to that last straw; the last straw which *Siti* is letting go.

Siti's Story

Siti has always been the subdued one. She only spoke when spoken to. She mustered the strength to put on a demure smile, nevertheless. Her dialogue had always been limited to worries about her *'masa depan, bayar hutang rumah dan makan'* which summarised all their concerns (going into the future, paying their debts, and having food on the table). Her lacklustre expressions and her struggle to verbalise her sorry situation without choking up epitomised a broken woman on the verge of a complete breakdown. Here alone with employers who wanted to get their money's worth, she has endured some heavy workload over the years. A long sigh ensued, almost sounding like one taking their last breath.

The imposed lockdowns in Malaysia resulted in her employers losing their jobs. This escalated their financial woes which were already heading into the red in the last few years. They decided to cut the cord and send *Siti* back to Indonesia. To add salt to the wound, *Siti* has recently developed a heart condition that does not work in her favour for continued employment in Malaysia. *Siti* is not ready to go. With a house loan to pay for, a host of children and grandchildren to feed and clothe, the men of the house are nowhere in sight. She is seen making calls, renewing connections, and asking for favours from *Ibu Sumi* who she has always looked up to as a mentor. She attempts to salvage what only she knows relationships can do. Her final words resonate clearly, *'tuhan akan lindungi, semoga cucu jagan susah macam nenek, jagan bodoh macam nenek'* (Her final prayer is that God bless her grandchildren with a better life; she wishes for them to not be as silly as she has been). A deafening silence follows.

Findings and Discussion: Perspectives and Possibilities

These are the parts of the stories that these women tell us. What they do not tell us is what truly captures how these damsels in distress operate. Through observation and participation in their daily lived experiences, it is eye-opening to see how gender, identity, and culture are negotiated through the contemporary manifestation of historical tensions of the relationship between economy and society as espoused by Adam Smith. These narratives offer a set of lenses and references that can help to understand the diverse but interconnected nature of these participants in this ecosystem. These women are defined by their cultural norms, values, and status. What is observed is an organised social life bound by a sense of belonging from a previous context of community in their homeland. This is entangled in a cultural mindset that negotiates roles entrenched in patriarchy and inequality of power relations. Nayati and Puri (2021) elaborate on this ideology where women are supposed to be good mothers and wives while husbands do not have such expectations from society. What is observed here seems to mock the men folk and their entitled ways.

There is a community like spirit, nevertheless, because of shared physical space and beliefs (Toennies & Loomis, 1988). We see why this happens here almost by default in this context. These women through groupthink are in fact a think tank of sorts. We get a glimpse of Social Constructivism in action as this form of interaction between these women does more than create themes that we can study as researchers but in fact outlines some of the key community development practices that showcase structure, power, and shared meaning. These findings parallel that of Wijaya, Watson, and Bruce (2022) when their study revealed that these engagements and interactions secure their well-being. On top of that it re-affirms their self-efficacy and self-esteem all of which enhance their capabilities to take control over the migration processes.

Symbiotic Relationships

These women are a society on their own terms. They form a 'society' that represents what they stand for. An institution that defines relationships, roles, and norms in a specific way that together constitutes a society that serves to uphold its individual agendas during the pandemic. While acting in silos from their own households, each is indispensable for the continued existence of the other. We learn that *Irum* and *Yati* are interdependent on a more literal level because they live next to each other, but with *Ike*'s constant prodding of the rest into sharing sessions imposes a structure on their behaviour. *Ike* not only became the agent of change wanting to honour the bond, so to speak, but also took over the lead from *Ibu Sumi* in initiating action. This sense of negotiations falling into place through intervention and mediation suggests an integrated system with life characteristics of its own, exterior to individuals yet driving their behaviour. This symbiosis captures Durkheim's (1984) notions of mechanical solidarity and organic solidarity.

The mechanical solidarity is motivated vis-à-vis their roles as domestic helpers. The sentimental attraction of this social unit that performs similar functions of facilitating home chores of their employers automatically drew the group together on the surface. However, organic solidarity is far more complex as this interdependence is based on their differentiated functions in their families, their employer's families, and their social roles here and at home. Their stories capture what each is in their own situations versus what each is collectively as a group. The division of labour is intrinsic in how each uses the other's expertise to service one another during the pandemic. *Siti* is seen resorting to this when she seeks advice from *Ibu Sumi*, the supposed leader of the team, who is on her way out to find another job.

Ibu Sumi's connections with the social world are seen as superior to the rest in this situation. However, *Siti* is seen consulting *Irum*, the only other grandmother in this society that they have built on issues regarding managing the young ones at home. As interdependent but differentiated individuals, what can be understood here is that the focus is more on regulating relationships so that the ecosystem is like a well-oiled mechanism that keeps the peace during the pandemic. This scenario parallels the interdependence that Watson, Harris, and Iwabuchi (2020) discuss when they bring to light the Nepalese domestic workers' system of reconstructing multicultural power structures. In this study, *Ibu Sumi*'s cordial relations with the local domestic helpers' privies her to both 'insider' and 'outsider' information; her assimilation of 'other' cultural values and the dissemination of these within the group is weighed in.

Women Empowerment in Disguise

The working woman of the house often is seen as the epitome of the modern career woman who is the multi-tasker cum all-rounder when it comes to running a household and achieving that same balance at the workplace. While this is the scenario in many Malaysian homes today, the other women in their lives, namely the domestic helpers, especially in the context of this study, continue to remain in their shadows. *Ibu Sumi, Yati, Irum, Ike,* and *Siti* are seen as backdrops in a stage where they are not the main players for logical reasons. Being so, it continues to feed our preconceived notions about who and what they are, given the situation they were brought into the country in the first place. Further to that is the complexities that inherently lie in the perception of inequality of social class which conflict theory stands to challenge (Marx & Engels, 1998). Straddling somewhere in between are these individual Indonesian women that are not ever really seen for who they are and what they know.

Being amongst them brought to the fore a shade of what Functionalism is perhaps about looking at the situation at a micro-level. The pandemic was a stimulus, or rather a simulation of what these women are potentially capable of achieving in a less controlled environment. Pushed to the edge, we see these women battling it out in a concocted social system that they must meet to survive. In the least expected ways, *Irum* is seen coordinating and managing her family affairs in Indonesia with minimal technology at hand. Her Skype sessions with her children involve her mobilising food and other necessities from one relative to another, calling out delivery instructions, and allocating food rations in an authoritative manner. Elsewhere, *Yati* and *Ike* are in decision-making positions attempting to solve the issues brought on by their men. Suddenly, their voices are louder; they have grown in stature and are now calling the shots, seemingly belittling the men folk along the way who have either escaped to marry other women or gotten caught by the law. Nayati and Puri (2021) acknowledge this new identity construction that is suppressed in the homeland founded on the grounds that only the men are capable of these things directly impacting wage differences and other forms of inequality. The role reversal which this study observes is noteworthy.

Studies on migrant domestic workers have shown that migrant women's bodies are constructed through the narratives of the global economy, nation, and gender (Pratt, 1988; Stiell & England, 1997; Anderson, 2007). They are not only empowered to act in the situations highlighted in this study, but they seem to also have the gumption and cognition to expedite processes to set others in motion. Between working with each other and working alone, we see them mediate and moderate their finances and working conditions in a way that is akin to performing functions that are aligned with keeping social order and stability.

Acculturation for Survival

Being a part of Malaysian society for more than 10–15 years, these women have begun to understand that their roles are not merely confined to what their society has meted out to them. While on the one hand, they belong in a society made up of the five of them, on the other hand, they are also part and parcel of the dynamics created in the households they are employed in. Being so, they have re-constructed their notions of gender, identity, and culture in relation to the women they work for via interaction, observation, and inclusion. Their reliance on verbal and non-verbal cues is essential as they learn to navigate the needs and wants of their employers. This is akin to the symbolic interactionism theory that highlights this as a necessity to arrive at a shared understanding of interactions and engagement (Blumer, 1969).

What is learnt in the context of this study is that these domestic helpers adopt, adapt, and adjust their bearings to 'speak' the language. They see this attempt to socially situate themselves as part of the family. The acclimatisation in terms of choice of words, especially that of those that displease their employers with impressionable young children, is seen as a strategic one. In fact, it shows the complexity of power relations. Sharp et al. (2000) point out that the local status of power can be negotiated through one's skill and quick-wittedness. Similarly, their sense of foresight and initiative coupled with their sense of accountability and rigour is worth understanding. There is an attempt to unlearn, relearn, and forsake their own ways of doing things and saying things. This echoes what Lukman, Othman, and Sulaiman (2009) point out about their tendency to practise the avoiding or integrating style when managing conflict. This is seen not only in their dealings with their employers but also amongst themselves which suggest a deeply rooted understanding of an intimate level of co-existence and sense of belonging to a family (Killias, 2014).

Irum narrates the value of these sacrifices as one that saw her through the pandemic. By giving up her own beliefs and practices over the last 17 years, her employers came to her aid in the recent two years of the pandemic. She was able to send large boxes of necessities through shipment for her family who are in dire straits. In addition, *Yati, Ike, Ibu Sumi*, and *Siti* were also beneficiaries of what they believe is due to getting on the same page where verbal and non-verbal cues are concerned.

Conclusion: Moving Forward

As promised, this is a story of resilience. It is one that forces us to re-consider, re-evaluate, and re-visit our perceptions and preconceived stigmas against this sect of society that can be more than meets the eye. The pandemic perhaps brought out a side of them that they themselves were not aware they had especially in the absence of the men. There was no struggle for power, as in most modern societies, but this episode unleashed a power that they had from within. These are not weak women despite their skeletal bodies. Their grip on reality far outweighs those of us who claim to be grounded in essence. As women have so much to offer, both countries must pave the way forward for them and their families post-pandemic. While there have been initiatives and strategies in place such as educational measures and the use of local entertainment culture to inject awareness of the issues discussed, appropriate dissemination of information is still being developed. Orange, Seitz, and Kor (2012) have outlined extensively the needs of this group and recommended policy-shaping endeavours with pilot projects as stepping stones. Nayati and Puri (2021) have also suggested measures to reduce the gender impact which will be beneficial post-pandemic. What is clear is that action is underway, but the hurdles are manifold.

From this study, one would gather that the first step would be to fully legalise domestic helpers whose spouses have already been in Malaysia for over a decade and working in construction sites contractually. It serves little purpose to send them back and add to the psychological turmoil faced by both parties. Granted that entering foreign waters without proper documentation is not desirable, but during the pandemic, these illegal immigrants ran into hiding out of fear of being caught when authorities started to enforce the law. This only increased the spread of Covid-19. To what end does this benefit any party is questionable. Secondly, there should be avenues for these domestic helpers to seek counselling and advice in the name of promoting mental health awareness. These services should be extended to this group who are vulnerable, lonely, and traumatised by various happenings in their own families at home.

Octavianus and Lin (2021) shed light on Hong Kong's initiatives to scale up interventions with regard to supporting the migrant domestic workers, particularly the Indonesians. The storytelling networks offered various types of social support, including informational, emotional, and instrumental or tangible assistance. Such solicitation is needed if we intend to genuinely elevate these individuals. Licensed social workers alongside clinical sociologists should be mobilised without having to deal with too much red tape and bureaucracy that hinders goodwill and reduces the capacity for the right people to do what they are trained for. On the same note, Pasaribu (2021) draws attention to how '*Perempuan Berkisah*,' a community group that was mobilised to offer support that uplifted Indonesian women during the pandemic by instilling feminist knowledge, promoting self-empowerment, encouraging sisterhood, and providing a safe space for sharing. Feasible initiatives as such are often more fruitful than large-scaled policy-changing endeavours.

There should not be double standards when it comes to these basic healthcare services. These are women who keep our homes together, nurture our children, and support us in ways we sometimes cannot express. These women are enablers in a sense that they allow many Malaysian women to build a career for themselves. In extension, these domestic helpers are contributing to the country's shared prosperity. On a final note, this study has revealed five spirited women who have great potential. While they may not be representative of all domestic helpers out there, they do in fact give us a glimpse of what they could be if channelled correctly. Taking from this, employers should empower these women through the acquisition of new skills and leverage their capabilities through education. Let this story create a ripple in the way we see them.

References

Anaf, A., Ibnu, F., Romdiati, H., & Noveria, M. (2022). "Indonesian Migrant Workers: The Migration Process and Vulnerability to COVID-19." *Journal of Environmental and Public Health*, 2022, p. 2563684. DOI: 10.1155/2022/2563684. PMID: 35755883; PMCID: PMC9217585.

Anam, M. Z., Pribadi, U., Warsito, T., Sugito, & Al-Fadhat, F. (2021). Pandemics and its aftermath in Southeast Asia *Sociology & Technoscience / Sociología y Tecnociencia*, 11(2), pp. 160–194.

Anderson, B. (2007). "A Very Private Business: Exploring the Demand for Migrant Domestic Workers." *European Journal of Women's Studies*, 14(3), pp. 247–264. DOI: 10.1177/1350506807079013.

Blumer, H. (1969). *Symbolic Interactionism: Perspective and Method*. Englewood Cliffs, NJ: Prentice Hall.

Cheah, W. L. (2022). "CEDAW and Transformative Judicial Obligations: The Vulnerable Migrant Domestic Worker and Root Causes of Abuse." *Michigan Journal of International Law*, 43, p. 129. Retrieved from https://repository.law.umich.edu/mjil/vol43/iss1/4.

Department of Statistics Malaysia. (2020). Retrieved from https://dosm.gov.my/. Site accessed on 10 December 2021.

Durkheim, E. (1984). *The Division of Labour in Society*. London: Macmillan.

Flambonita, S., Novianti, V., & Febriansyah, A. (2022). "Preventive Protection for Indonesian Migrant Workers as Part of an Effort to Prevent Human Trafficking in Johor Bahru Malaysia." *Journal La Sociale*, 3(3), pp. 111–116. DOI: 10.37899/journal-la-sociale.v3i3.659.

Hierofani, P. Y. (2021). "Productive and Deferential Bodies: The Experiences of Indonesian Domestic Workers in Malaysia." *Gender, Place and Culture*, 28(12), pp. 1738–1754. DOI: 10.1080/0966369X.2020.1855121.

Killias, O. (2014). "Intimate Encounters: The Ambiguities of Belonging in the Transnational Migration of Indonesian Domestic Workers to Malaysia." *Citizenship Studies*, 18(8), pp. 885–899. DOI: 10.1080/13621025.2014.964550.

Llewellyn, A. (2021, December 28). "Indonesian Migrants Brave Treacherous Seas for Malaysian Dream." Aljazeera. Retrieved from https://www.aljazeera.com/economy /2021/12/28/indonesian-migrants-brave-treacherous-seas-for-malaysian-dream

Lukman, I. B., Othman, J., Hassan, M. S., & Sulaiman, A. H. (2009). *Intercultural communication and conflict anagement among Malaysian mployers and Indonesian omestic Workers in Kuala Lumpur.Malaysia Labor Review*, 3(2), 27–38

Marx, K., & Engels, F. (1998). *The Communist Manifesto*. New York: Penguin.

Nayati, W., & Puri, V. Y. (2021). "The Impact of the COVID-19 Pandemic on Indonesian Women Workers Is Based on a Social-Cultural Perspective." *International Journal for Studies on Children, Women, Elderly and Disabled*, 12, pp. 20–25.

Oktavianus, J., & Lin, W. Y. (2021). "Soliciting Social Support from Migrant Domestic Workers' Connections to Storytelling Networks during a Public Health Crisis." *Health Communication*, 386pp. 1179–1188.DOI: 10.1080/10410236.2021.1996675

Orange, G., Seitz, V., & Kor, A. (2012). "Information Dissemination Needs of Indonesian Migrant Domestic Workers in Malaysia." *Journal of Southeast Asian Research*. DOI: 10.5171/2012.492902.

Pasaribu, R. (2021). "Feminist Knowledge, Self-Empowerment and Sisterhood, and Safe Space: How the 'Perempuan Berkisah' Community Group Empowers Indonesian Women in the Pandemic Era." *Journal of International Women's Studies*, 22(12), Article 10. Retrieved from https://vc.bridgew.edu/jiws/vol22/iss12/10.

Pratt, G. (1998). "Inscribing Domestic Work on Filipina Bodies." In *Places through the Body*, edited by Nast, H. and Pile, S., pp. 211–226. London: Routledge.

Sharp, J., Routledge, P., Philo, C., & Paddison, R. (2000). "Entanglements of Power: Geographies of Domination/Resistance." In *Entanglements of Power: Geographies of Domination/Resistance*, edited by Sharp, J., Routledge, P., Philo, C., and Paddison, R., pp. 1–42. London: Routledge.

Stiell, B., & England, K. (1997). "Domestic Distinctions: Constructing Difference among Paid Domestic Workers in Toronto." *Gender, Place and Culture*, 4(3), pp. 339–360. DOI: 10.1080/09663699725387.

Tandos, R., Zhu, R., & Krever, R. (2022). "The Protection and Empowerment of Indonesian Female Migrant Domestic Workers: Proposals from a Multi-Stage Analysis." *Asian Journal of Women's Studies*, 28(2), pp. 205–227. DOI: 10.1080/12259276.2022.2051818.

Toennies, F., & Loomies, C. P. (1988). *Community and Society* London, United Kingdom:. Routledge.

Walton, J., Harris, A., & Iwabuchi, K. (2020). "Introduction: Everyday Multiculturalism in/ across Asia." *Ethnic and Racial Studies*, 43(5), pp. 807–815.

Wijaya, S. W., Watson, J., & Bruce, C. (2022). "A Virtual Ethnography Study of Indonesian Migrant Domestic Workers' Empowerment in Online Communities." *Behaviour & Information Technology*. DOI: 10.1080/0144929X.2022.2052184.

10 Deaf Women in Malaysia

The Unspoken Truth about Their Experiences and Challenges Amidst COVID-19 Pandemic

Wan Puspa Melati

Understanding the Context: Malaysia and the COVID-19 Pandemic

The COVID-19 pandemic has taken the world by storm, affecting global citizens physically, economically, psychologically, and socially. The battle against the 'unknown' created a sense of anomie among the community members and demanded commitment by the government as well as relevant authorities to ensure that the country remained safe and stable. Additionally, the prolonged 'battle' does not only see the accumulated impact on the people and the nation, but it also poses a challenge for individuals and countries to 'recover' from such impact and to gain momentum back to some form of normalcy.

In the case of Malaysia, the development of the COVID-19 pandemic can be categorised into three waves. The first wave was between 25 January and 15 February 2020. During this phase, 22 reported cases were declared, and they were mainly infected outside of Malaysia or what is termed the imported cases. The second wave can be linked to the congregations and meetings during that period. As a result, significant clusters were identified, including the Sri Petaling Tabligh Cluster – a religious congregation that took place between 27 February and 3 March 2020. It was reported that 14,500 Malaysians and 1,500 global participants took part in that event; hence, many infected individuals were not surprising. Then, the nation saw the third wave – increased cases in Sabah (8,082), followed by Selangor (3,357), Kuala Lumpur (2,853), and Kedah (1,940) (The Star, 2020). In Sabah, the infections were linked to the Lahad Datu District Police Headquarters as well as the Tawau prison subclusters. In September 2020, there was also another spike as many politicians travelled to Sabah to campaign and support the Sabah state election without allegedly not observing the standard operating procedures (SOPs) (Ministry of Health [MOH], 2020). Upon their return, these politicians were believed to have spread the COVID-19 infections.

The lockdown, curfew and movement control orders were introduced by the government around the world to manage the pandemic by limiting the exposure of individuals to others. This is based on the belief that the virus can spread between people during close contact interactions namely through small droplets produced through coughing, sneezing, or talking (World Health Organization, 2022). In Malaysia, the government implemented a two-week Movement Control Order

DOI: 10.4324/9781003267133-13

(MCO), which started on the 18th of March 2020 and was then extended twice between the period of 1–14 April and 15–28 April 2020. During the initial lockdowns and MCO, Malaysia has closed its borders, shut down non-essential businesses, schools, and universities as well as closed off places for religious worship. Later between 13 May and 9 June 2020, Malaysia moved into the Conditional Movement Control Order (CMCO) with more services and businesses back in operation to support the economy of the country. By 9 June, Malaysia moved into the Recovery Movement Control Order (RMCO) which ran until 31 August 2020 and later extended to January 2021. On 11 January 2021, the Prime Minister announced that Movement Control Order restrictions would be reintroduced in the states of Malacca, Johor, Penang, Selangor, Sabah, and the Federal Territories of Kuala Lumpur, Putrajaya, and Labuan between 13 and 26 January 2021 and later extended to 18 February 2021 (MOH, 2020).

The MCO has been further extended in the Federal Territories of Kuala Lumpur, Selangor, Johor, and Penang until 4 March 2021. Though there were periodic slots of Conditional and Recovery Movement Control Orders, 2020–2021 has largely been a controlled environment. Malaysians, especially, those living in areas with high infection cases have been concerned about social interaction beyond close circles and try to avoid unnecessary exposure. Thus, many engaged in self-isolation – adults were working from home, students were doing online classes, and food necessities were getting delivered to the doorsteps. External help for household chores and childcare was also limited due to the closure of businesses and national borders. At the later stage, though some services are available, i.e., daycare centres and house cleaning services, many were hesitant to use such services due to the increased number of cases and community spread. As a result, this pandemic has exacerbated the existing challenges and obstacles faced by individuals and the nation in addition to being tested in ways that have never been challenged before.

Focusing on the Deaf: The Impact of COVID-19

Previous research has discussed the different impacts of COVID-19 on different segments of society, including the Deaf (Almeida et al., 2014; Hub Editorial, 2020; Rose, 2020; Shew, 2020). The Deaf was chosen as the subject focus of this chapter as they are the oppressed majority among the people with disabilities. Statistics indicated that 1.6 billion people are affected by the loss of hearing globally, either by birth or later in their lives (Tonelli & Warick, 2022). In Malaysia, about 44,500 individuals with hearing impairment have registered with the welfare department (Jabatan Kebajikan Masyarakat [JKM], 2018). Some may choose not to register as they do not consider their condition as a form of disability, or they do not need any assistance from the welfare department. Moreover, research in a global setting has shown that the Deaf are negatively affected by the pandemic, but not much is known in the context of Malaysia especially based on qualitative data.

Among the negative impacts on the Deaf during the pandemic is the limited access to COVID-19-related information (Murray, 2020). A study by Panko et al. (2021) found that the Deaf are 4.7 times more likely than their hearing counterparts to report difficulty in obtaining COVID-19-related information. Others have highlighted that for those who do have access, the information was reportedly inconsistent which in turn placed them at more risk during the pandemic (Abuelgasim et al., 2020; Piller et al., 2020). The limited health literacy and health information are also linked to the preventive health measures that individuals take (McKee et al., 2011; Tamaskar et al., 2000; Wollin & Elder, 2003). Thus, it is not surprising to learn that 60% of the Deaf studied by Panko et al. (2021) were less likely to stay at home during the pandemic and they were also not likely to call their doctors when they experienced any COVID-19 symptoms.

Additionally, there was evidence that the Deaf tends to have a lower reading proficiency level, which in turn affects their understanding of the communicated messages and ability to assess the situation that they were facing (McKee et al., 2015). Thus, many of the Deaf tend to rely on their friends and families for information rather than on their healthcare providers before and during pandemics (McKee et al., 2011; Valentine & Skelton, 2009; Lima et al., 2020). Though the issue of lower reading proficiency and reliance on significant others is not new, the issue was heightened during the pandemic – to lack and delayed access to information related to COVID-19 (Engelman et al., 2020). Another raised concern about access to COVID-19 information is linked to the limited communication between the Deaf and the medical personnel due to the inability to sign among professionals (Al Majali & Alghazo 2021). Thus, the anxiety and worry were arguably more intense among the Deaf community than in the hearing counterparts during the pandemic.

Communication among the Deaf was also affected due to the obligation to mask-wearing as part of the pandemic SOPs. For the Deaf, the ability to express and observe both gestures and facial expressions is imperative for effective communication. The mask affected communication among members of the Deaf community as well as between the Deaf and the interpreters. There have been initiatives to manage this – the creation of clear face masks which were considered safe and Deaf-friendly (Chang & Lipner, 2020). However, not many Malaysians are aware of such products as they are not readily and widely available in Malaysia. For those who were aware and able to purchase online, many questioned the effectiveness and safety of such masks as they have not been endorsed by Malaysian health agencies or the government, in addition to the relatively high cost compared to conventional masks.

Another major impact that concerns social scientists as the repercussion of the COVID-19 pandemic is the well-being of global citizens. The home confinement, the uncertainties, the lack of information, the change of norm, and the restricting SOPs were all linked to the state of psychological well-being of individuals (Al Majali & Alghazo, 2021). This is in addition to the change of lifestyle and leisure time spent by the individuals (Asmundson & Taylor, 2020; Kadam & Atre, 2020). Scholars have highlighted the reports of confusion, increased anxiety, stress, and depression as well as the feeling of helplessness due to the pandemic (Dong & Bouey, 2020; Duan & Zhu, 2020; Wang et al., 2020). This concern was not only applicable to their self and well-being but extended to the worry about the safety and well-being of their significant others and the nation (Al Majali & Alghazo, 2021). Other worries include their food sustainability, educational performance, and social connections (Engelman et al., 2020). Previous research findings have found that living with others could reduce the levels of anxiety, worry, and depression (Al Majali & Alghazo, 2021).

To support the Deaf during the pandemic, mechanisms to allow them to get access to medical professionals should have been provided, namely using visual online platforms, and having free interpreter services (Al Majali & Alghazo, 2021). Scholars have also emphasised the use of captions on online platforms as well as the amplification of devices as part of the inclusive initiative to manage the pandemic. Other strategies include having trusted agents and social media channels that can reach and be better received by the Deaf community (Panko et al., 2021). However, as evident, these sensitivities were sidelined in most countries (Tonelli & Warick, 2022).

Highlighting the Concern: COVID-19 Pandemic and Deaf Women

As illustrated above, the realities of the pandemic as well as its impact are evident and have been discussed by previous researchers. Taking them together, the current author highlights the need to understand and consider the complexities of multiple identities and social roles that individuals have, which adds to the layers of intricacy in our understanding of COVID-19. This includes the intersection of age, marital status, number of household members, education level, economic standing, race, and religion, and the list continues.

The impact of the COVID-19 pandemic is further exacerbated for Deaf women due to the additional intersections of gender and disability. Evidence of the lived challenges that Deaf women faced daily has been well-established before, but these pre-existing challenges are topped by the severe impact of the COVID-19 pandemic. The report by United Nations Population Fund (UNFPA) and Women Enabled International (WEI) (2021) entitled "The Impact of COVID-19 on Women and Girls with Disabilities: A Global Assessment and Case Studies on Sexual and Reproductive Health and Rights, Gender-Based Violence, and Related Rights" highlighted the limited access to information on sexual and reproductive health among women and girls with disabilities as well as access to other disability-related needed goods, services, employment, education, and bodily autonomy during the pandemic. They were also limited in terms of the ability to have an interpreter to support them during the pandemic because of social distancing and Movement Control Order.

The Movement Control Order and home confinement also meant that disabled women are unable to get further support beyond their homes including getting help when confronted with psychological, social, and sexual violence. Unlike hearing women who may be able to call any helpline, welfare, or police officers, the Deaf women in Malaysia are limited as such services are not made easily accessible to the Deaf. There was also evidence that even in instances where such mechanisms are available, the mechanisms were not efficient and slow during the pandemic (UNFPA & WEI, 2021). Therefore, it is not surprising to note that researchers have found a higher group of depression and anxiety among women and that the increase is also faster among women than among men. In addition, the Deaf has also been found to be severely affected by prolonged home confinement (Al Majali & Alghazo 2021)

The concept of intersectionality has been introduced by earlier scholars and has been used to discuss various social realities. Intersectionality refers to 'the complex, cumulative way in which the effects of multiple forms of discrimination (such as racism, sexism, and classism) combine, overlap, or intersect especially in the experiences of marginalized individuals or groups' (*Merriam-Webster Dictionary*, 2022, 'Intersectionality'). This is an important and powerful concept as issues are being discussed in a unidimensional manner and failing to look at the interplay between variables will not provide the much-needed understanding of the issues at hand. Many studies considered multiple variables in their research studies, but the intersection and the simultaneous impact it has have not been widely discussed. The current author agrees with Pratima, a Nepali advocate for persons with disabilities who once said,

> I would say that the issue of gender, the issue of intersectionality has almost remained in a vacuum. So, it's always in a single linear model and that single linear model is not working for women with disabilities and other marginalised groups.
>
> (UNFPA & WEI, 2021, p. 5)

One of the earlier works that championed this lens was the work of Patricia Hill Collins (2002) in her book, *The Black Feminist Thought*. The intersectionality discussed was on multiple axes of oppression which is reflected through a complex systematic challenge that individuals face due to their multiple social identities and social structures. Though her discussion centres on various social identities affecting 'Black women,' this frame helps to discuss the intersectionality of other social identities, such as Deaf women. Besides highlighting the need to consider the intersections as a myriad of challenges to understand the complexities of lived experiences, this model also emphasises the need to empower individuals to rise against dominance and oppression through knowledge and consciousness as well as to push for the social transformation of institutions.

Like any other social group, there is also variation within the Deaf women category. One could find some highly empowered women with a strong sense of Deaf identity and who are determined to see the rise of other Deaf women in various spheres. In terms of communication, some women are better communicators than others in terms of both signing and expressing themselves to others. However, one of the salient characteristics that the author has encountered over 15 years of interaction with the Deaf is that most of the women that she has met do not consider being Deaf a condition that limits themselves, but rather the limits are often defined and imposed by others upon them. The experience of Deaf women may not only differ based on their attitude towards their conditions and ability to communicate but their other identities as defined by their marital status, educational level, occupational role, familial support, and financial standing, among others. Thus, this chapter aims to discuss the lived experiences and challenges faced by Deaf women in Malaysia amidst the COVID-19 pandemic using the intersectional lens.

Researching the Target Group: Methodology of Research

This chapter is based on qualitative research with Malaysian Deaf women. Ten respondents were interviewed using Malaysian Sign Language. The researcher also received assistance from a Deaf informant who can verbalise/speak and helped clarify some responses. The respondents were recruited from Deaf associations and through the snowball sampling method. The interviews were conducted online, via the Zoom platform, as preferred by the respondents who were concerned about the COVID-19 situation during the data collection phase (January–July 2021). Since this is exploratory research, minimal criteria were imposed. Women, regardless of their age, religion, race, and educational background, could be selected as part of this research. However, these women must have access to the internet and possess a device that allows them to be interviewed online.

A semi-structured interview was selected as it provides the structure to the research and simultaneously allows for further exploration beyond the lens of the researcher. The interview method is also a better approach for the Deaf as the questions could be better elaborated and supported with relevant examples compared to the survey. Interviews also allow the respondents to be able to understand the questions better and for the researcher to seek further clarification or elaboration. The interview sessions were recorded and later transcribed in consultation with a Deaf expert. A pilot study with two respondents was conducted and the procedure and questions were retained.

Revealing the Findings: Discussion on Lived Experiences and Challenges Faced by Malaysian Deaf Women during the COVID-19 Pandemic

The lived experiences and challenges reported by Deaf women during the pandemic can be categorised into four main categories, namely (1) communication during the time of the pandemic, (2) financial constraints and well-being, (3) socialising and social support, and (4) interpersonal conflict. For each of these categories, different social identities were also discussed to provide a better understanding of the raised concerns.

Communication in the Time of the Pandemic

Communication among the Deaf in Malaysia is arguably one of the sensitive topics of discussion. The arguments can be traced to the debate between the Deaf community and the policymakers on Bahasa Isyarat Malaysia (BIM), the sign language used in their daily conversations, and Kod Bahasa Tangan Malaysia (KTBM), the sign language used in schools to communicate using the Malay language. The community has been pushing for the recognition of BIM as their official language and to be used in schools and official interaction, which have been making progress but have not been widely institutionalised. The Deaf members have also highlighted the need for them to have a strong language fundamental in BIM before they embark on other language acquisition (Haziah Sa'ari, 2009).

Thus, as one could imagine, this lack of recognition in the social institution is not a new thing and affected the Deaf. However, the lack of a solid language foundation impacts the language proficiency among the Deaf, which was exacerbated during the pandemic. One of the main issues highlighted was the communication on COVID-19 itself. The informants expressed the lack of clear communication on COVID-19, including official and credible sources regarding what is COVID-19, how COVID-19 is transmitted, who are at higher risk, and what can be done to keep them and their families safe, why they need to get vaccinated and the like. They cited the heavy use of medical jargon or complex concepts that are unfamiliar to the Deaf population as one of the main communication barriers that they experienced. Earlier scholars have also highlighted the struggle that the Deaf has within medical centres in other parts of the world (Basu, 2020; Tan, 2020). Thus, like the earlier findings (Engelman et al., 2020), most informants shared that they had to rely on family members who could elaborate on the issue of COVID-19, which helped them to understand the situation better. In addition, those who are educated were also able to understand the written communication materials by the government and non-governmental organisations better than others. A few highlighted that not all Deaf members are fortunate to have concerned and supportive family members who were able to keep them informed in a timely manner. Thus, some of them claimed to have initiated efforts to try and clarify some concerns among their Deaf peers.

Though the Malaysian government showed initiatives to create 'bit size' and visual information to enable an easier grasp of information such as infographics and campaign posters, the government also used a few platforms such as the official website and social media accounts. However, as shared by the informant, not all would be able to interpret the visuals accurately, and it is still best to have individuals who can explain them using Malaysian Sign Language. In cases where news channels and special announcements included BIM interpreters (JBIM), some informants noted that the JBIM tended to be placed in a small box at the bottom corner of the screen – either not visible when viewing from their smartphones or the running titles of the news would affect the visibility of the sign language done.

When asked about respondents' experiences in the hospital, a few mentioned that they have heard of the availability of a Deaf liaison who was tasked to communicate some vital information about COVID-19 to the Deaf community, as well as be part of collaborative talks between medical experts and the Deaf community. However, these are pocketed efforts that would benefit specific Deaf communities due to their locality, social network, and accessibility (Tan, 2020). Instead, efforts to properly communicate with the Deaf should have been formally institutionalised and done systematically to ensure that no one is left behind (Al Majali & Alghazo, 2021).

Another aspect of communication that the Deaf women highlighted was communicating with the doctors and nurses. They claimed that it has always been a challenge communicating with hospital personnel even before COVID-19, but during COVID-19, it has gotten worse (Al Majali & Alghazo, 2021). Unable to communicate their health status, medical history, ongoing medication, or the effect they feel during the process of COVID-19 infection may have affected the diagnosis or prescriptions of these individuals (Tan, 2020). Moreover, the lack of understanding of the virus and its effect on individuals made them anxious and unable to engage in effective two-way communication with the doctors and nurses, making the experience worse for them. Two of them spoke about their lack of clarity on the link between pregnancy as well as severe menstrual cramps and COVID-19. These communication issues exemplify the complexity of the COVID-19 impact on Deaf women.

The respondents also highlighted the communication breakdown that happened due to mask-wearing during the pandemic. Since the mask covers most of the face as well as the mouth, these coverings affect the effectiveness of the communication as facial expression plays an essential role in delivering meaning and intention as well as accentuating the sign words (sords) (Haile, 2021; Saltsman, 2020; Water for Women, 2020). The mask also may affect those wearing the hearing aid as both the mask ear loop and the hearing aid are worn around the ear (Saltsman, 2020). There are Deaf-friendly masks that expose the lip area and most parts of the face in the market and are accessible to the Malaysian population (Basu, 2020). However, it has not been a norm among the Deaf, let alone among the frontliners who need to communicate with the Deaf population.

Deaf women who are mothers also mentioned that the challenge lies in communicating with others during the quarantine phase. They were worried about their children, especially those with younger children, to feed and care for them. Due to single-income household arrangements, significant others may not take on this role or need to work. Any additional support needed either to employ an interpreter to communicate with the hospital personnel or to support their child at home means additional costs that they would have to bear. Thus, the lived experience of Deaf women surrounding the issue of communication can also be linked to their educational background, sign language proficiency, available support from significant others, work, and household arrangements, as well as access to interpreters.

Financial Constraints and Well-Being

Besides exploring the effective communication factors and role of the support system of the respondents, financial constraints also affected Deaf women substantially during the COVID-19 pandemic. To begin with, some of the informants highlighted that the Deaf community members tend to engage in low-paying jobs, work on a project basis or commission basis, as well as part-time work arrangements. It is also not uncommon for the Deaf to be unemployed and live on a single household income with their husbands (who may also be Deaf) serving as the primary breadwinner. Thus, for these Deaf women, financial constraints are felt immensely for those who categorise themselves as 'poor' and make ends meet daily for the couple and their children.

Statistics in the US, as reported in 2016 by National Deaf Centre, highlight this issue – only 53.3% of Deaf are employed, which can be contrasted to 75.8% of hearing people. Out of those employed, about 60% of them are male, and 50% are female (Garberoglio et al., 2019). Unemployment rates increased with each additional intersection of marginalised identities, including race or additional disabilities. Unfortunately, in Malaysia, there is no official published data on the labour force participated by the Deaf population.

The concerns lie in, first, the loss of jobs or sources of income during the pandemic. The low-paid work, part-time work, or project-based work is most susceptible to losing their income during the trying times. Statistically, during the first year of the pandemic, Malaysia saw a 40% increase in unemployment (711,000 people) with more women than men affected by this (Free Malaysia Today, 2022). Some Deaf individuals are small business owners, again impacted by the affected economy. These individuals then find it difficult even to get other jobs, and the single-income household arrangement translates into the inability to support the household. Some of the women also shared that their husbands only gave them a small amount of money to manage the bills and groceries for the entire family during this pandemic due to the current conditions. These women then resorted to borrowing money from their parents or friends.

The pressure then adds to the second issue of these financial constraints – women as wives and mothers are often obliged to feed and maintain the well-being of the family members given the financial constraints. Though some sought help from associations and friends that they know, one of the respondents shared that many members of the Deaf do not generally open up about their personal or familial issues to others. This adds to the pressure experienced by these Deaf women, and some may resort to borrowing money with high interest or affect their mental well-being by not being able to manage their home well.

The pandemic also restricts physical and recreational activities. This affects their well-being due to a lack of exercise or endorphin release into the system. This is coupled with their increase in weight because of the lack of physical activity, which affects their physical and psychological well-being. These findings are also in line with previous studies that the COVID-19 pandemic has caused much stress and anger among the respondents and affected their well-being severely (Al Majali & Alghazo, 2021; Asmundson & Taylor, 2020; Dong & Bouey, 2020; Duan & Zhu, 2020; Haile, 2021; Kadam & Atre, 2020; Wang et al., 2020). Therefore, the financial status of these Deaf women alongside their financial social network, socioeconomic background, and social roles adds to the intersectionality experienced by the Deaf women.

Socialising and Social Support

A sound social support system often mediates one's well-being. Though it may not necessarily be due to support for finances, social support has been known to contribute to the better well-being of individuals. The importance of socialising is amplified in Malaysia due to the '**Mamak**' and '**lepak**' cultures. The 'Mamak' culture refers to the 24-hour restaurants, which are affordable, easily accessible, often have open-spaced areas, and may even have TV and screens for communal viewing of football or other sports. People often head to Mamak to '**lepak**' or hang out until the wee hours. Of course, this is not the only form of socialising site for Deaf Malaysians, but it is common and preferred by many.

This social norm was affected substantially during the pandemic, especially during the government's different phases of a Movement Control Order. In the first phase, the restaurants were not allowed to operate, and the residents were required to stay at home. In the second phase, the restaurants are open, but no dine-in was allowed – only takeaways/delivery services. In the third phase, the restaurants were allowed to have dine-ins, with strict standard operating procedures (SOPs) and a limited number of customers. The tables and seating arrangements were also highly regulated; failing to observe would mean a high penalty, and the fourth phase enabled the restaurants to operate with more members within each table while still observing the SOPs.

In addition, the Movement Control Order also affected the physical movement of individuals and the congregation of individuals within the enclosed vicinity, including the citizens' homes. During the Movement Control Order (MCO), individuals were not allowed to travel within more than a 10 km radius of where they resided. The number of members in the car was limited to one person unless those travelling to the hospital or for emergencies. Then the regulation enables two individuals within the same household to travel within a 10 km radius. To move beyond requires approval from the Malaysian government and/or a police support letter. In the later phase, travelling beyond the 10 km radius was lifted but restrained from interstate movement. During these movement control phases, big festivities celebrated by Malaysians were also affected. Strict SOPs and the control of only 15 people within the household translate into immense despair among members of the society.

Again, these were experienced by all residing in Malaysia at that point – not specifically among Deaf women. However, as mentioned above, these restrictions negatively impacted the social well-being of the respondents. One of the informants shared that as someone who is physically expressive, this restriction affected her emotionally in addition to socially. Similar findings were found in earlier research findings (Haile, 2021), and having others around during the pandemic, such as living with others or having family members around, tends to reduce the risk of fear, anxiety, and depression of the Deaf during the pandemic (Al Majali & Alghazo, 2021). Relating to the author's informant, the control movement order was complicated when she was going through a hard time and just wished to express herself in person. There were efforts to manage such a social gap; for example, some of them resorted to scheduled online meetings with their significant others. However, it is rather challenging when the internet is unstable. Unlike their hearing counterparts, who could choose to switch off the video and rely on verbal communication during internet instability, the Deaf community are not able to do so.

Their hanging out sessions with others also are essential as they are often the source of information. The informant hypothesises that a *lepak* session is possible during the earlier pandemic, of course, by observing the required SOPs, the Deaf community may have a better understanding of the pandemic and/or be able to cope with the pandemic better emotionally and psychologically. They will not feel disconnected, irrational, and unnecessary fear and have their support system to keep them at bay.

Interpersonal Conflict

Interpersonal conflict was one of the issues faced by Deaf women during the pandemic. Statistics in Malaysia regarding physical and sexual violence saw a sharp rise during this period with a 57% increase in 2021 compared to that in 2020 (Suwannarat, 2021). The global trend, as highlighted by the United Nations in April 2020, warned that the consequences of six months of quarantine resulted in increased domestic violence globally, while the National Deaf Domestic Violence hotline in the US showed an increase of 200% within the first quarter of 2020 in Katz, 2020). Though there is no available data reflecting the Deaf women per se, the data also suggest the link to financial difficulties, job insecurities, and mental stress as the contributing factors, which are not uncommon experiences by Deaf women. They, too, are the statistics of women suffering during the pandemic.

Like the issue of finances mentioned above, abuse is another topic that is often being suffered in silence among Deaf women. The informants shared that they avoid discussing this openly with others, but they also hardly sought professional help. It was reasoned that these women tend to be ashamed of what they are experiencing and worry that the word gets around. Since the community is relatively small, they loathe the idea that others know what happened in the bedroom and would be ashamed of what happened. Getting professional help is relatively tricky because some of them do not know where to seek such help, or they are not financially able to seek help. Even if they go to governmental-based assistance or non-governmental organizations (NGOs), they believe that assistance will not be Deaf-friendly. They would still need to fork out money to pay for interpreting services, a luxury during the pandemic.

Similar reasoning was also given when they were asked why not seek assistance from the police to report abuse cases. That was a case where the Deaf lady wanted to lodge a report with the help of a hearing family member who could sign, which was denied by the police because the family member may not report the case as it is stated by the person reporting. Instead, she was asked to find another interpreter, who was not a family member. This does not only make the process more complicated but also the financial burden for her to record her case. Though the issue of abuse is not a unique issue faced by Deaf women during the pandemic, the communication breakdown and the required interpretation made it harder for Deaf women to seek assistance and may end up suffering in silence. Other Deaf women in the US have reported a similar experience – it is challenging for Deaf women to report their abuse cases due to communication breakdown. An effort has been made in the

US to encourage the full-on usage of text-to-911, which is more accessible to the Deaf community (Katz, 2020). Hence, the safety of Deaf women and their bodies was also among the concerns and challenges that confronted the respondents of this research, showcasing the importance to recognise the intersectionality when analysing the impact of COVID-19.

Moving Forward: A Final Thought

The pandemic has affected Deaf women in terms of their communication with others, financial constraints and well-being, socialising, and social support, as well as interpersonal conflict. As indicated above, these issues may not necessarily be unique experiences or only realised during the pandemic. However, the intersection of social identity based on their disability, gender, marital status, occupation, and socioeconomic status, among others need to be considered to understand the multifaceted impact of the COVID-19 pandemic. Some of the issues may not be new, but these issues are exacerbated due to the pandemic. Given the reactive nature (rather than preventive) of the authorities and policymakers, these issues may be quickly 'forgotten' once the pandemic is over. Hence, the author argues that it is imperative to take note of and improve on these issues as soon as possible. This is to avoid the prolonged impact which in turn may have serious repercussions on the individuals, society, and the nation.

The Deaf concerns may not be given much emphasis due to the fetish with the majority (hearing people), the inability to empathise with the Deaf, or that their plight is easily silenced. Of course, the Deaf have been doing 'okay' all along and survived well, but their well-being and life chances may be affected because of this lack of sensitivity. The respondents have informed that even basic access to employment has been a challenge prior to and now heightened before the pandemic. Some Deaf were not hired because most jobs require them to 'speak,' or the employers are not confident in hiring disabled persons. With the narrow-mindedness of the employers and structural barriers, Deaf members are more likely to remain unemployed, unable to secure full-time jobs, and be hired only for specific 'suitable' work. Those jobs oftentimes are low-paying ones, i.e., data entry, driver, delivery person. This is coupled with employers neither being able to sign nor understand the Deaf culture. Thus, many initiatives that were done at the organisational and national levels are often not Deaf-friendly as they are based on baseless assumptions that the hearing majority have towards the Deaf. Therefore, the author argues that though training for the Deaf is imperative to increase the life chances of the Deaf, training for the hearing is also imperative to truly achieve an inclusive society.

The lack of openness among Deaf women to talk about their issues, be it financial or abuse, is not surprising but rather worrying. These discussions do not come naturally but instead would have undergone a cultural transformation due to ideological and paradigm shifts. How can society educate Deaf women on keeping them safe, what can be done when confronted with issues like this, why it is okay for them to ask for help, and whom they can seek help from are among some vital questions that these women should be able to answer? Should they be well informed and choose to keep to themselves, that is their personal choice. However, authorities should have a fundamental obligation to ensure that the Deaf are given the necessary knowledge, skills, and opportunities to understand and manage the situation accordingly when confronted (Yao et al., 2020; Zhai & Du, 2020).

This is especially when earlier data shows that Deaf women are more at risk than their hearing counterparts to be victims of relationship violence, sexual assault, forced sex, and physical abuse in their lifetimes (Pollard et al., 2014). Compared to a sample of hearing female undergraduates (Sabina & Straus, 2008), twice as many Deaf respondents (52%) reported experiencing past-year IPV. In this Gallaudet sample's responses to past-year IPV, 91% reported experiencing psychological aggression, 61% sexual coercion, and 52% physical assault.

Various movements and initiatives have been carried out by the government to inform and prepare women better, but these efforts tend to sideline Deaf women. The current support system and activities are not inclusive or Deaf-friendly. Their lack of knowledge does not reflect their inability to comprehend but rather the systematic marginalisation of Deaf women. It is time for a targeted initiative to ensure that Deaf women possess the relevant information about financial and interpersonal conflict challenges (among many others) as well as skills to manage them. They should also have access to support systems and professional services with more professionals to be proficient in BIM or train the Deaf to possess the necessary skills to be in the helping profession.

It is hoped that this chapter provided much-needed insights on Deaf women during the COVID-19 pandemic. The author would like to reiterate the importance of understanding the intersections of social identities and realise that Deaf women do not experience daily lives and challenges similarly. The author believes that training individuals and providing institutional support are imperative to support the professional development of the Deaf community and ensure that equal educational, social, physical, and psychological support opportunities are observed, which in turn can benefit the community.

References

Abuelgasim, E., Saw, L. J., Shirke, M., Zeinah, M., & Harky, A. (2020). COVID-19: Unique public health issues facing Black, Asian and minority ethnic communities. *Current Problems in Cardiology*, *45*, 100621. Advance online publication. https://doi.org/10.1016/j.cpcardiol.2020.100621. PMID:32448759.

Almeida, R. C. N., Schiaffino, R. S., & Rumjanek, V. M. (2014). Access and comprehension of information by profound deaf youngsters in Brazil. *Journal of Media and Communication Studies*, *6*(11), pp. 174–178. https://doi.org/10.5897/jmcs2014.0411.

Al Majali, S. A., & Alghazo, E. M. (2021). Mental health of individuals who are deaf during COVID-19: Depression, anxiety, aggression, and fear. *Journal of Community Psychology*. https://doi.org/10.1002/jcop.22539.

Asmundson, G. J., & Taylor, S. (2020). Coronaphobia: Fear and the 2019-nCoV outbreak. *Journal of Anxiety Disorders*, *70*, 102196. https://doi.org/10.1016/j.janxdis.2020.102196.

Basu, T. (May 28, 2020). The pandemic made life harder for deaf people. The solutions could benefit everyone. https://www.technologyreview.com/2020/05/28/1002314/clear-mask-captioning-live-transcription-deaf-coronavirus-pandemic/.

Chang, M. J., & Lipner, S. R. (2020). Caring for deaf and hard-of-hearing patients in dermatology during the COVID-19 pandemic. *Dermatologic Therapy*, *33*(6), e14185. https://doi.org/10.1111/dth.14185.

Collins, P. H. (2002). *Black Feminist Thought: Knowledge, Consciousness, and the Politics of Empowerment*. New York: Routledge.

Dong, L., & Bouey, J. (2020). Public mental health crisis during COVID-19 pandemic, China. *Emerging Infectious Diseases*, *26*, pp. 10–3201. https://doi.org/10.3201/eid2607.20240.

Duan, L., & Zhu, G. (2020). Psychological interventions for people affected by the COVID-19 epidemic. *The Lancet Psychiatry*, *7*, pp. 300–302. https://doi.org/10.1016/s2215-0366(20)30073-0.

Engelman, A., Paludneviciene, R., Wagner, K., Jacobs, K., & Kushalnagar, P. (2020). Food worry in the deaf and hard-of-hearing population during the COVID-19 pandemic. *Public Health Reports*, pp. 1–6. https://doi.org/10.1177/0033354920974666.

Free Malaysia Today. (2022). *Malaysia's Unemployment Levels Rose by 83% in 2020, Asean Stats Show*. https://www.freemalaysiatoday.com/category/nation/2022/06/02/Malaysia-fourth-largest-in-unemployment-in-2020-ASEAN-stats-show/.

Garberoglio, C. L., Palmer, J. L., Cawthon, S. W., & Sales, A. (2019). Deaf people and employment in the United States: 2019. National Deaf Center on Postsecondary Outcomes. https://www.nationaldeafcenter.org/sites/default/files/Deaf%20People%20and%20Employment%20in%20the%20United%20States_%202019%20(7.26.19)(ENGLISH)(WEB).pdf.

Haile, L. (2021). Hearing loss, social isolation, and the COVID-19 pandemic. *Think Global Health*. https://www.thinkglobalhealth.org/article/hearing-loss-social-isolation-and-covid-19-pandemic.

Hazian Sa'ari. (2009). The effectiveness and efficiency in the usage of software e-MySL© in Learning Malaysian Sign Language (MySQL). Conference on Scientific & Social Research. A' Famosa Resort Hotel Malacca, 14–15 March 2009.

Hub Editorial. (April 23, 2020). COVID-19 poses unique challenges for people with disabilities. *HUB, Johns Hopkins Magazine*. https://hub.jhu.edu/2020/04/23/how-covid-19-affects-people-with-disabilities/.

Jabatan Kebajikan Masyarakat [JKM]. (2018). *Pendaftaran orang kurang upaya*. https://www.jkm.gov.my/jkm/index.php?r=portal/left&id=UnN2U3dtUHhacVN4aHNPbUlPayt2QT09.

Kadam, A. B., & Atre, S. R. (2020). Social media panic and COVID-19 in India. *Journal of Travel Medicine*, *27*, taaa057. https://doi.org/10.1093/jtm/taaa057.

Katz, S. (June 22, 2020). Many deaf women aren't safer at home. https://www.bitchmedia.org/article/deaf-women-domestic-violence-pandemic.

Lima, C. K. T., de Medeiros Carvalho, P. M., Lima, I. D. A. S., de Oliveira Nunes, J. V. A., Saraiva, J. S., de Souza, R. I., Lian da Silva, C. G., & Neto, M. L. R. (2020). The emotional impact of coronavirus 2019-nCoV (new coronavirus disease). *Psychiatry Research*, *287*, 112915. https://doi.org/10.1016/j.psychres.2020.112915.

McKee, M., Schlehofer, D., Cuculick, J., Starr, M., Smith, S., & Chin, N. P. (2011). Perceptions of cardiovascular health in an underserved community of deaf adults using American Sign Language. *Disability and Health Journal*, *4*(3), pp. 192–197. https://doi.org/10.1016/j.dhjo.2011.04.001. PMID:21723526.

McKee, M. M., Barnett, S. L., Block, R. C., & Pearson, T. A. (2011). Impact of communication on preventive services among deaf American Sign Language users. *American Journal of Preventive Medicine, 41*(1), pp. 75–79. https://doi.org/10.1016/j.amepre.2011.03.004. PMID:21665066.

McKee, M. M., Paasche-Orlow, M. K., Winters, P. C., Fiscella, K., Zazove, P., Sen, A., & Pearson, T. (2015). Assessing health literacy in deaf American Sign Language users. *Journal of Health Communication, 20*(Suppl. 2), pp. 92–100. https://doi.org/10.1080/10810730.2015.1066468.

Merriam-Webster Dictionary. (2022). *Intersectionality.* https://www.merriam-webster.com/dictionary/intersectionality.

Ministry of Health Malaysia. (2020). *Laporan Kluster COVID-19 Yang Aktif di Malaysia (sehingga 29 April 2020).* Putrajaya: Ministry of Health Malaysia.

Murray, J. J. (2020). Improving signed language and communication accessibility during COVID-19 Pandemic [online exclusive]. *The Hearing Journal.* https://journals.lww.com/thehearingjournal/blog/onlinefirst/pages/post.aspx?PostID=66.

Panko, T. L., Contreras, J., Postl, D., Mussallem, A., Champlin, S., Paasche-Orlow, M. K., Hill, J., Plegue, M. A., Hauser, P. C., & McKee, M. (2021). The deaf community's experiences navigating COVID-19 pandemic information. *Health Literacy Research and Practice, 5*(2), pp. e162–e170. https://doi.org/10.3928/24748307-20210503-01.

Piller, I., Zhang, J., & Li, J. (2020). Linguistic diversity in a time of crisis: Language challenges of the COVID-19 pandemic. *Multilingua, 39*(5), pp. 503–515. https://doi.org/10.1515/multi-2020-0136.

Pollard, R. Q. Jr, Sutter, E., & Cerulli, C. (2014). Intimate partner violence was reported by two samples of deaf adults via a computerized American sign language survey. *Journal of Interpersonal Violence, 29*(5), pp. 948–965. https://doi.org/10.1177/0886260513505703.

Rose, B. (April 28, 2020). Coronavirus: Lack of sign language interpreters leads to legal case against government. *BBC News.* https://www.bbc.com/news/disability-52323854.

Sabina, C. & Straus, M. (2008). Polyvictimization by Dating Partners and Mental Health Among US College Students. Violence and victims, 23, 667–82.

Saltsman, L. (2020). How COVID-19 impacts the deaf & hard-of-hearing community. *Health Hive.* https://hive.rochesterregional.org/2020/10/covid-impact-on-deaf-community.

Shew, A. (2020). Let COVID-19 expand awareness of disability tech. *Nature, 581*(7806), p. 9. https://doi.org/10.1038/d41586-020-01312-w.

Suwannarat, S. (September 24, 2021). COVID-19 sparks a pandemic of domestic violence. *PIME Asia News.* https://www.asianews.it/news-en/COVID-19-sparks-a-pandemic-of-domestic-violence-54137.html.

Tamaskar, P., Malia, T., Stern, C., Gorenflo, D., Meador, H., & Zazove, P. (2000). Preventive attitudes and beliefs of deaf and hard-of-hearing individuals. *Archives of Family Medicine, 9*(6), 518–525. https://doi.org/10.1001/archfami.9.6.518. PMID:10862214.

Tan, M. Z. (October 28, 2020). Covid-19: To help the Deaf, Malaysian academics translate screening questions into sign language (VIDEO). *Malay Mail.* https://www.malaymail.com/news/life/2020/10/28/covid-19-to-help-the-deaf-malaysian-academics-translate-screening-questions/1917168.

The Star Online. (October 14, 2020). Turning the tide on Malaysia's third COVID-19 wave. https://www.thestar.com.my/news/nation/2020/10/14/turning-the-tide-on-malaysias-third-covid-19-wave.

Tonelli, M., & Warick, R. (2022). Focusing on the needs of people with hearing loss during the COVID-19 pandemic and beyond. *JAMA, 327*(12), pp. 1129–1130. https://doi.org/10.1001/jama.2022.3026.

United Nations Population Fund United Nations Population Fund (UNFPA) and Women Enabled International (WEI). (2021). *The Impact of COVID-19 on Women and Girls with Disabilities: A Global Assessment and Case Studies on Sexual and Reproductive Health and Rights, Gender-Based Violence, and Related Rights.* https://www.unfpa.org/featured-publication/impact-covid-19-women-and-girls-disabilities.

Valentine, G., & Skelton, T. (2009). An umbilical cord to the world. *Information Communication and Society, 12*(1), pp. 44–65. https://doi.org/10.1080/13691180802158573

Wang, C., Pan, R., Wan, X., Tan, Y., Xu, L., Ho, C. S., & Ho, R. C. (2020). Immediate psychological responses and associated factors during the initial stage of the 2019 coronavirus disease (COVID-19) epidemic among the general population in China. *International Journal of Environmental Research and Public Health, 17*, p. 1729. https://doi.org/10.3390/ijerph17051729.

Water for Women. (December 1, 2020). *Supporting the Deaf and Hard of Hearing to Communicate during COVID-19.* https://www.waterforwomenfund.org/en/news/supporting-the-deaf-and-hard-of-hearing-to-communicate-during-covid-19.aspx.

Wollin, J., & Elder, R. (2003). Mammograms and pap smears for Australian deaf women. *Cancer Nursing, 26*(5), pp. 405–409. https://doi.org/10.1097/00002820-200310000-00010 PMID:14710803.

World Health Organization. (2022). Integrated people-centred ear and hearing care: policy brief. https://apps.who.int/iris/handle/10665/339957.

Yao, H., Chen, J. H., & Xu, Y. F. (2020). Rethinking online mental health services in China during the COVID-19 epidemic. *Asian Journal of Psychiatry, 50*, 102015. https://doi.org/10.1016/j.ajp.2020.102015.

Zhai, Y., & Du, X. (2020). Mental health care for international Chinese students affected by the COVID-19 outbreak. *The Lancet Psychiatry, 7*, e22. https://doi.org/10.1016/s2215-0366(20)30089-4.

Part IV
Education

11 Female Academics' Career Progression and Motivation during COVID-19

An African Perspective

Rashmi Watson, Upasana G. Singh and Chenicheri Sid Nair

Introduction

The current chapter reports on a small snapshot of experiences of female academics working in African higher education institutions (HEIs) as a summary of their perceptions about career progression, workload, and motivation since the start of the global pandemic in early 2020. The study provides data to HEIs for possible future adaptations and opportunities to continue integrating and supporting the female academic workforce. To ensure the gender gaps, disparities, biases, or hardships are not made even greater during this COVID-19 pandemic period, where females have been uniquely impacted, and work–life balance (WLB) issues can be addressed by HEI policies (Okeke-Uzodike and Gamede, 2021). Adjusting to remote work or working from home (WFH) and having WLB are new and evolving factors. Academics have responded positively and negatively to both WFH and WLB and have realigned themselves, home duties and families/others they reside with whilst continuing work in the remote, and online distance work as a *new normal* way of being an academic in 2022.

The increasingly rapid changes faced by academics across the globe to adapt and adopt new ways of working remotely whilst maintaining a balanced work and home life has proved challenging. New and emerging literature is regularly being published providing Higher education institutions (HEIs) with evidence-based data about how they may better understand and respond to academics to support them in the best possible way. Such research includes the reshaping of digital teaching and learning pedagogies and the use of new online, video conferencing formats (Lalani et al., 2021), issues with digital equity issues (Costello et al., 2020), supporting academics to work in remote modes, gather feedback on their own teaching, and maintain a secure online environment (Heitz et al., 2020).

Additional support specifically for female academics through and post-pandemic is also an emerging body of research in providing support to maintain work and life balance (Watson et al., 2022a) reducing the increased anxiety, social isolation, challenges of communicating with colleagues and benefits of working from home (Watson et al., 2022b, Couch et al., 2021). Female academic experiences provide

DOI: 10.4324/9781003267133-15

deeper insight into the additional responsibilities that COVID-19 has required by all academics but additionally for females as the primary carers and home managers. Benefits from the shift to remote learning have been viewed through opportunities to enhance teaching through flexible, blended, hybrid, and a blend of synchronous and asynchronous methods of learning (Marinoni et al., 2020).

Female academics are experiencing greater global hardship at a time when female academics are already constantly facing reduced gender disparity (Malisch et al., 2020) and recognition for skills and contribution as academic teachers and published researchers (Walters et al., 2022). The underrepresentation of females in academia and leadership roles is well published (Deryugina et al., 2021, Krause, 2017, Gabster et al., 2020). Academic progression is an important component of academic life. Recognition of success from early-career academics through to senior levels such as Associate Professor/Professor, usually take many years to achieve through formal and rigorous higher education, academic promotional processes with a high level of evidence of research and teaching quality output. However, research output for females has taken a hit with a high reduction of papers across many disciplines including health and humanities (Amano-Patiño et al., 2020, Gabster et al., 2020). It is reported that career progression has stalled for almost 40% of academics and equally around the same reporting that it has progressed well for them during the COVID pandemic (Kolakowski et al., 2021).

A New Way of Working

Like everywhere else across the globe, academics across Africa had to pivot to a working-from-home model from 26 March 2020 and learn/apply new technological teaching and learning and ways to interact remotely with colleagues and students. Technological competence and preparedness for online, remote teaching practices and response to isolation from others were factors to acceptance and adaptability. The transition has created new collaborations and opportunities such as the ability to attend remote conferences and open access to resources and increased collaboration globally (Fernandez and Shaw, 2020). The boundaries of work and home life in this current pandemic period have now become somewhat blurred (Anwer, 2020) as a new model of working since 2020 has been the remote, offline, virtual world of work bringing new challenges and stresses. Walters et al. (2022) reported on the high increase in balancing academic workloads with the 'traditional family roles assumed by females while working from home,' (p. 2) and the decline in research activity among female academics in public universities.

Academics are not new to working from home or taking work home as a regular part of an academic life (Anwer, 2020); however, components that could be outsourced such as childcare, school, domestic work, and meals outside of the home have now all become key responsibilities of the home carers, namely females. In 2021, a global report where 5,000 females across ten countries, including 500 respondents from South Africa, were surveyed suggests that gender equality has regressed during the pandemic, workloads increased (77%), and care responsibilities have increased for their own children/others (79%) (Deloitte, 2021).

Work–Life Balance

The figures are slightly higher (67%) for females 'of colour' (Deloitte, 2021) holding the responsibility for household tasks. Implicit in work–life balance often lies work–family balance, and where high-powered females manage to balance a 'spectacularly successful career with a satisfying home life' (Rottenberg, 2014, p. 428). Higher workloads may lead to work-related stress causing negative physical and emotional impacts on employees (Kotteeswari and Sharief, 2014). Due to the continuing pandemic unpredictability and ongoing evolving virus strains, organisational support and job stress are key factors influencing the acceptance of the 'new way' of working online.

The rapid changes to having to work remotely and independently online with the forced adoption of using technology to conduct routine tasks have posed a challenge for many employees causing academic stress (Hadiwijaya and Sentanu, 2021). All the stress can thus lead to less motivation and less productivity. Motivation was difficult to maintain with remote teaching and an increased workload requiring attending to additional tasks leading to exhaustion (Oliveira et al., 2021).

Method

Context and Rationale

The world has been facing a pandemic known as the novel coronavirus disease (COVID-19) since late 2019 and the higher education sector has had to rapidly adjust, pivot, adapt, create, and adopt new ways of working and relating to each other (García-Morales et al., 2021) to respond to changes thrust on academics globally. The context of this study is important in the future support of females in the academic workforce in the continent of Africa, the focus of this chapter. The authors acknowledge how the pandemic has affected *all* academics regardless of gender; however, the pandemic has brought to light the gender differences in the lived experiences of female academics with additional care and home responsibilities. The authors recognise that global experiences amongst female academics can be vastly different based on but not limited to the pandemic extensiveness, its impact, pre-pandemic policies, and approaches to supporting female academics and economic status and affordances.

The researchers are based in Africa and Australia and as such have conducted collaborative research exploring experiences across both continents about the pandemic, remote teaching (Singh et al., 2022), working from home (Watson et al., 2022a), and the female academic experience (Watson et al., 2022b). This current study, as a small sample where broad generalisations cannot be definitively made, is instead viewed as a sample and insight into the context of experiences of African female academics. This study may provide an insight for continued attention and response by HEIs for future support of female academics to ensure sustainability and renewal as valued members of academia. This chapter also draws on Burger and Luckmann's social construction of knowledge (Dreher, 2016) whereby respondents are the power structures experiencing the pandemic through the lens of female academics in their own African context. A new narrative and social discourse or phenomenology are being developed about new ways of being, working, interacting (Gergen and Wortham, 2001), and what it means to be a female academic in 2022 (Couch et al., 2021).

Research Questions, Collection, and Analysis

Ethics approval was received through the University of Western Australia (REF: ET000781). The questions being reported are as follows:

1. How motivated do African female academics feel about career progression since the pandemic and what are the factors contributing to their stated level of motivation?
2. How the respondents perceived their level of opportunities to progress as a female academic, the status of the female academic at their institution, and the level of support by their HEI for work–life balance.
3. How do African female academics perceive their workload since the start of the pandemic and their ability to manage?

Data were collected through an online survey using a mixed-method approach with both open qualitative questions and closed quantitative questions. The authors were spread across Africa and Australia and this chapter was prepared from previously collected data from female academics' experiences through the pandemic, hence the connection between the University of Western Australia (UWA) and the African context. There were 33 questions in total (24 closed and nine open-ended) asking perceptions about academic workload, career progression, support, motivation, and academic leadership. Numerous means were used to encourage participation. Due to the pandemic, social distancing, and travel bans, the main source of invitation came from email distribution lists within each author's university in which the authors are based in Africa and Australia. As per the university design and ethics protocol, the researchers were able to request participation via formal processes within their HEIs and personal, academic networks using the approved ethics' communication for academic mailing lists, individual email, or social media requests including LinkedIn, Twitter, Facebook, and WhatsApp. From July to October 2021, data were collected from respondents spanning across the globe.

Thematic analysis has been used for the open-ended questions and descriptive statistical analysis for all closed questions. The specific thematic analysis applied was inductive thematic analysis, often used in mixed-method designs, as the theoretical flexibility of thematic analysis makes it a more straightforward choice than approaches with specific embedded theoretical assumptions (Creswell, 2003). Thematic analysis is a commonly used tool in qualitative research adopted to identify, analyse, describe, organise, and report themes found within a data set (Terry et al., 2017, Nowell et al., 2017b, Kiger and Varpio, 2020). An inductive thematic approach allows research findings to emerge from frequent, dominant, or

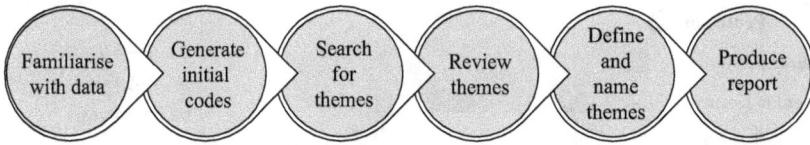

Figure 11.1 Thematic analysis process.

significant themes inherent in raw data (Liu, 2016). The thematic analysis model was adapted from Nowell et al. (2017a) and is illustrated in Figure 11.1.

Results

Demographics

From an online survey of female academics globally, there were 260 responses with 27 specifically from African female academics (10%) which provide the basis of data for this chapter. Whilst the response rate from African-specific female academics can be considered low, the qualitative data from the open-ended questions still provide a rich set of responses which can be shared amongst the academic community. Most African respondents (66%) stated they were married, (30%) were single, and one in a de facto relationship, and overall, most had at least one child under their care (89%) and (26%) with care responsibilities for an elderly parent/s living with them regardless of marital status. A smaller number (22%) stated they had no additional care responsibilities (see Figure 11.2). All respondents (100%) stated they had worked remotely at least once since February 2020 and the majority (78%) worked in a public HEI. Most respondents were in the 35–44 age range (37%) and at least in the 25–34 age range (14%). Respondents were in the early to mid-career level at lecturer or senior lecturer level (85%) with only one respondent in the (55–64 age range) at the highest academic ranking of Professor (see Figure 11.3).

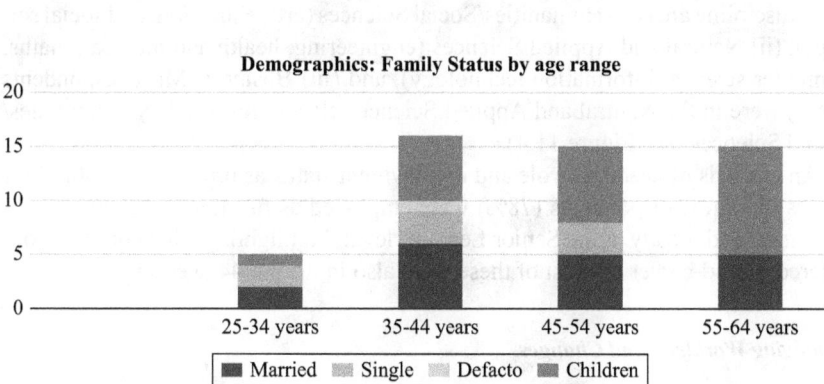

Figure 11.2 Demographics (family status by age range).

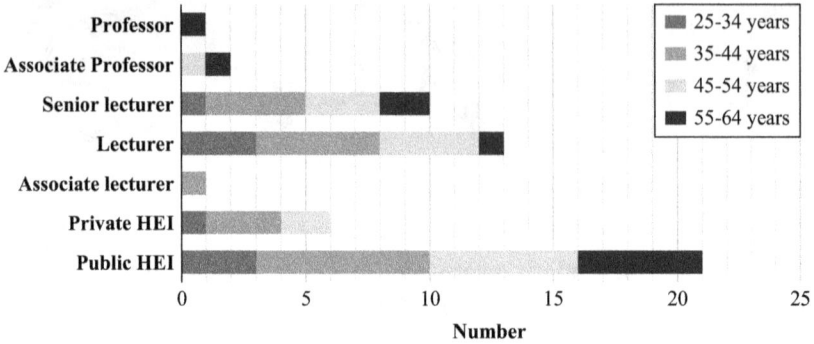

Figure 11.3 Demographics (academic level, age range, and HEI type).

Demographic (by discipline area)

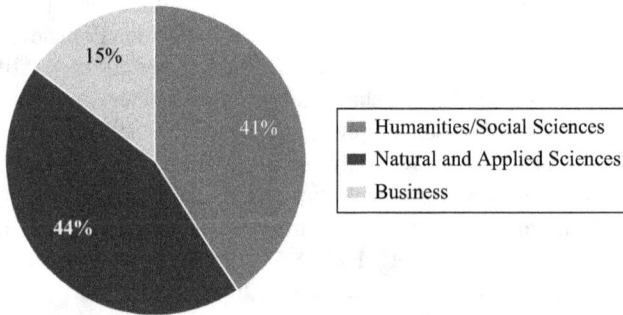

Figure 11.4 Demographics by discipline area/s.

The discipline areas selected by respondents have been categorised into three main discipline areas (i) Humanities/Social Sciences (arts, education, and social science), (ii) Natural and Applied Sciences (engineering, health and medical, maths, computer science, information technology), and (iii) Business. Most respondents (44%) were in the Natural and Applied Sciences closely followed by Humanities/ Social Sciences (see Figure 11.4).

An analysis of academic role and employment status as provided in Table 11.1 shows that most respondents (78%) were employed as full-time, ongoing permanent staff, and mostly at the Senior Lecturer level, highlighting what could be considered as mid-career as most of these were also in the 35–44 age range.

Managing Workload and Changes

In the online survey (i.e., 14 closed questions), respondents were asked to comment about workload changes since the start of the pandemic; how they perceived

Table 11.1 Demographics by employment status

Employment status N (%)				
Position type:	Adjunct (paid/ stipend)	Contract (part-time)	Full-time (contract)	Full-time (permanent)
Total Breakdown by level	1 (4%) Lecturer 1 (4%)	2 (7%) Lecturer 2 (7%)	3 (11%) Associate Lecturer 1 (33%) Lecturer 2 (67%)	Total =21 (78%) Lecturer 8 (38%) Senior Lecturer 10 (48%) Associate Professor 2 (9%) Professor 1 (5%)

managing their workload and how they perceived managing their workload with others in the home during the remote work. The results show that the highest response from the African female respondents stated their workload had *increased a great deal* (48%) followed by increased somewhat (9%) and equal (7%) stated *increased at the start/stayed approximately the same.* Only one respondent stated their workload had *decreased somewhat* and nil stated *decreased a great deal.* Overall, 88% of responses were related to any increase, 8% to staying the same and 4% to decreasing in any way.

When examining the age ranges in responses to workload, both the 45–64 age range and 55–64 age range had the highest equal response stating their work-load had increased a great deal (31%). The 35–44 age range had the highest response (33%) to an increase (to any degree) to their workload, followed by the 45–54 age range (30%). The one respondent who stated their workload had decreased somewhat was in the highest age bracket (55–64 years). Figure 11.5

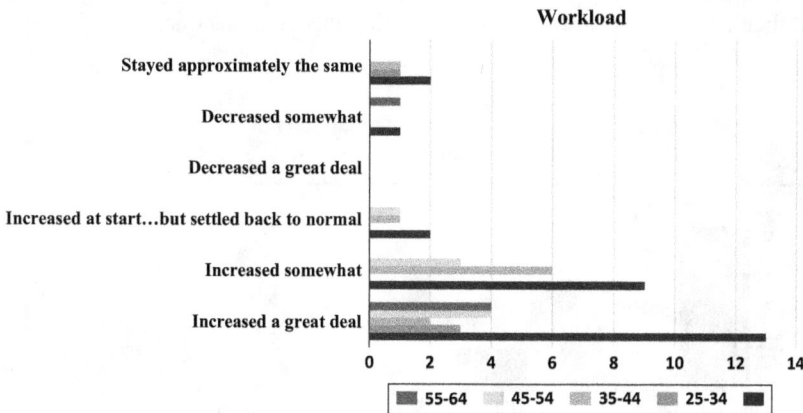

Figure 11.5 Perceptions of workload change.

shows that the data is based on qualitative, verbatim responses related to managing workload.

Although the question of workload was a closed question, there were numerous comments related to an increase in workload in the open-ended questions about the challenges that they perceived during COVID-19 as a female academic which have been provided below as supporting statements to the quantitative data in Figure 17.5.

> I cannot work around the clock and yet the university management seems to expect it.
>
> [ID_260]

> Employment duties have increased.
>
> [ID_9]

> Teaching workloads increased significantly in 2020 in relation to teaching and assessing undergraduate modules online, yet this was not considered when conducting performance assessments for 2020, with the same workload formula being applied as in previous years.
>
> [ID_160]

> Ridiculous deadlines and demands. At work they forget that if you are working from home, you are juggling work, home, and school.
>
> [ID_28]

Most respondents (74%) stated it was 'more difficult in managing home and work duties since the start of the pandemic'; a smaller number of respondents (18%) stated it was easier and 7% stated there was no difference (see Figure 11.6).

The respondents stated a higher proportion of agreement that managing working from home was 'easy to manage …' with a partner/family/children/other members (67%) partner/family/children/other members (67%) with just 33% stating it was difficult to manage with others. Supporting this sentiment are the following

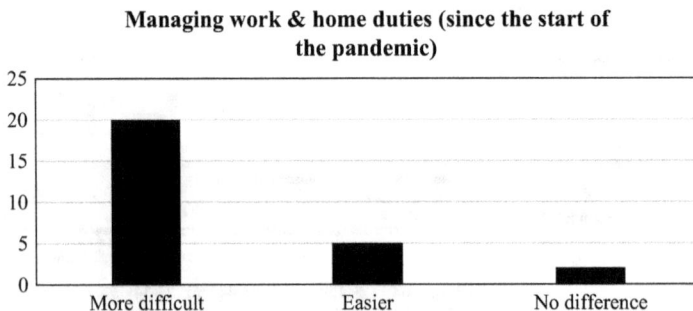

Figure 11.6 Perceptions of workload home change.

comments showing high agreement and positivity with the WFH approach providing benefits for increased family time, management, and ability to focus and find new opportunities such as attending conferences. See supporting comments below for the variations in responses.

> Working online is more economical; Flexibility to attend family duties; Giving quality time to children; Devoting additional time to my students.
>
> [ID_8]

> Managing your own time
>
> [ID_24]

> Working from home attending online conferences I would not be able to attend easily as a single parent.
>
> [ID_260]

> Uninterrupted chunks of time.
>
> [ID_26]

> Working from the comfort of my home. Spending more time with family. And I got time to see my daughter grow and was there for each milestone.
>
> [ID_27]

Motivation

The survey asked two questions about career motivation, one closed question and one open-ended question. A slightly higher portion of the African female respondents stated that they felt *less motivated* to progress in their career (48%): 44% stated feeling more motivated and one respondent (4%) stated feeling no difference in their motivation for career progression.

The motivation levels were the highest from the youngest to the oldest. The age range group of 25–34 years was the most positive with 100% saying they felt *more* motivated in their career progression. There were nil respondents in the youngest age range who felt less motivated and the 35–45 age range had the highest responses (70%) feeling *less* motivated in their career progression. The one respondent who stated no change in motivation was in the 45–54 age range (see Figure 11.7).

More Motivated

On further analysis of which academics felt more motivated by age range and academic status: the highest majority (33%) were in the youngest age range (25–34 years) and 50% were in the junior academic role of lecturer regardless of age range.

Motivation level (age range)

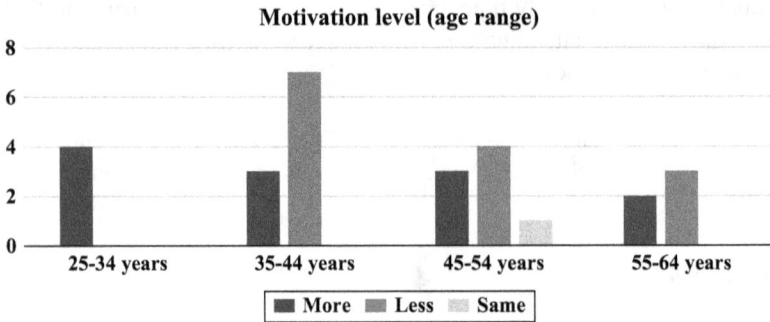

Figure 11.7 Motivation level by age range.

The motivation level percentage decreased by age range with the lowest motivation in the oldest age range (55+ years see Table 11.2).

In the open-ended question asking respondents about their response, see comments in the following related to feeling more motivated.

Less Motivated

Overall, the respondents who indicated as being *less motivated* (48%): there were 46% in the 35–44 age range making it the youngest age range as there will be nil in the 25–34 year range. The majority (46%) were in a junior academic role (lecturer). As can be seen in Table 11.3, there was a decreasing number who stated as being less motivated as the academic role levels increased to the higher levels.

Factors Contributing to Motivation Levels (Career Progression)

In the open-ended question asking respondents about their response to their motivation level, see comments in the following related to feeling less motivated, followed by more motivation and the contributing factors to greater motivation.

Less Motivation

The key theme to emerge from the respondents who stated they felt 'less' motivated was workload balance (62%), the others (31%) stated 'less opportunities' and (8%) stated their 'age' as a factor. Examples of feedback comments (verbatim) from participants highlight their reasoning for less motivation for career progression:

> Teaching loads have grown – staff numbers remain the same, but students grow. Balancing teaching and research have become close to impossible. At one time, I was only getting 4–5 hours sleep, to handle the demand. I have

Table 11.2 Motivation by age and academic level (more motivated)

Age range	Associate lecturer	Lecturer	Senior lecturer	Associate Professor	Professor	Total number of respondents
25–34 years	0 (0%)	3 (75%)	1 (25%)	0 (0%)	0	4 (33%)
35–44 years	0 (0%)	2 (67%)	1 (33%)	0 (0%)	0	3 (25%)
45–54 years	0 (0%)	1 (25%)	2 (50%)	0 (0%)	0	3 (25%)
55–64 years	0 (0%)	0 (0%)	1 (100%)	0 (0%)	1 (50%)	2 (17%)
Total	0	6 (50%)	5 (42%)	0	1 (8%)	12 (44%) of respondents

Table 11.3 Motivation by age and academic level (less motivated)

Age range	Associate lecturer	Lecturer	Senior lecturer	Associate Professor	Professor	Total (number)
25–34 years	0 (0%)	0 (0%)	0 (0%)	0 (0%)	0 (0%)	**0**
35–44 years	1 (8%)	3 (50%)	3 (50%)	0 (0%)	0 (0%)	**6 (46%)**
45–54 years	0 (0%)	3 (50%)	0 (0%)	1 (25%)	0 (0%)	**4 (31%)**
55–64 years	0 (0%)	1 (14%)	1 (50%)	1 (0%)	0 (0%)	**2 (23%)**
Total	1 (8%)	6 (46%)	4 (31%)	2 (15%)	0 (0%)	Total = 13 (48%) of total respondents

found it difficult to balance taking care of my children and family and doing work.

[ID_21]

I cannot work around the clock and yet the university management…expect it. Home life demands (children, mother) are constantly present…makes me despair.

[ID_28]

The first three comments are related to gender perceptions:

As a female one must work extra hard for recognition as compared to our male counterparts.

[ID_8]

Getting my husband to realise that I am working albeit online.

[ID_149]

Fewer opportunities for women; lack of response from professors; age discrimination … i.e., fewer opportunities for women over 35 yrs.

[ID_15]

The following comments are related to work–life balance issues:

I have had the flexibility to research and publish.

[ID_6]

The fact that there is more flexibility to teaching and learning. Now, we can employ various means to achieve maximum results. I feel less motivated as I find it difficult to balance career and home life.

[ID_75]

I moved from South Africa to the UK in the middle of the pandemic. In South Africa I could afford to hire a domestic worker to help at home. In the UK, this is too expensive. It was a huge adjustment, especially when children were at home due to lockdown. All this was not considered by our university. My husband is also an academic, and he helped a bit. However, the majority of managing the family and household were on me.

[ID_141]

The following statement is reflective of people reconsidering their employment status or role change considering lockdown periods and time spent at home:

I am nearing retirement and this time from home has motivated me to perhaps retire sooner than previously thought.

[ID_45]

More Motivation

The open responses by the respondents regarding positive motivation levels showed two *equal* top themes to emerge as (i) research and collaboration and (ii) flexibility (of time/access/self-management) at 48%, followed by online skills in teaching and a small percentage (11%) stated they could not foresee any new opportunities from the pandemic period (see Figure 11.8).

A sample of comments (verbatim) supporting the themes are: '*The flexibility and comfort of my job [ID_8];*' '*Seeing my baby while I work from home intermittently, being able to notice milestones, not having to commute to and from work [ID_44];*' '*The possible collaborative opportunities [ID_7.].*'

Opportunities for Career Progression

In response to the closed question about respondents' perceptions about their perceived *opportunities for career progression* since the start of the pandemic, 40% stated they felt there was *less* opportunity and 30% stated *equally* that they felt *more/same level* of opportunity for career progression. The following responses exemplify respondents' feelings:

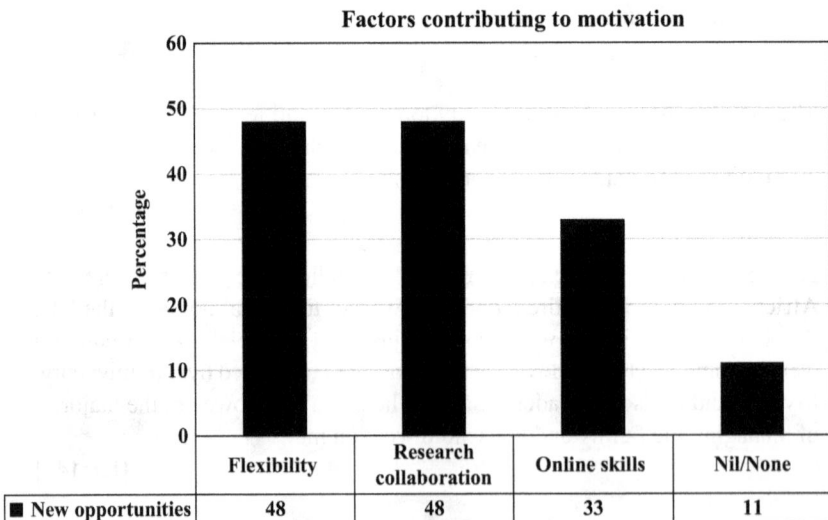

Factors contributing to motivation

	Flexibility	Research collaboration	Online skills	Nil/None
■ New opportunities	48	48	33	11

Figure 11.8 New opportunities.

Opportunities for career progression

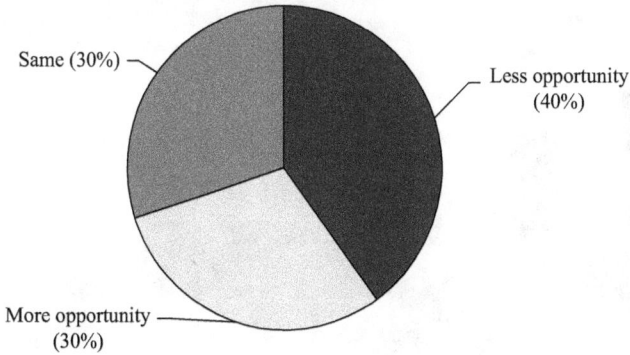

Figure 11.9 Perceptions for career progression.

(Less opportunities): 'Fewer opportunities for women; lack of response from professors; age discrimination ... i.e., fewer opportunities for women over 35 yrs ... [ID_5].'(More opportunities): 'The possibilities of what can be achieved [ID_259];' 'I take better care of myself. I enjoy virtual meetings. Less people politics [ID_27].'(No change): 'Intrinsic drive that I have irrespective of the pandemic [ID_26].'

See Figure 11.9.

Support Levels

In Figure 11.10, in the closed-response question, there were relatively equal responses as to how female academics perceived their HEI support level as a female academic for WLB. As can be seen, the results were 41% in agreement, 40% in disagreement, and 19% as unsure or neutral.

Academic Status

Respondents were asked to select their perception about female academic status (since the start of the pandemic). The highest response was in 'no difference' (52%) followed by 'unsure' (26%) and equal numbers of 'greater status' and 'less status' (see Figure 11.11).

Discussion

Managing Workload

Respondents in this study have stated it has been *more difficult* to manage home and work duties (74%); however, they also responded that it was *easy to manage*

Support from HEI (for WLB)

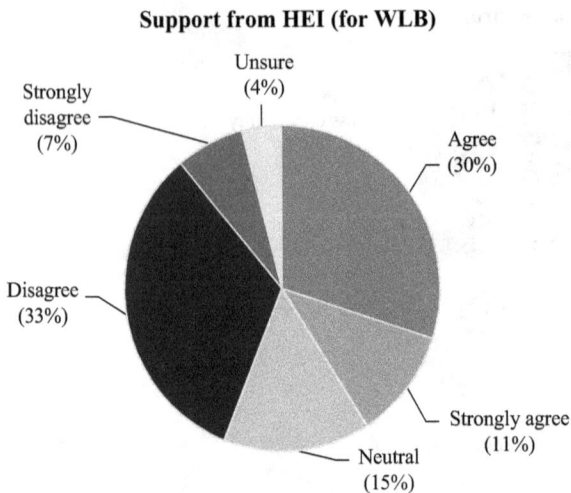

Figure 11.10 The HEI is responsive to the needs of the female academic (work–life balance).

Academic status

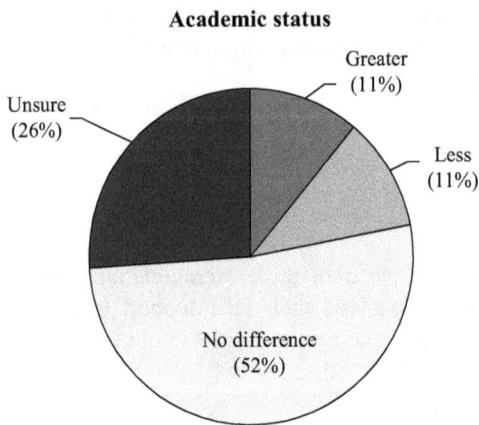

Figure 11.11 Perceptions about academic status.

(with others) 67% whilst working from home. This data in this study suggests that most of the female academic respondents were able to adapt to the changing environment in WFH and it is perhaps the flexibility that WFH offered that has contributed to the majority response.

The increased workload for regular routine tasks slowly generates professional wear and tear. Those who stated it was more difficult, made comments such as:

I find life overwhelming … I find online teaching alien and disconnected I miss the stimulation and encouragement of work colleagues I feel isolated and not sure what is happening in the academic world home demands feel dominating and restrictive.

[ID_260]

Backing this finding is the academic literature reporting that there has been an increase in the workload by about 50% of academics during remote lockdowns, and a statistically significant correlation between professional burnout, and the increase in hours dedicated to work. This is further correlated with emotional exhaustion and depersonalisation (Gonzalez et al., 2021).

Exhaustion has taken a toll and I feel like I am trying to stay afloat.

[ID_161]

Of the academics who stated they felt *less motivated* in their career progression, this was mainly due to increased workloads and struggle in balancing home and work life. Again, these respondents perceived it was 'easy to manage' working from home *with others* at home and all had children over the age of 15 years. Whilst the data may appear somewhat contradictory, it *may* be due to the increased flexibility that has attributed respondents' agreement in managing with others at home or perhaps that help from others whilst WFH has been helpful. Motivation is personal and with many factors impacting an individual's circumstances, each will experience their work life in a different manner within the structural constraints they experience.

Workplace Stress

The World Health Organization (WHO) identified the lack of management of chronic workplace stress resulting in employees feeling depleted or exhausted and with reduced professional efficacy (Organization, 2018) and female employees face increased stress with caring for themselves and loved ones (Boserup et al., 2020). This study has reinforced the increased stress being felt or placed on academics during the pandemic:

Poor participation and attendance of students in live online lectures/tutorials, the lack of face-to-face contact, and my concerns around students cheating in assessments means that my enjoyment of teaching and the sense of accomplishment that it used to bring has declined.

[ID_24]

It is therefore critical that HEIs now must consider ways to best support staff remotely and to minimise possible work-related stress. An increase in workload since the pandemic started has been noted, with the ever-increasing encroachment of digital technologies into private lives, raising the expectations that employees are always available and contactable. The typical academic tasks which are completed in the office environment in higher education, away from home, such as teaching, when conducted from home are assumed to take longer. This can be attributed to a few reasons including the requirement of training in or working in the online space to be able to respond to the changes resulting from confinement (Gonzalez et al., 2021).

Increased Flexibility

The pandemic has highlighted opportunities for academics including online teaching, greater flexibility, and ability to collaborate, time for research and ability to attend global professional conferences (Duncanson et al., 2021). These were reported as positive outcomes in this study as part of the motivating factors for continued career progression. The African HEIs can consider how they continue to motivate and retain female academics in the workforce with greater flexible work-from-home policies. The current study has highlighted that female academics can work effectively from home whilst enjoying their family/personal self-care and self-management of time when given the option to do so. This study suggests the locus of control gained from working from home as a motivator for greater career progression is a key benefit allowing flexibility in hours and proving to be an intrinsic motivator for female academics (Othman et al., 2021, Watson et al., 2022b). However, the difficulties of managing WFH that 74% of respondents reported must be acknowledged.

The concept of remote working is two pronged for females – firstly it may potentially disadvantage females, as they typically must shoulder both childcare and household chores as well as paid employment.

> I have seen that working from home with children schooling from home, life is a nightmare. With pre-school children, it is even more nightmarish.
>
> [ID_143]

However, alternatively, it may help academics to facilitate their desired work–life balance (Papandrea and Azzi, 2020). This was true in this study where respondents noted that workloads had increased, yet the increased flexibility was viewed as a highly motivating factor in females' ability to manage with others at home whilst in lockdown, remote work. The increased flexibility has provided many females with greater WLB positively associated with productivity and is directly correlated with job satisfaction (Ravi and Anulakshmi, 2021). Human resource (HR) policies can adapt to promote family-friendly policies and measures, focusing on encouraging men to share the responsibilities of unpaid care and domestic chores equally with females. The OECD further suggests that HR policies should allow for flexibility, ensuring that the WFH option remains a choice and is not overdone and address aspects such as hidden work beyond work hours.

> Flexibility happened de facto during the pandemic and needs to continue.
>
> [ID_143]

Career Progression Opportunities

In this current, small sample study, motivation for career progression since the onset of the pandemic was viewed as being *less* (40%) and (30%), indicating that career progression *increased somewhat*, and another (30%) perceived *no differ-ence* in career progression since February 2020. This finding supports the work of Kolakowski et al. (2021) that academics' careers had progressed well, but for only around 40% during the COVID pandemic and this study shows around 30% saying some increase was perceived. Watson et al. (2022) also found that career progres-sion of female academics in the Australian context was less with a 69% agreement. 'I still have the same progression motivation. With the pandemic, it may take a little longer than planned due to a slowdown in research conducted and therefore research outputs [ID_46].'

Gender Bias

This chapter adds to the growing research literature about the challenges being faced by female academics during the COVID-19 pandemic including a belief that the pandemic will further increase the existing gender inequalities (Alon, 2020). 'As a female one has to work extra hard for recognition as compared to our male counterparts [ID_8].' The comment below highlights a respondent's negative per-ception of gender bias and a lack of support for career progression.

> Few opportunities *in Africa* for women to get real practical IS skills … most organisations want men … thus women shy away from the deeply tech-nical IT stuff and stick to _soft IT/IS_ … yet women have other duties to do … housework, childcare etc … thus, divided attention.
>
> [ID_14]

> Give women opportunities (esp financial … i.e., scholarships …) without insisting too much on age limits … older women in Africa are more stable and focused.
>
> [ID_15]

Many respondents perceived no difference in female academic status at their insti-tution. Supporting female academics and their prominence in academia are critical in ensuring career progression and in overcoming the many challenges faced by females in the pre-COVID period (Gabster et al., 2020). It is important that HEIs support females at all stages of their careers.

Limitations

The authors acknowledge that the current chapter reports on a small data set which is a subset of a larger study. As such, it is a small-scale sample and thus gener-alisations about African female academic voices cannot be made as absolute but instead placed in the context of the sample size. It is, however, a sample of the African female voices which can add value to other studies being conducted in the future. The current chapter has, however, captured the voices of females in a unique period which cannot be replicated even though the current pandemic will continue and evolve over the coming years. The authors acknowledge that whilst the study focuses on the female academics' experiences, many of these may also have been experienced by male and non-binary gendered academics and have not been represented in this chapter. The authors hope though that the specific gender focus can provide a reflection for readers on their academic experience.

Summary

The current study has reported on a small cohort of female academics in the African HEI context and has provided a focused, gendered account about their motivation to progress in their career and associated factors contributing to motivation levels and perceptions of academic status. This study provides a narrative with rich text descriptions of female voices which are unique to a context and yet are mirrored across the globe of academic experiences. The current chapter can provide insight for policy administrators in the higher education sector that though institutions had to move fast in a pandemic there is a need to recognise the additional and ongoing challenges faced by females. Such recognition by institutional policy will support the development of females in academics acknowledging the responsibilities associated with home-based work. Continued research is needed to ensure the ongoing academic female voices across the globe are captured to enable and foster academic motivation, progression, and encourage new and early-career females into the world of academia. Females' contribution to academia is an important area of work and any research that contributes to the growing body of literature is valuable in promoting female advocacy and the lived experiences of African females in the higher education context as this chapter has offered. Female academics' lives have now been exposed and have become known through the pandemic, hopefully bringing about greater understanding through institutional policies in how they acknowledge and support quality female academics.

On a final note, the quote below from one academic sums up many female academic experiences during this current global pandemic:

A female academic in 2021, is like being a female superhero - a very demanding and challenging task. The struggle goes on.

[ID_62]

References

Alon, T., Doepke, M., Olmstead-Rumsey, J. & Tertilt, M. 2020. *The Impact of COVID-10 on Gender Equality* [Online]. National Bureau of Economic Research (NBER). Available: https://www.nber.org/papers/w26947 [Accessed October 4 2021].

Amano-Patiño, N., Faraglia, E., Giannitsarou, C. & Hasna, Z. 2020. The unequal effects of Covid-19 on economists' research productivity. Cambridge-INET Working Paper WP2022 doi: 10.17863/CAM.57979

Anwer, M. 2020. Academic labor and the global pandemic: Revisiting life-work balance under COVID-19. *Susan Bulkeley Butler Center for Leadership Excellence and Advance Working Paper Series*, 3, 5–13.

Boserup, B., McKenney, M. & Elkbuli, A. 2020. Alarming trends in US domestic violence during the COVID-19 pandemic. *The American Journal of Emergency Medicine*, 38, 2753–2755.

Costello, E., Brown, M., Donlon, E. & Girme, P. 2020. 'The pandemic will not be on zoom': A retrospective from the year 2050. *Postdigital Science and Education*, 2, 619–627.

Couch, D. L., O'Sullivan, B. & Malatzky, C. 2021. What COVID-19 could mean for the future of "work from home": The provocations of three women in the academy. *Gender, Work & Organization*, 28, 266–275.

Creswell, J. W. ed. 2003. A framework for design. In *Research Design: Qualitative, Quantitative, and Mixed Methods Approaches*, (2nd edn.). Thousand Oaks, CA: Sage. 9–11.

Deloitte. 2021. Women@Work. A global outlook.

Deryugina, T., Shurchkov, O. & Stearns, J. 2021.Covid-19 disruptions disproportionately affect female academics. *AEA Papers and Proceedings*,111 164168DOI: 10.1257/pandp.20211017.

Dreher, J. 2016. The social construction of power: Reflections beyond Berger/Luckmann and Bourdieu. *Cultural Sociology*, 10, 53–68.

Duncanson, K., Weir, N., Siriwardhane, P. & Khan, T. 2021. *How COVID is Widening the Academic Gender Divide in Australia* [Online]. Australia: OCUFA Journal of Higher Education. Available: https://academicmatters.ca/how-covid-is-widening-the-academic -gender-divide-in-australia/ [Accessed November 3 2021].

Fernandez, A. A. & Shaw, G. P. 2020. Academic leadership in a time of crisis: The Coronavirus and COVID-19. *Journal of Leadership Studies*, 14, 39–45.

Gabster, B. P., Van Daalen, K., Dhatt, R. & Barry, M. 2020. Challenges for the female academic during the COVID-19 pandemic. *The Lancet*, 395, 1968–1970.

Garcia-Morales, V. J., Garrido-Moreno, A. & Martin-Rojas, R. 2021. The transformation of higher education after the COVID disruption: Emerging challenges in an online learning scenario. *Frontiers in Psychology*, 12, 616059 doi: 10.3389/fpsyg.2021.616059.

Gergen, K. J. & Wortham, S. 2001. Social construction and pedagogical practice. *Social Construction in Context*, 115–136.

Gonzalez, E. P. R., Otalvaro, A. M. R., Argel, M. N. M. & Urzola, A. U. 2021. Professional burnout and increased workload during covid-19 in higher education teachers in monteria-colombia. *European Psychiatry*, 64, S267–S268.

Hadiwijaya, H. & Sentanu, I. G. E. P. S. 2021.Effects of WFH (Work from Home) policies, perceived organizational support, job stress, and the ability to use technology on lecturer performance during the new normal. *3rd Annual International Conference on Public and Business Administration (AICoBPA 2020)*, Atlantis Press, 263–271.

Heitz, C., Laboissiere, M., Sanghvi, S. & Sarakatsannis, J. 2020. Getting the next phase of remote learning right in higher education. *McKinsey Insights*.

Kiger, M. E. & Varpio, L. 2020. Thematic analysis of qualitative data: AMEE Guide No. 131. *Medical Teacher*, 42, 846–854.

Kolakwski, H., Shepley, M. M., Valenzuela-Mendoza, E. & Ziebarth, N. R. 2021. How the Covid-19 pandemic will change workplaces, healthcare markets and healthy living: An overview and assessment. *Sustainability*, 13, 10096.

Kotteeswari, M. & Sharief, S. T. 2014. Job stress and its impact on employees' performance a study with reference to employees working in Bpos. *International Journal of Business and Administration Research Review*, 2, 18–25.

Krause, S. F. 2017. *Leadership: Underrepresentation of Women in Higher Education.* Arizona: Northcentral University.

Lalani, K., Crawford, J. & Butler-Henderson, K. 2021. Academic leadership during COVID-19 in higher education: Technology adoption and adaptation for online learning during a pandemic. *International Journal of Leadership in Education,* 1–17doi: https://doi.org/10 .1080/13603124.2021.1988716.

Liu, L. 2016. Using generic inductive approach in qualitative educational research: A case study analysis. *Journal of Education and Learning,* 5, 129–135.

Malisch, J. L., Harris, B. N., Sherrer, S. M., Lewis, K. A., Shepherd, S. L., McCarthy, P. C., Spott, J. L., Karam, E. P., Moustaid-Moussa, N., Calarco, J. M., Ramalingam, L., Talley, A. E., Cañas-Carrell, J. E., Ardon-Dryer, K., Weiser, D. A., Bernal, X. E. & Deitloff, J. 2020. Opinion: In the wake of COVID-19, academia needs new solutions to ensure gender equity. *Proceedings of the National Academy of Sciences,* 117, 15378.

Marinoni, G., Van't Land, H. & Jensen, T. 2020. The impact of Covid-19 on higher education around the world. IAU Global Survey Report.

Nowell, L. S., Norris, J. M., White, D. E. & Moules, N. J. 2017a. Thematic analysis: Striving to meet the trustworthiness criteria. *International Journal of Qualitative Methods,* 16, 1609406917733847.

Nowell, L. S., Norris, J. M., White, D. E. & Moules, N. J. 2017b. Thematic analysis: Striving to meet the trustworthiness criteria. *International Journal of Qualitative Methods,* 16, 1609406917733847.

Okeke-Uzodike, O. & Gamede, V. 2021. The dilemma of unrelenting workload amidst Covid-19 pandemic: An agenda for university female academics. *Journal of Research in Higher Education,* 5,12–46.

Oliveira, G., Greha Teixeira, J., Torres, A. & Morais, C. 2021. An exploratory study on the emergency remote education experience of higher education students and teachers during the COVID-19 pandemic. *British Journal of Educational Technology,* 2021 Jul; 52(4): 1357–1376. doi: 10.1111/bjet.13112. Epub 2021 May 18. PMID: 34219758; PMCID: PMC8237053.

Othman, S., Awis, M. L., Samad, S. A. & Harun, A. F. 2021. Consolidating work from home as the new norms: Internal vs external factors among UiTM staff. *Advances in Business Research International Journal,* 7, 65–80.

Papandrea, D. & Azzi, M. 2020. Managing work-related psychosocial risks during the COVID-19 pandemic. *International Labour Organization,* 6–35.

Ravi, N. & Anulakshimi, M. R. 2021. Work from home and employee productivity during COVID-19. *Asian Basic and Applied Research Journal,* 3, 14–21.

Rottenberg, C. 2014. The rise of neoliberal feminism. *Cultural Studies,* 28, 418–437.

Singh, U. G., Watson, R. & Nair, C. S. 2022. Across continents: A comparison of African and Australian academics' online preparedness. *Perspectives in Education,* 40, 39–61.

Terry, G., Hayfield, N., Clarke, V. & Braun, V. 2017. Thematic analysis. *The SAGE Handbook of Qualitative Research in Psychology,* 2, 17–37.

Walters, C., Mehl, G. G., Piraino, P., Jansen, J. D. & Kriger, S. 2022. The impact of the pandemic-enforced lockdown on the scholarly productivity of women academics in South Africa. *Research Policy,* 51, 104403.

Watson, R., Singh, U. & Sid Nair, C. 2022a. Pandemic, disruption and adjustment in higher education. In Gonçalves, S. & Majhanovich, S. (eds.), Chapter 11 *Higher Education Academics' Perspectives: Working from Home during COVID-19.*Netherlands: Brill.

Watson, R., Singh, U. G. & Nair, C. S. 2022b. Experiences of female academics in Australia during COVID-19: Opportunities and challenges. *Journal of University Teaching & Learning Practice*, 19 (1), 176–198, https://doi.org/10.53761/1.19.1.11.

World Health Organization. 2018. *Digital Technologies: Shaping the Future of Primary Health Care*. Geneva: World Health Organization.

12 The Impact of Japanese Schools' Policy Responses to COVID-19 on Filipino Women Assistant Language Teachers

Tricia Abigail Santos Fermin and
Johanna O. Zulueta

Introduction

COVID-19 has brought about unprecedented disruptions in everyday life, especially in the field of education. As the disease presented itself in various parts of the world, governments ordered school closures, affecting 91% of learners worldwide (Nugroho et al. 2020). In Japan, then-Prime Minister Shinzo Abe requested on 27 February 2020 for the closure of all elementary, middle, and high schools from March until early April. As infection rates began to increase, the central government then declared a 1-month nationwide state of emergency on 7 April, effectively extending the school closure to a total of 3 months. This caused confusion and worry among parents, as it seriously impacted childcare arrangements (Saito et al. 2020). The move was also met with criticism from ministry officials and opposition lawmakers for its lack of 'consideration for people at schools,' for it did not provide any clear directives on how schools should deal with classes and ceremonies during the period (Kyodo News 2020a).

These abrupt changes in education delivery methods amid a global health crisis negatively affected the occupational health of teaching staff. Iwahori et al. (2020) examined Japanese school teachers' perceptions and concerns regarding the pandemic's effects on their work environment during the closure and after reopening in July 2020. Results of the study revealed that while the school closure led to an overall decrease in teachers' workload compared to the same period in the previous year, older and more experienced teachers reported an increase in their workload, as they are generally given more decision-making and crisis management responsibilities. On the other hand, teachers' workload increased after schools reopened compared to the same period in the previous year. This was attributed to significant changes made in the academic calendar to catch up on lessons and the addition of hygiene management tasks.[1] Three main sources of teachers' anxiety identified were changes in workload, maintaining workplace hygiene, and implementing pandemic response measures. Moreover, 18% of part-time teachers surveyed cited the lack of employment security as another contributing factor to anxiety during the pandemic. Wakui

DOI: 10.4324/9781003267133-16

et al. (2021) examined the causes of anxiety post-school reopening among teachers in Tokyo. It noted similar patterns that teachers primarily experience education-related (e.g., managing lesson delays and learning loss, dealing with students' parents) and infection-related (e.g., vaccine availability, personal and family security, infection among students, facing discrimination if one is found to be infected) anxiety.

The emerging body of literature has identified factors that negatively impact teaching staff in Japan. However, there are two significant gaps. First, current studies have yet to investigate the specific challenges women in the educational profession face during the pandemic, despite women comprising over 90% of full-time teaching staff in early education institutions and 62% in elementary schools (Ministry of Education, Culture, Sports, Science, and Technology [MEXT] 2021). Moreover, they focus only on Japanese nationals, effectively obscuring the experiences of foreign teaching staff, particularly the Assistant Language Teachers (ALTs), who are part of everyday life in Japanese schools. Public health researchers have highlighted the importance of intersectionality as a critical lens to expose the heterogeneity in people's lived experiences of the pandemic. Intersectionality serves as a compelling reminder that any clinical intervention, social advocacy work, or activism using simplistic, catch-all categories such as 'women' would likely end up merely perpetrating current systems of inequalities (Harris and Leonardo 2018).

This chapter discusses the impact of Japanese schools' responses to COVID-19 on the occupational health of foreign teaching staff during the first 6 months of the pandemic. It investigates the experiences of women Assistant Language Teachers (ALTs) from the Philippines employed through the Japan Exchange and Teaching (JET) Programme. First, it will examine their positionality and status in the Japanese education system and discuss how their experiences during the school closure revealed critical vulnerabilities that have put their well-being at risk. Results show that while the ongoing pandemic has not endangered Filipino women ALTs' livelihood and immigration status in the country, it has exacerbated the problems they have been experiencing due to their marginal position in the Japanese education system, thus rendering them particularly vulnerable to mental health risks. This chapter also investigates the important role of online platforms and digital media in addressing these women migrant teachers' mental and emotional well-being as they navigate and mitigate the risks posed by the current pandemic.

Data was collected through semi-structured interviews conducted with eight Filipino JET ALTs via Zoom from late February to mid-March 2021. Interviewees were recruited from the participants of a study on the profiles and motivations of Filipino ALTs one of the authors conducted in 2019 (see Fermin 2020). It was then analysed using an inductive thematic approach. All names have been changed to protect the privacy of the interviewees. Any references to individual interviewees' age, location of work, or years of service in the JET Programme have also been removed. Filipino ALTs comprise merely 2% of the total ALT population in the programme,[2] so providing any additional personal information aside from their gender expression may be enough to extrapolate their identities.

Filipino Women ALTs in the JET Programme

In Japan's English language classrooms, the term 'ALT' refers to English language speakers who team-teach with Japanese Teachers of English (JTEs) in elementary, middle, and high schools. In terms of rank, ALTs serve as assistants to JTEs, but they are, in theory, on equal footing with JTEs in the classroom and are expected to play a full role in communicative activities with the students and JTEs (Wada 1992). Team-teaching with ALTs in foreign language classes was incorporated into Japan's education policy in 1987 through the establishment of the JET Programme, which aims to promote international exchange in local communities and help develop foreign language education. The Council of Local Authorities for International Relations (CLAIR) manages the JET Programme in partnership with three other government ministries, which includes the Ministry of Education, Culture, Sports, Science, and Technology (MEXT).

The JET Programme mainly recruits young college graduates from 57 participating countries. Candidates must hold at least a bachelor's degree by their arrival in Japan. They are neither required to have teaching qualifications nor a high proficiency level in the Japanese language, although additional consideration is given to those who do (CLAIR n.d.). Fermin (2020) notes, however, that Filipino JET ALTs tend to be qualified professionals who specialise in English language, literature, or education, with an average of 7 years teaching experience in the Philippines and/or abroad before coming to Japan. She also observes that many of the successful candidates are female, which suggests that more women apply and/ or are chosen for the programme and are usually between 21 and 35 years old at the time of arrival in Japan. They are all selected after a rigorous screening process that closely examines applicants' teaching backgrounds and abilities. Their high educational attainment and record of overseas travel also suggest a middle-class background. However, economic factors such as low pay and less-than-ideal working conditions for teachers in the Philippines pushed them to seek better work opportunities in Japan. In addition, the chance of being able to live in a country they admire and participate in the country's internationalisation efforts were pull factors in Filipino teacher migration as ALTs through the programme.

Upon successful application, an ALT is placed by CLAIR in a local government organisation (i.e., prefectural boards of education or government-designated cities), which, in turn, assigns them to local schools. The number of schools and education levels they are assigned to vary depending on their contracting organisation.[3] Furthermore, each ALT is assigned to a supervisor, usually a member of their local school board tasked with overseeing ALTs' needs, work performance, and contract renewals. JET ALTs are employed on a 1-year contract, renewable annually up to a maximum of 5 years. As full-time government employees, they are entitled to 20 days of paid time off and are covered with health, pension, employment, and accident insurance.

ALTs' Marginal Status in Japan's Education System

JET ALTs are the official members of school staff and local education boards. They are, in principle, expected to be as fully engaged in working towards improving

Japanese students' communicative language competencies as the JTEs. However, ALTs are limited by Japan's education law and the JET Programme's directives on their qualifications, roles, and responsibilities as teaching staff.

As assistant teachers, ALTs merely play a supporting role in the classroom and are not normally allowed by Japan's education law to teach on their own.[4] They assist JTEs in conducting communication activities and help with the teaching workload based on the teaching and lesson plan prepared by the JTE (MEXT 2011). While they may propose lesson plans and activities for team-taught classes, the JTE ultimately decides whether their suggestions make it to the day's lesson. As a result, ALT involvement varies greatly across classrooms. Some JTEs actively involve ALTs in their lesson preparation and classroom instruction. Yet contrary to MEXT directives, some ALTs are left to conduct classes on their own, with little to no team-teaching done (Ohtani 2010), while others merely serve as mechanical models of pronunciation. ALTs not required to take an active role in classroom instruction would have very limited to almost no student engagement. On the other hand, while some JTEs actively engage ALTs in lesson planning and classroom instruction, the content and type of classes they are tasked to teach are not always fully integrated in an exam-focused curriculum. Oral communication classes with the ALT are generally expected to be 'fun' rather than educational, as they are not geared towards entrance exam preparations (Roloff Rothman 2012; Geluso 2013). This tends to give students the impression that communicative language classes with the ALT are irrelevant or lead them to see ALTs as mere 'entertainers,' compared to JTEs, who are the 'real teachers' (Falout 2013).

Furthermore, ALTs tend to be treated as 'temporary guests' (Hasegawa 2008) or 'foreign guests' (Komisarof 2010) rather than regular members of the school staff. Since their term of stay is limited, their 'host' organisations set up policies and systems in place that are deemed appropriate for temporary visitors. This usually means that they are given lighter workloads and are exempted from certain duties that other full-time teachers are required to fulfil, such as attending faculty meetings and other non-teaching responsibilities. However, as they are not fully integrated with the school community, this leads to a general feeling of isolation and exclusion among ALTs. Several researchers have suggested ways on how to make ALTs feel more included and valued in their respective communities (see Hoogenboom and Uehara 2006; Komisarof 2010; Lawrence 2016), but these merely emphasise their position as outsiders in the Japanese education system.

The foregoing discussion demonstrates how ALTs' ambiguous and marginal role in the Japanese school system makes them vulnerable to disempowerment and exploitation. In the following sections, we will see how problems stemming from their positionality are brought into relief and exacerbated by schools' COVID-19 policies, especially during the first few months of the pandemic

Role Ambiguity and Prolonged 'Desk Warming'

Despite Japan's reputation as a global leader in technology, the 2018 Teaching and Learning International Survey (TALIS) showed that information and communications technology (ICT) use in Japanese schools is extremely low compared to other OECD countries. Less than 18% of teachers surveyed allowed students to use ICT for projects or class work (OECD 2019). Thus, Japanese schools were unprepared to suddenly shift to online instruction. According to a status report released by MEXT (2020b), student learning during the school closure centred on home study using paper-based textbooks and other learning materials provided to them by the schools. Only 10% of local school boards produced video lessons for students to study at home, and merely 5% of public schools conducted synchronous instruction during the said period. Close to 40% of schools required students to have to come to school about once a week for teachers to check on their learning progress and distribute class materials for the succeeding week (Ministry of Education, Culture, Science, and Technology 2020b). Japanese teaching staff were occupied with preparing and distributing study materials and checking on the students' well-being online or in person.

On the other hand, ALTs interviewed in the study report that the school closures left them with very little to almost nothing to do since their work primarily involves facilitating oral communication activities in English. Out of the eight interviewees, only one was constantly engaged by her employers and was tasked to make specific learning materials such as lesson videos, handouts, and worksheets that were used by the students during the said period. Four reported being asked by their local school boards to make videos introducing themselves only during the first month of the school closure. All interviewees proposed to their JTEs that they make interesting videos or fun online lessons that can be posted on the school's website or YouTube channel to motivate students to learn English at home, but only one employer went with their suggestions. They were not given any specific duties to perform but were still expected to report to work either in their base school or in the city hall where the local Board of Education's (BOE) office is located.

The result of this role ambiguity is commonly referred to by JET ALTs as 'desk warming,' where one is required to sit at one's desk for long periods of time without any specific work-related duties to perform. Majority of ALTs experience a certain amount of desk warming during school holidays, but this becomes a significant problem during the school term, when a JTE decides to teach classes alone for a number of reasons, which leaves the ALT with nothing to do.[5] Occupational health research shows that there is a moderate, yet significant positive relationship between role ambiguity and negative mental health outcomes, such as depression (Papastylianou, Kaila, and Polychronopoulos 2009; Schmidt et al. 2014). Borg (2020) points out that desk warming has a negative effect on ALTs, leaving many feelings marginalised and exhausted from a lack of physical and mental stimulation. Our interviewees corroborate this, relating that desk warming is one of the biggest causes of job dissatisfaction among ALTs, as they feel that they are not doing any meaningful work. The pandemic, however, only prolonged the period of desk warming for the ALTs and finding teaching-related tasks to do to keep them occupied during the school closures proved to be challenging because there were no students they could interact with, both in person and online.

Other than school closures, teleworking has also been one of the mobility interventions suggested to minimise COVID-19 community transmission. In early April 2020, MEXT forwarded to school boards and educational institutions nationwide a memorandum from the Ministry of Internal Affairs and Communications requesting that all workplaces implement various infection prevention measures, which included staggered working hours and teleworking (MEXT 2020a). The decision on whether to allow school staff to work remotely rested on the local education boards. Telework policies in schools therefore depended on the directives issued by their respective local education boards and varied greatly across the country. Several local education boards allowed ALTs to work from home because they did not have any class-related duties to perform on campus. They were required to check in and out with their supervisors every day, as well as submit periodic reports on the work-related tasks they have been performing at home. Tasks considered relevant to their duties were lesson planning and teaching materials creation, learning about language teaching methods, and studying Japanese. All interviewees viewed the submitted reports as a mere formality, since their supervisors reportedly almost never checked their output. There generally was no guidance given either by their superiors regarding the specific form or content of their expected output during that period, effectively extending their experience of desk warming at home. Some were still required to periodically come to school without any formal duties to perform.

Interviewee narratives highlight the negative impact of ALT role ambiguity on work stress and satisfaction. For example, in the following excerpt, Maria relates how this sort of situation led her to feel isolated and lost during this period:

It's understandable [that the schools didn't know what to do with us] because they also don't know exactly what's going on. They're just waiting for directives from above. After all, it's the first time everyone has experienced a pandemic … but if something like this were to happen again, I think there should be direct contact with ALTs, and we should be given roles. We can be foreign translators or be involved in a community. Around that time, everyone seemed to be moving. The Japanese people seemed to know what to do. As an ALT, I was, like, where is my place in all this? I felt lost at that time.

(Maria, Personal communication, 8 March 2021)

Another interviewee, Cristina, reports that she felt pressure from the local school board to find ways to keep herself busy to justify the pay that she continued to receive:

I felt more pressured to work and be productive [despite not being given specific tasks to do]. I kept thinking of things to do. The BOE told us, especially the ALTs, to make sure that we don't do anything that would ruin, I think, the reputation of [the prefecture's] ALTs. It basically said, make sure you work. I've heard reports that some ALTs at that time would just be eating together and going out during their work hours, and basically not doing their jobs. I

felt that I had to set myself apart from that … and prove that I'm working
because we get paid for that

(Cristina, Personal communication, 21 March 2021).

This type of work style has also resulted in some ALTs quitting their jobs. One
of the interviewees did not renew her contract and went back to the Philippines in
August 2021 because she found her job as an ALT unfulfilling.

These ALTs' experiences illustrate how role ambiguity tends to exacerbate the
uncertainties brought about by the pandemic as well as job dissatisfaction. Schmidt
et al. (2014) argued that clearly defined roles and job objectives are factors that
would contribute to employee health. The foregoing ALT narratives show us that
these are especially important in promoting worker productivity and well-being
during a global health crisis.

Management Resistance to Employee Telework

Despite government directives, some local education boards did not allow ALTs to
work from home. Analyn and Gloria both work for such a local education board.
Analyn shares the reasons they requested permission to telework:

Teachers still had to come in for work. That's when the ALTs asked the
BOE to allow us to telework, because they didn't want to risk sitting in a
staff room with the desks close to each other. People were still eating in pubs
and weren't taking it seriously yet. Us ALTs, we were really worried about
catching the virus. The fears weren't unfounded because, us foreigners, if we
caught the virus, that would have bad consequences for us, being a foreigner
in a small city …. At first, the BOE said that we shouldn't work from home
because we were still considered civil servants …. And being 'teachers' –
that's the only time they considered us as teachers – we had to follow what
the other full-time teachers were supposed to do, which was to go to work

(Analyn, Personal communication, 3 March 2021).

She also reported the struggle they had to face and the need to organise and negoti-
ate with their employer as a group to be allowed to telework.

They were eventually allowed to do so if they use their sick leave to telework
due to mental health reasons, a compromise that many ALTs did not agree with but
had no choice but to accept:

Our BOE finally relented and said that we could use our sick leave if we
wanted to work from home. That was the compromise. But that didn't sit
well with us because the explanation would be that because us foreigners,
our mental health is, well, not weak, but very fragile. That didn't sit well with
us because [it was made to appear that] our mental health was fragile so we
could use our sick leave to not come to work.

(Analyn, Personal communication, 3 March 2021)

Gloria surmises that the resistance to employee telework is an indication of a wider cultural belief that one's physical presence at work is a sign of discipline and industriousness. She explains:

> I have an impression that they believe people who work from home are lazy. I remember, my JTE once asked me what a good topic for our small talk activity would be. I suggested 'Which is better, online or in-person classes?' Of course, I was for online classes. I said online classes are better because it's safer, especially at a time like this. Also, when you wake up in the morning, you just log in and there you are in the classroom! The JTE then told me that that's so lazy. (laughs) What was the word used? '*Wagamama*' [self-indulgent]. They said, 'That's so lazy!' to everyone in the classroom. They were just joking, but of course, if they reacted as such, I think that that's their impression of teleworking.
>
> (Gloria, Personal communication, 4 March 2021)

The above narratives suggest several vulnerabilities that are specific to ALTs' status as foreigners in Japan. First, many education boards and contracting organisations tend to treat JET ALTs as 'civil servants' and full-time teaching staff only in name and would invoke such status only when it suits their purposes. Her remark that they were referred to as 'teachers' only when the dispute over their work-from-home request came up implies a perceived double standard in the way they are treated compared to other Japanese full-time teaching staff. As previously discussed, JET ALTs are technically government employees and full-time teaching staff but are often treated as temporary visiting staff with minimal responsibilities, teaching or otherwise. In fact, they are usually not included in staff meetings, especially those where COVID-19 updates and measures are brought up and discussed, leaving them largely uninformed on the current situation in their schools unless they deliberately seek out information and ask their JTEs.

Also, ALTs are cognisant of COVID-19-related discrimination in Japan, especially against foreigners. Discriminatory remarks and behaviours have been primarily targeted against COVID-19 patients, patients' families, and healthcare workers (24Ministry of Health, Labour and Welfare 2020a, 2020b) due to persistent social pressures to prevent bringing the disease into local communities (Suzuki, Iizuka, and Lefor 2021). However, foreigners also become easy targets of discrimination,[6] especially in small, rural communities. Analyn's narrative reveals that COVID-19-related discrimination was a real and constant worry among ALTs, and not being able to access teleworking options to mitigate infection risk for the sake of following rules merely compounded their anxieties.

The school board's decision to make ALTs use their sick leave to be able to work from home also points to a gross misuse of the sick leave policy, especially during a pandemic. Not only does this take away paid leaves that should be used for future health emergencies, but ALTs were still expected to be working despite being on leave. Both reported that they still had to call in twice a day to log in and out of work, as well as submit progress reports like teleworking ALTs in other local school boards, although they were technically on leave. Moreover, the decision can also be regarded as prejudicial, as it pathologises ALTs' concerns about their working conditions by framing them as the result of having a 'fragile mental health condition.'

Social Isolation

Perhaps the most critical vulnerability that ALTs had to face during the school closure period was social isolation. All the ALTs interviewed report that they had been carefully following social distancing measures and stay-home requests, especially given the negative social repercussions they may face if they were to contract COVID-19. Several interviewees talked about the negative psychological effects they experienced during the early months of the pandemic. For instance, Maria explains how social isolation negatively impacted both her physical and mental health:

> I think there was a time I overate chocolate. I think I didn't realise I was stress-eating, so I was surprised how high my blood sugar was after my health check last year .... And then everybody's leaving, you can't travel, which is worse because I'm outdoorsy! I couldn't meet my friends. They are my only support system here in Japan, so it's very easy to feel isolated. So yeah, I went crazy last year.
>
> (Maria, Personal communication, 8 March 2021)

Being apart from relatives and worrying about their well-being also causes anxiety among ALTs. Maria shares that several ALTs she knew quit in the middle of their contract period due to extreme anxiety about their families back home. Also, Gabriela reports experiencing extreme anxiety attributed to worries about her family in the Philippines and high hormonal activity from her pregnancy that she had to seek professional counselling:

> I suffered a bit of mental issues before giving birth, and I had to see a psychologist a few times. Well, the analysis was because I was pregnant, my hormones were going up and down. Luckily after giving birth, the maternity blues eventually went away. I didn't imagine myself calling the JET mental helpline, but I did. Early last year [January 2020] Taal Volcano erupted.[7] From that time, I developed anxiety, add the hormones, so it was terrible. You asked me how I dealt with it? Keeping myself busy helped a lot. I'm lucky because I have a family [in Japan], and I have something to be busy with. But how about the ALTs with a lot freer time? I can't imagine myself being a single ALT, who would stay at home, do nothing and wait for the day to be over, you know?
>
> (Gabriela, Personal communication, 17 March 2021)

Research conducted prior to the pandemic consistently demonstrates that social isolation and loneliness are closely related to worse cardiovascular and mental health (Leigh-Hunt et al. 2017). Brooks et al. (2020) report that periods of isolation, even those less than 10 days, bring about negative psychological effects such as post-traumatic stress syndrome, confusion, and anger. Their study also identified stressors that contribute to negative psychological effects, which include the length of isolation period, infection fears, frustration, boredom, inadequate information, and stigma. With the onset of the pandemic, enforced isolation brought about by social distancing and mobility interventions is most likely exacerbating the effects of ALTs' outsider status in their respective communities. In addition, most ALTs are single and live alone, so the government's request for self-restraint meant that they cannot meet with friends they rely on for emotional and psychological support or engage in outdoor leisure activities.

Support and Intervention

Even prior to the pandemic, the JET Programme has been providing various mental health support services. For instance, CLAIR's JET Online Counselling Service offers free professional counselling services through Skype (up to seven sessions per year) and Web Mail (unlimited use). Moreover, through the JET Mental Health Counselling Assistance Programme, participants can claim partial subsidies of 50%, up to 30,000 yen for professional mental health counselling costs incurred in Japan or abroad that are not covered by health insurance. However, since the onset of the pandemic, CLAIR added a toll-free telephone counselling service twice a month to the programme's mental health resources. The service does not require advance reservation and has no annual limit but is limited only to one call per person for each day the service is available. Three telephone lines are dedicated for this service (CLAIR 2021). ALTs are strongly encouraged to make use of this service whenever they experience anxiety or any other mental health burden. Professional mental health counselling services in English are not only limited but can also be rather expensive. CLAIR's toll-free counselling service, therefore, makes a much-needed health service more accessible to ALTs. As mentioned in the previous section, Gabriela made use of this service when she developed anxiety in the early months of the pandemic. The counselling she received helped her identify the causes of her problem and find ways to deal with her anxiety.

Digital media and online platforms have also been a source of mental and emotional support. Lisista et al.'s (2020) study shows that while overall social media use is associated with increased loneliness among young adults during the pandemic, those who actively used social media with support-seeking motives tend to experience no increase in loneliness. Since effective interventions for reducing loneliness involve adaptability, community development, and active engagement (Gardiner, Geldenhuys, and Gott 2018), young adults should be encouraged to access online social connections and communities that provide opportunities for contribution, such as volunteering, joining workshops, or participating in musical or writing communities in various online platforms. They suggest that these activities may be more useful for countering loneliness than passive social media use.

ALTs interviewed all reported that connecting regularly with family, friends, and other fellow ALTs through video conferencing tools such as Zoom and Skype, or social media applications with built-in instant messaging and video call functions such as Facebook (FB) have been helping them feel less isolated. They note that Filipino ALTs have a private FB group, where they can regularly update each other on their respective work situation, as well as provide emotional support. They would offer encouraging words and try to help each other find humour in negative situations as they face each day of the pandemic. In addition, Analyn, Gloria, and their other colleagues used FB to communicate with each other and get organised to collectively request for permission to telework when infection rates began increasing in their city.

While the private FB group has made it possible for these Filipino women ALTs to vent and share their problems and experiences before and during the pandemic, the challenges that these ALTs currently face during the pandemic are exacerbated by structural factors that tend to amplify existing inequalities in the ALT system.

Based on ongoing observations of interactions of these ALTs in the FB group, and with the alarming situation that brought a rapid increase of COVID cases in the country due to the Omicron variant, the authors are designing a model that could assist and empower these ALTs as they navigate their current situation. This model of intervention will utilise video conferencing technology such as Zoom, which would enable these ALTs to join and be part of a small private group, where they can discuss, examine, and share experiences in a safe, comfortable, and non-judgmental environment. These group discussions will be facilitated by a clinical sociologist using the language these ALTs are most comfortable in, i.e., Filipino (Tagalog). Groups of these kinds are important to address the specific needs of women ALTs who are not 'white' and are considered to be 'native speakers' of English. This will also assist these women to be more aware that their troubles are deeply embedded in their positionality as women ALTs in Japan, as well as very much linked to structural forces.

The group sessions would be 1 hour per week and would be facilitated like focus group discussions. It would start with having the participants lay out the problems they have faced before the pandemic, and then discuss the issues they have faced from its onset leading to the present day. Based on the interviews, the authors anticipate several concerns to come up, such as dealing with career transitions and social isolation, as well as those of an interpersonal (e.g., discord and understanding in the workplace) or socio-structural (e.g., sexism, racial discrimination) nature. The facilitator will help participants recognise how these are reflective of the sociocultural context that they are in as women ALTs and guide them in identifying courses of action that would encourage them to better adapt to the ongoing pandemic. The results of the sessions would be used to map out a plan to address the psychosocial challenges faced by ALTs who may have different needs from Japanese teachers as well as other JETs and ALTs who come from more privileged backgrounds due to their race, nationality, and gender.

Clinical sociology, as a creative and humanistic specialisation (Fritz 2008), aims to enable change that would lead to better outcomes and facilitate adaptive responses to challenges. It is the hope that with the adoption of an intersectional approach to clinical practice, interventions such as those proposed by the authors would lead women towards empowerment, self-awareness, and positive connections to others that are very much needed to ride through this unprecedented global health crisis.

Conclusion

This chapter focused on the experiences of women Assistant Language Teachers or ALTs in Japan during the early years of the COVID-19 pandemic. These teachers are migrants, with many of them coming from the Philippines. As assistants to Japanese Teachers of English (JTEs), they reportedly are in a marginalised position, often having a minimal role in English classrooms, as 'entertainers' or as mechanical models of pronunciation. The marginality of the ALTs' role in a Japanese classroom was further exacerbated during the pandemic when many of them became 'desk warmers,' where they had to stay at their desks for long periods of time without doing anything. Some of those interviewed also spoke of management's resistance towards telework, and for those who decided to work from home, they were asked to use their sick leaves for this purpose.

The ALTs also reported experiencing social isolation, anxiety, and loneliness during the pandemic. Many of them sought mental and emotional support from social media and communication tools such as Zoom and Skype. The JET Programme itself offers counselling services for ALTs. However, the authors propose creating interventionist measures to address the problems experienced by these ALTs, that are more tailored to the needs of these Filipino ALTs, recognising their sociocultural background as well as their position as foreign teachers and migrants in Japan.

Notes

1 Iwahori et al. defined 'changes in the school calendar' as shortened school holidays and reduced number of school events. 'Hygiene management tasks' cited in the study were disinfection of school premises, temperature checks, and checking on and responding to documents from the government.
2 Based on the statistics provided by the JET Programme, there are only 136 Filipino ALTs out of a total of 5,234 participants from all eligible countries for the academic year 2019–2022 (CLAIR 2019).
3 ALTs are usually assigned to a 'base school,' typically a junior or senior high school, where they spend most of the time teaching. They may also be assigned to periodically teach at 'visit schools,' which include elementary schools, night schools, and special needs schools. The frequency of their visits depends on the needs of the schools. Some ALTs are reported to teach at as many as 11 visit schools in a contract year.
4 Act No. 26 of 1947 of the School Education Act or *Gakkō Kyōikuhō* stipulates that the assistant teachers' role in elementary, middle, and high schools is to provide support to the lead teacher in their duties. They are allowed to teach their own class only in special circumstances.
5 Borg cites several reasons for JTEs wanting to teach alone. Some JTEs deem the communicative language classes with the ALTs as a distraction from entrance exam preparations, and thus try to keep ALT involvement in their class to a minimum. Dysfunctional relationships with JTEs or being in a school culture that is unreceptive to foreigners are also possible reasons. ALTs are relegated to desk warming even during the regular semester.

6   There had been several reported cases in the media of COVID-19-related discriminatory remarks and behaviour against foreigners in Japan. Even government health institutions have been the source of discriminatory remarks, such as the case of the Itako Health Centre in Ibaraki Prefecture. It sent out a document to agricultural cooperatives and the city hall, warning people against eating with foreigners and advising them wear masks when speaking with foreigners because there were many COVID-infected patients in the city 'that likely caught it from foreigners' (Nihon Hōsōkyoku [NHK] 2021). See Kyodo News (2020b) for more examples of COVID-related discrimination against foreigners.

7   Taal Volcano, located in Batangas province, erupted three times from 2020 to 2022. The first eruption occurred from January 12-22, 2020 as COVID-19 was starting to spread around the world. The explosive eruption resulted in wet ashfall raining north towards the direction of neighboring provinces Cavite and Laguna, even as far as Metro Manila. Gabriela's immediate family was residing in one of the neighboring provinces affected by the ashfall at that time.

References

Borg, P. (2020). 'The JET Programme's de facto ESID policy and its consequences: Critical perspectives from the online ALT community,' *Gifu Kyōritsu Daigaku Ronbunshū*, 53(3), pp. 41–59.

Brooks, S. K., Webster, R. K., Smith, L. E., Woodland, L., Wessley, S. & Greenberg, N. 2020. The psychological impact of quarantine and how to reduce it: Rapid review of the evidence. *Rapid Review*, 395(10227), 912–920. https://doi.org/10.1016/S0140 -6736(20)30460-8.

Council of Local Authorities for International Relations. (n.d.). 'Eligibility,' *The Japan Exchange and Teaching Programme*, viewed 4 March 2021, http://jetprogramme.org/ en/eligibility/

———. (2019). 'Participating countries,' *The Japan Exchange and Teaching Programme*, viewed 14 August 2022, http://jetprogramme.org/en/countries/

(2021). 'Mental health resources,' *CLAIR News*, December, viewed 17 January 2022, http:// jetprogramme.org/en/clairnewsdecember2021/

Falout, J. 2013. Forming pathways of belonging: Social inclusion for teacherse abroad. In Houghton, S. A. and Rivers, D. J. (eds.), *Native-speakerism in Japan: Intergroup Dynamics in Foreign Language Education*. Bristol: Multilingual Matters, pp. 105–115.

Fermin, T.A.S. (2020). 'Profile and motivations of Filipino JET ALTs in the JET Programme: An exploratory study,' *The Bulletin of the Graduate School of Josai International University*, 23, pp. 313–328, viewed 6 October 2021, https://www.jiu.ac.jp/files/user/ education/books/pdf/2019-23-015.pdf

Fritz, J.M. (2008). 'Introduction,' in Marie Fritz, J. (ed.), *International Clinical Sociology*, New York, Springer, pp. 1–6.

Gakkō Kyōikuhō, Shōwa 22-nen Hōritsu dai-26-gō. (1947), viewed 13 August 2021, https:// elaws.e-gov.go.jp/document?lawid=322AC0000000026

Gardiner, C., Geldenhuys, G., & Gott, M. (2018). 'Interventions to reduce social isolation and loneliness among older people: An integrative review,' *Health and Social Care in the Community*, 26, pp. 147–157. doi: 10.1111/hsc.12367

Geluso, J. (2013). 'Negotiating a professional identity: Non-Japanese teachers of English in pre-tertiary education in Japan,' in Houghton, S.A. and Rivers, D.J. (eds.),

Native-Speakerism in Japan: Intergroup Dynamics in Foreign Language Education, Bristol, Multilingual Matters, pp. 132–146.

Harris, A., & Leonardo, Z. (2018). 'Intersectionality, race-gender subordination and education,' *Review of Research in Education*, 42(1), pp. 1–27.

Hasegawa, H. (2008). 'Non-native and native teachers' perceptions of a team-teaching approach: Case of the JET programme,' *The International Journal of Language, Society and Culture*, 26(1), pp. 42–54.

Hoogenboom, R.B., & Uehara, K. (2006). 'Primary and secondary school English: How we can succeed in working with our ALT,' *Gunma Daigaku Kyōikubu Kiyō Jinbun Shakaigaku-hen*, 55, pp. 133–141.

Iwahori, S., Omata, K., Watanabe, Y., Ari, Y., & Imamura, K. (2020). 'Koronaka no kinmu kankyō ni taisuru kyōshi no ninshiki: zenkoku web ankēto chōsa wo moto ni,' *Tōkyō Daigaku Daigakuin Kyōikugaku Kenkyūka Kiyō*, 60, pp. 581–603.

Komisarof, A. (2010). 'Five keys to improving assistant language teacher and Japanese teacher relations on the JET program,' *Reitaku Journal of Interdisciplinary Studies*, 18(2), pp. 1–9.

Kyodo News. (2020a). 'Abe's abrupt call to close schools amid virus triggers confusion,' *Kyodo News*, 28 February, viewed 8 December 2021, https://english.kyodonews.net /news/2020/02/ce71c062614b-abes-abrupt-call-to-close-schools-amid-virus-triggers -confusion.html

———. (2020b). 'Foreigners in Japan becoming target of discrimination due to virus,' *Kyodo News*, 12 September, viewed 29 December 2021, https://english.kyodonews .net/news/2020/09/b7a412698d9e-feature-foreigners-in-japan-becoming-target-of -discrimination-due-to-virus.html

Lawrence, L. (2016). 'Responsibility without power: Native-speaker experiences of team teaching in Japanese secondary schools,' in Copeland, F., Garton, S., and Mann, S. (eds.), *LETs and NESTs: Voices, Views and Vignettes* [eBook edition], London, British Council, pp. 20–36, viewed 7 September 2019, https://www.teachingenglish.org.uk/sites /teacheng/files/pub_BC_Book_VVV_online_screen_res_FINAL.pdf

Leigh-Hunt, N., Bagguley, D., Bash, K., Turner, V., Turnbull, S., Valorta, N. & Caan, W. 2017. An overview on systemic reviews on the public health consequences of social isolation and loneliness. *Public Health*, 152, 157–171. https://doi.org/10.1016/j.puhe .2017.07.035.

Lisista, E., Benjamin, K.S., Chun, S.K., Skalisky, J., Hammond, L.E., & Mezulis, A.H. (2020). 'Loneliness among young adults during COVID-19 pandemic: The mediational roles of social media use and social support seeking,' *Journal of Social and Clinical Psychology*, 39(8), pp. 708–726.

Ministry of Education, Culture, Sports, Science, and Technology. (2011). 'Monbukagakushō ga ippanteki ni kangaeru gaikokugo shidō joshu (ALT) to tīmu tīchingu ni okeru ALT no yakuwari,' *Ministry of Education, Culture, Sports, Science and Technology-Japan*, viewed 13 August 2021, https://www.mext.go.jp/a_menu/kokusai/gaikokugo/1304113 .htm

———. (2020a). 'Shingata koronauirusu kansenshō no daikibo na kansen kakudai bōshi ni muketa shokuba ni okeru taiō ni tsuite (tsūchi),' *Ministry of Education, Culture, Sports, Science and Technology-Japan*, 6 April, viewed 5 January 2022, https://www.mext.go.jp /content/20200407-mxt_kouhou01-000004520_4.pdf

———. (2020b). 'Shingata koronauirusu kansenshō taisaku no tame no gakkō rinji kyūgyō ni kanrenshita kōritsu gakkō in okeru gakushū shidō nado no torikumi jōkyō ni tsuite,' *Ministry of Education, Culture, Sports, Science and Technology-Japan*, 21 April,

viewed 17 November 2021, https://www.mext.go.jp/content/20200421-mxt_kouhou01
-000006590_1.pdf

———. (2021). 'Monbukagaku tōkei yōran (Reiwa 3-nenban), 1. Gakkō kyōiku sōkatsu,'
Ministry of Education, Culture, Sports, Science and Technology-Japan, viewed 2 January
2022, https://www.mext.go.jp/b_menu/toukei/002/002b/1417059_00006.htm

Ministry of Health, Labour and Welfare of Japan. (2020a). 'Iryō jūjisha ni taisuru hokenjo
nado ni okeru shingata koronauirusu he no taiō ni tsuite,' *Ministry of Health, Labour and
Welfare of Japan*, 17 April, viewed 3 January 2022, https://www.mhlw.go.jp/content
/000622822.pdf

———. (2020b). 'Shingata koronauirusu kansenshō ni tatchimukatteiru iryō jūjisha he no
gorikai to ōen wo onegai shimasu,' *Ministry of Health, Labour and Welfare of Japan*,
1 May, viewed 3 January 2022, https://www.mhlw.go.jp/stf/newpage_11124.html

NHK News Web. (2021). 'Gaikokujin to shokuji shinai yō ni: Kansen yobō keihatsu bunshō
ni hokenjo ga kisai,' *NHK*, 22 May, viewed 5 January 2022, https://www3.nhk.or.jp/
news/html/20210522/k10013044921000.html

Nugroho, D., Pasquini, C., Reuge, N., & Amaro, D. (2020), 'How are countries preparing
to mitigate the learning loss as schools reopen? Trends and emerging good practices to
support the most vulnerable children,' *Innocenti Research Briefs*, no. 2020-20, pp. 1–8,
viewed 19 August 2021, https://www.unicef-irc.org/publications/1119-covid-19-how
-are-countries-preparing-to-mitigate-the-learning-loss-as-they-reopen.html

OECD. (2019). 'TALIS 2018 data,' *Organisation for Economic Co-operation and
Development*, viewed 23 August 2020, https://www.oecd.org/education/talis/talis-2018
-data.htm

Ohtani, C. (2010). 'Problems in the assistant language teacher system and English activity
at Japanese public elementary schools,' *Educational Perspectives*, 43(1&2), pp. 38–45.

Papastylianou, A., Kaila, M., & Polychronopoulos, M. (2009). 'Teachers' burnout,
depression, role ambiguity and conflict,' *Social Psychology of Education*, 12(3), pp.
295–314.

Roloff Rothman, J. (2012). 'Looking for common ground: An investigation of motivational
strategies valued by ALTs and JTEs,' *Accents Asia*, 5(2), pp. 1–20.

Saito, B., Mimata, T., Homma, H., & Honda, T. (2020). 'Parents speak of pressure, concern
after sudden school closure request by Japan gov't,' *The Mainichi*, 28 February, viewed
8 December 2021, https://mainichi.jp/english/articles/20200228/p2a/00m/0na/036000c

Schmidt, S., Roesler, U., Kusserow, T., & Rau, R. (2014). 'Uncertainty in the workplace:
Examining role ambiguity and role conflict, and their link to depression—A meta-
analysis,' *European Journal of Work and Organizational Psychology*, 23(1), pp. 91–106.

Suzuki, R., Iizuka, Y., & Lefor, A.K. (2021). 'COVID-19 related discrimination in Japan:
A preliminary analysis utilizing text mining,' *Medicine (Baltimore)*, 100(36), p. 327105.
doi: 10.1097/MD0000000000027105

Wada, W. (1992). 'Tīmu tīchingu no kihonteki na kangaekata to igi,' in Suzuki, K (ed.),
Eigo Kyōiku Jissen Kōza Dai-1 Maki: AET to no Tīmu Tīchingu, Tokyo, ECOLA Eigoka
Kyōiku Jissen Kōza Kankōkai, pp. 8–12.

Wakui, N., Abe, S., Shirozu, S., Yamamoto, Y., Yamamura, M., Abe, Y., Murata, S.,
Ozawa, M., Igarashi, T., Yanagiya, T., Machida, T., & Kikuchi M. (2021). 'Causes of
anxiety among teachers giving face-to-face lessons after the reopening of schools during
the COVID-19 pandemic: A cross sectional study,' *BMC Public Health*, 21(1), pp. 1–10.
doi: 10.1186/s12889-021-11130-y

13 The Educational Impact of COVID-19 on Lone Mothers in the Global South

Aradhana Ramnund-Mansingh and Mariam Seedat-Khan

Introduction

The COVID-19 pandemic has severely impacted women, specifically lone mothers. Scientific research globally exposes a significant gap in research between South Africa (SA) and the Global South. Lone mothers, particularly those in lower socio-economic circumstances, do not merely experience the triple burden of work, family, and community but more profound challenges that underpin this triple burden. Although the chapter focuses on the experiences of lone mothers and the educational trajectory of their children during the pandemic, a holistic picture is portrayed, contextualising socio-economic and structural inequalities. It is vital to understand the background and context of the challenges faced. The chapter will explore pre-pandemic circumstances and intersecting challenges to COVID-19 about the educational journey of children from lone mothers. The content evaluates different countries within the Global South.

Contextualising the Environment

Countries in the Global South have been severely affected by the COVID-19 pandemic due to already entrenched historical vulnerabilities and contexts. These include a lack of or limited housing and access to essential services, healthcare, and formal employment. Other vulnerabilities which increase the risk are disability and poor mental health (Lancet, 2020). Lone mothers face most, if not all, of these vulnerabilities in different communities. In SA, for example, the living conditions of many rural lone-parent (mother) families result from the historical–political landscape of men taking up migrant jobs in other provinces. Current statistics during the COVID-19 pandemic are unavailable, with 2018 statistics being the latest published. The reported figures are likely to have increased significantly because of the pandemic. Women are more vulnerable to poverty, and in SA, for example, 74.8% of women-led households fall below the upper-bound poverty line (UBPL), which is indicative of a monthly income of 1,183 Rand ($70.90) (Stats SA, 2018). Geographic locations wedge more profound inequality as it differentiates access to fundamental services. 46% of children live with a lone mother, and 12% live with

DOI: 10.4324/9781003267133-17

neither of their parents. Limited access to electricity, water, sanitation, and housing intersects the impact on families. In 2017, 25.5% of children aged 0–6 years in female-headed households skipped one meal a week (Bittar, 2020; Stats SA, 2018). 'Poverty patterns continue to be gendered, and female-headed households are more likely to have low incomes, to be dependent on social grants, and less likely to have employed members' (Parry & Gordon, 2021, 797). The pandemic has exacerbated these conditions of hunger, food insecurity, lack of basic services, and loss of employment (Bittar, 2020).

Lone Mothers

The United Nations Women (2020) statistics reveal 1,01.3 million lone mothers globally. 'Family, the smallest social unit, is experiencing the impact, particularly for the woman as single parent. Being a single parent is either a choice, decision, or condition that must be accepted due to the spouse's passing or other condition' (Febrianto, 2021, p. 19). Lone mothers are a vulnerable group, who face social stigma and are therefore hesitant to reach out for support or financial assistance (Diaz-Serrano & Flamand, 2020). Lone mothers in Global South countries have been the most vulnerable group during the COVID-19 pandemic. 127,000 lone mothers globally are under the age of 18, while 3.8 million are under the age of 25 (Bhatt, 2020).

The context of the lone mother in SA engages several complexities, including conducting work on a migrant basis, reliance on neighbours and extended family for childcare, the loss of employment, instances of working from home and having to contend with challenges of securing internet connectivity and sharing small home spaces with homeschooled children during the pandemic. Lone mothers are responsible for childcare, schooling, and elder care in the home and community (Carli, 2020). 'Women in single-adult households experienced tremendous pressure and were haunted by the fear that they were failing in all the roles they had taken on' (Hertz, Mattes & Shook, 2021, p. 2041). The socially constructed expectations allow lone mothers to seek help from girl children, which continues the cycle of gender inequality (Parry & Gordon, 2021). This is clearly articulated in the Brazilian study by Leavy and Shabel (2022), where girls and young women aged 8–19 years were co-opted for their participation in childcare and other duties in and outside of the home. This also included girl children walking long distances to collect water for the house (Silva, Sales, Lanza, Heller & Rezende, 2020).

In India, approximately 45 million households are headed by lone mothers, of which 32 million live in extended families (Ghosh, 2020; United Nations Women, 2020). Assets and monies are controlled by male heads of the extended household, which disempowers women who are legally underage and living within a patriarchal constructed traditional family. However, in certain countries and communities, lone mothers are not permitted to engage in paid work, as they are responsible for domestic household chores and caring for elders and children (United Nations Women, 2020). In Korea, lone mothers experience severe discrimination and stigmatisation, as they are defined and measured against definitions of traditional family conceptualisations. These exclusions were specifically for lone mothers and not as much for lone fathers (Choi, Byoun & Kim, 2020).

Family Structures, Home Environment, and Childcare

A significant relationship between family structures and the educational attainment of children is evident (Asgari & Jazayeri, 2019; Bose-Duker, Henry & Strobl, 2020; Meng & Yamauchi, 2017; Schneider & Coleman, 2018; Grawe, 2018; Munje & Mncube, 2018). While definitions of family in the Global North and the Global South are evident, lone mothers in the Global South remain vulnerable. Schneider and Coleman (2018) found a parent's race, income, ethnicity, and education are linked to children's successful education. Supporting children academically via institutional activities impact positively on their success, career, and success as an adult.

The socio-economic narratives of lone mothers fail to align with traditional roles. Lone mothers are sole breadwinners, with multiple jobs, sustaining migrant labour. Lone mothers' limited education and finances fail to provide academic support. Time dedicated to both paid and unpaid employment limits the support required by children (Grawe, 2018; Munje & Mncube, 2018). Lone mothers can mobilise resources and support in marginalised communities for childcare and fundamental education resources. The impact of lone parenting and the absence of a dual income create physical and mental health strain, making academic support more difficult (Hall & Sambu, 2019).

Methodology Approach

This research provides a systematic review of literature on lone mothers' experiences during the COVID-19 pandemic. The focus is on countries in the Global South, and the context is the educational achievement of children in families with lone mothers during the pandemic. The authors make use of secondary desktop resources because of COVID-19 safety protocols. Additionally, access to vulnerable communities is limited, and with the burden of activity on the lone mother, qualitative interviews or narratives may be challenging and time constraining. Common methodological approaches during pandemic times include high-speed scoping reviews, strengths of recommendations, evaluation of various studies' raw data, and standards of research and reporting (Knottnerus & Tugwell, 2020). Data sources for this study were accessed online via scientifically recognised academic websites, including Google Scholar, SCOPUS, and EBSCO Host Research Platform. An extensive literature search was conducted in August 2021. The search included scientific, academic articles, media articles, and books about lone mothers' experiences during COVID-19. A general search of this nature gave the author context through the lens of a lone mother.

Eligibility Criteria

The challenges faced by mothers globally were somewhat similar but with varying intricacies depending on the geographic location of residence. It was important to understand the holistic experiences of lone mothers before attaching specific eligibility criteria. The constantly changing nature of the COVID-19 virus transformed knowledge production regarding government strategies and rollout, and socio-economic complexities, rapidly. Therefore, themes, keywords, and key phrases surrounding the essential concepts were highlighted in considering the eligibility criteria. These include *single mothers and COVID-19, Global South single mothers, children at university during COVID-19, women and COVID-19, and single mother challenges during COVID-19*. The words *lone* and *single* were used interchangeably. To contextualise the study, vulnerable groups of women and their challenges before and during the pandemic were also explored.

Selection Process

The researchers screened titles and abstracts. Literature review themes were split and independently reviewed by both researchers. Several discussions took place among the researchers to present reviews to each other. Articles, academic content, and studies were deselected based on a lack of suitability. This included shared parenting or traditional family models and studies from the Global North and developed countries.

Data Extraction

Data extraction focused on a comprehensive and systematic literature framework and outcomes related to lone mothers and educational experiences during the COVID-19 pandemic. Most of the studies had varied information, not all of which were pertinent to the study. Essential data were extracted and presented accordingly. The researchers extracted data addressing the criteria of these themes. An in-depth reading of data was explored, followed by abstracting and identifying themes to form the basis of the study.

Lone Mothers: Stressors and Challenges during COVID-19

Economic stress and food security were high among the stressors experienced by lone mothers in developing countries. For lone mothers in the Global South, job loss was a fear, especially since the unemployment rates were high, even before the COVID-19 pandemic in countries like SA (Fisher, Languilaire, Lawthom, Nieuwenhuis, Petts, Runswick-Cole & Yerkes, 2020; Graham, 2020). For example, lone mothers in Malaysia experienced severe challenges during the pandemic, which included the more significant burdens of 'financial insecurity, equity of children's education, job security, comfortable place to stay, utilities and food supply, in addition to other kinds of social protection aspects' (Rahman, 2021, p. 294). The studies on challenges experienced by lone mothers during the COVID-19 pandemic focus heavily on countries in the Global North. Abundant studies are available for Canada, the United Kingdom, Hungary, Germany, Italy, and various geographic locations in Europe and the United States (Council of Europe, 2021; Clark, McGrane, Boyle, Joksimovic, Burke, Rock & O'Sullivan, 2021; Kallitsoglou

& Topalli, 2021; Langmeyer, Guglhör-Rudan, Winklhofer, Chabursky, Naab & Pötter, 2022). While many challenges are mirrored for women in the Global North and South, the context is different. In developed countries, government policies and provisions are in place to support these women, such as social rented housing in the UK (Garthwaite & Patrick [eds.], 2022).

The themes identified as challenges for lone mothers in a Global South geographic location are isolation, home education, work stress, and the consequences of the virus.

Isolation

Isolation due to the initial lockdowns created challenges at various stages, as the lack of childcare support forced lone mothers to be parents primarily during this time (Daniels, 2020). Many lone mothers who worked from home had to perform unpaid domestic duties. Whilst children were at home, the lone mothers could not support their children from a comfort or resource perspective. The isolation circumstances negatively impacted the mental health of lone mothers, considering some mothers must work from home and perform domestic duties (Daniels, 2020). Lack of space in small dwellings and overcrowding also impacted negatively (Visagie & Turok, 2021). Families were living in homes or informal housing with sometimes two rooms to accommodate extended families. In certain situations, children who were based at university had to return home, and mothers had to also care for ailing and elderly parents or family members (Taylor, Bailey, Herrera, Nair & Adams, 2021). Lone mothers found their days exceedingly tricky, suffering from stress and anxiety and unable to create a boundary between paid work and domestic home duties. The lines between work and home have not been as blurred as during the pandemic and lockdown (Hertz, Mattes & Shook, 2021). Lone mothers expressed that they needed a break from the children to avoid conflicts of identity and the lash back from the children who were angered by what they viewed as a new competition for their mum's time and work (Hertz, Mattes & Shook, 2021). 'Disadvantaged families are the most severely affected, as they are at high risk of job loss and lack proper protection. The absence of institutional protections and interventions has created further economic and emotional hardships for these vulnerable families' (Lian & Yoon, 2020, p. 337). Jobs that were not compatible with online working were made redundant. This resulted in lone mothers who were the sole breadwinners losing their source of employment and income.

Home Schooling

Home schooling was a new concept to lone mothers and was *forced* upon them in a concise space of time. This proved challenging in two ways. Adult children also returned from higher education institutions, and lone mothers did not have the financial capacity to obtain resources to support their children in such a short time. Laptops or computers were shared between children or loaned from neighbourhood households and communities (Seedat-Khan & Ramnund-Mansingh, 2022). The latter was a COVID-19 infection risk leaving many mums with no alternatives.

Secondly, many lone mothers did not have the academic knowledge to support their children or to replace the teacher or lecturer for the specified time. Many vulnerable university students were the first generation in their families to attend university (Seedat-Khan & Ramnund-Mansingh, 2022). Therefore, the online school was one of the most significant strains on lone mothers as many did not have the educational capability to assist their children, the spatial divide between home schooling and working, and the lack or inability to secure resources.

Lone mothers experienced pandemic exhaustion while struggling to create boundaries between paid work and parenting (Taylor et al., 2021; Craig, 2020; Sahu, 2020; Hertz, Mattes & Shook, 2021). Therefore, lone mothers from vulnerable communities rely on an extended family support system for childcare and the school and university educators and infrastructure for support in this regard (Hertz, Mattes & Shook, 2021). 'Families differ in what they can offer, related to factors such as parental levels of education, poverty, physical and mental health, overcrowding, the availability of computers and adequate internet access to participate in distance learning' (Fisher et al., 2020, 250). Educational inequalities are stark in Global South countries. The study in Nigeria by Olaseni and Olaseni (2020) purports that children in households with lower socio-economic circumstances, lone mothers, or lack of parental education had little to no enforcement of educational tasks, thereby impacting children's educational attainment. Similarly, lone mothers had little to no education to support their children at home. Lone mothers view schools as enablers of socio-economic stability and growth. Lockdowns made it difficult to achieve this as children were held back a year or some completely dropped out of school (Daniels, 2020). In South Africa alone, the number of children who left school between March 2020 and July 2021 had tripled to 750,000 (Ndebele, 2022).

Some educational highlights are discussed below for varying countries in the Global South. This presents the context of lone mothers' challenges, recognising that lone mothers from vulnerable backgrounds do not know higher education systems, processes, or curriculum content to support their children. In Latin American countries, including Peru, Uruguay, Mexico, and Brazil, the experience of higher education transition was similar. Although varied legislation indicates preparedness for face-to-face, blended, and distance learning, the latter was not fully explored until the forced lockdowns. The challenges for students were a lack of poor digital infrastructure and a lack of knowledge of university academic requirements and processes. This fell on the shoulders of the lone mother, who was just as oblivious to this, creating feelings of maternal guilt and high-stress levels for both mum and child. Scenarios for countries in Asia, Russia, India, and China were like Latin America (Bozkurt, Jung, Xiao, Vladimirschi, Schuwer, Egorov, Lambert, Al-Freih, Pete, Olcott & Rodes, 2020).

Comparatively, countries in the Global North experienced the educational impact of the pandemic in a completely different manner. Challenges experienced by students and parents in these countries included the choice of online platforms or applications. They were supported by government-sponsored television channels and a network of family, friends, and community who had experience in higher education. These countries include the United States, the United Kingdom, Sweden, and Greece (Bozkurt et al., 2020). However, the challenges for education in Africa were more profound than those from the other Global South countries. 'Parents face (in normal times) disproportionate economic insecurity, difficulty meeting basic needs, and significant time and caregiving demands. 68% of parents of university students live in poverty' (Cruse, Contreras Mendez & Holtzman, 2020, p. 2). Although data infrastructure was a standard stumbling block, other associated challenges existed in SA and Namibia. Students relied on the National Student Financial Aid Scheme (NFSAS) for funding. In SA, this accounted for 730,000 students. The scheme provides a laptop for each student. Many students had not received funding when the countries locked down, and online deliverables were impeded. COVID-19 lockdown forced these children home with little to no support or infrastructure. Students in Ghana could not afford laptops or smartphones to continue with remote learning. Only private higher education institutions in Africa were prepared for the remote transition. In SA, of the 26 universities, 14 were unable to transition online due to infrastructure inadequacies (Bozkurt et al., 2020).

Young children and adults were stricken by fear and insecurity at the onset of COVID-19 and turned to lone mothers for support. Lone mothers negotiated for young adults to share community laptops. Financial insecurity and data costs in SA (Febrianto, 2021; Graham, 2020) intensified lone mothers' challenges. University attendance for first-year, first-generation students was daunting. The lone mother, unaware of university procedures and assessments with specialised modules, reduced their children's success. With over 11,000 rural schools in the country, many of these students feed into universities. These students are not computer literate as the rural schools are under-resourced, and language is also a barrier to learning (Seedat-Khan & Ramnund-Mansingh, 2022). All these factors exacerbated anxiety, stress, and depression for the lone mother and the children. The girl child university student had to make more sacrifices because boys were a preferred choice for using the community laptop. She also had to help with domestic chores. Lone mothers were ridden with guilt, severely impacting their mental health (Kallitsoglou & Topalli, 2021).

Work Stress

Lone mothers from vulnerable communities struggled the most in terms of paid employment. Women in part-time and temporary employment, including jobs like live-in domestic workers, found themselves without work and highly stressed. Lone mothers who worked from home experienced various challenges (Taylor et al., 2021) – finding a suitable workspace to set up a home office, navigating online platforms while fulfilling domestic chores, and supporting academics while working. A lone mother indicated,

> I am used to juggling as a single mom. You know, single moms, that's what we do, and we try to be good at it. But this pandemic forced me to juggle

even more. It felt like my personal and professional lives collided. And I felt stressed at times. And sometimes the day was not very smooth. And often there were headaches, and we would be finishing e-learning in the evenings or doing extra days.

Taylor et al. (2021, p. 6)

Lone mothers' distinct division of labour and historical financial insecurity demand constant management of paid and unpaid work (Clery, Dewar & Papoutsaki, 2021; Lu, Walker, Richard & Younis, 2020). Lone mothers experienced significant financial insecurity during the pandemic and became mentally and physically exhausted (Rahman, 2021).

Middle-class single mothers can pay for support, including domestic work and childcare assistance. These circumstances impacted lone mothers' mental health. They expressed anxiety, stress, and depression, which often manifested physically with headaches and body pain (Taylor et al., 2021). Choi, Byoun, and Kim (2020) advance that many lone mothers in South Korea had low-income jobs and experienced challenges working from home. Thirty-three per cent of women experienced little to no internet access. Depression and mental health were flagged as significant for women in South Korea, resulting from stigmatisation; they did not seek mental health support. 'Poorer parental mental health status is associated with the higher likelihood of child maltreatment' (Choi, Byoun & Kim, 2020, 678). Role overload and sleep deprivation will impact the lone mother's emotions and cognitive functioning (Gromada, Richardson & Rees, 2020).

Consequences of Contracting the Virus

Lone mothers had a grave fear of contracting the virus for several reasons. These included the risk of death, no support to assist with childcare, elder care, and domestic chores, and they were often the sole breadwinner in the home. This impact on mental health was for the same reasons in the event of a death. Countries with the highest deaths of lone parents were those in the Global South, including Brazil, India, and SA (Hillis, Unwin, Chen, Cluver, Sherr, Goldman, Ratmann, Donnelly, Bhatt, Villaveces & Butchart, 2021). This was attributed to limited healthcare and lack of access to basic services. This included little or no piped water in several areas with no infrastructure. This created a fear of contracting the virus and infecting the elderly and other family members.

Coping Mechanisms and Policy Recommendations

The virus's pervasive nature has negatively impacted people's mental health globally. Coping mechanisms were explained as optimism, happiness, and emotional closeness with family, friends, and romantic partners (Martínez, Valencia & Trofimoff, 2020). Lone mothers did not have the luxury of these coping mechanisms.

When strategies are advised from global levels, such as the United Nations, underdeveloped infrastructure, and conditions of countries in the Global South are not separately considered. 'Structural vulnerability determines where and how people live, extending beyond physical structures to shape the everyday conditions of labour and daily life produce ill-health, and social exclusion and discriminatory attitudes discourage access and undermine health care' (Team & Manderson, 2020, 672). The COVID-19 pandemic lay bare these differences with the underfunded and overburdened healthcare systems in these countries (Williamson, 2020). Lone mothers are invisible to policymakers and not consulted or included in policy-making processes. There needs to be a two-pronged strategy to support lone mothers. These include prioritising her mental health and reviewing her challenges via narratives to address them from a policy perspective. For example, suppose employees are allowed flexible-time arrangements. In that case, this 'might be insufficient for single parents during a pandemic. Child allowances or partly state-subsidised paid leave should be considered in such circumstances' (Gromada, Richardson & Rees, 2020, p. 9). The understanding of individual lived experiences will inform specific policy recommendations to support lone mothers in vulnerable environments.

Conclusion

This chapter focused on lone mothers from vulnerable backgrounds experiencing structural inequalities and gendered intersections. The debates on COVID-19 implications and impact on lone mothers are significant. They are stigmatised by communities, face financial challenges, work in more than one low-paid job, and manage unpaid domestic responsibilities. Inadequate access to suitable housing, running water, electricity, sanitation, and basic healthcare is common for lone mothers in the Global South. Their socially constructed gendered role sustains the subjugation of women. The pandemic, national safety protocol, and lockdowns intensified living conditions made worse by home schooling and childcare. Despite overwhelming evidence of resilience, evidence of declining mental health challenges, fear of contracting COVID-19, and physical illnesses intensified. Lone mothers experienced guilt, unable to provide academic support.

References

Abd Rahman, N.H. (2021). The impact of the COVID-19 pandemic and policy response on single-parent families in Malaysia. *Fulbright Review of Economics and Policy1*(2), pp.286–302

Asgari, Z. and Jazayeri, R.A. (2019). The parent-child relationship in high school girl students' academic achievement in mother-headed families: A qualitative research. *Journal of Family Psychology*, 5(2), pp. 3–14.

Bittar, A. (2020). 5 facts about poverty in South Africa, Borgen project. Retrieved [online] at: https://borgenproject.org/poverty-in-south-africa/

Bhatt, A. (February 2020). Expert's take: By undercounting single mothers, we underserve families. Retrieved [online] at: https://www.unwomen.org/en/news/stories/2020/2/experts-take-antra-bhatt-on-single-parent-households

Bose-Duker, T., Henry, M. and Strobl, E. (2020). Children's resource shares: Male versus female-headed households. *Journal of Family and Economic Issues*, 42pp. 1–13.

Bozkurt, A., Jung, I., Xiao, J., Vladimirschi, V., Schuwer, R., Egorov, G., Lambert, S., Al-Freih, M., Pete, J., Olcott Jr , D. and Rodes, V. (2020). A global outlook to the interruption of education due to COVID-19 pandemic: Navigating in a time of uncertainty and crisis. *Asian Journal of Distance Education*, *15*(1), pp. 1–126.

Carli, L.L. (2020). Women, gender equality and COVID-19. *Gender in Management: An International Journal* 35 (7/8), pp. 647–655.

Choi, S., Byoun, S.J. and Kim, E.H. (2020). Unwed single mothers in South Korea: Increased vulnerabilities during the COVID-19 pandemic. *International Social Work*, *63*(5), pp. 676–680.

Clark, S., McGrane, A., Boyle, N., Joksimovic, N., Burke, L., Rock, N. and O'Sullivan, K. (2021). "You're a teacher you're a mother, you're a worker": Gender inequality during COVID-19 in Ireland. *Gender, Work & Organisation*, *28*(4), pp. 1352–1362.

Clery, E., Dewar, L. and Papoutsaki, D. (2021). *Caring without Sharing: Single Parents' Journeys through the COVID-19 Pandemic – Final Report*. Gingerbread. Retrieved at: https://www.gingerbread.org.uk/policy-campaigns/publications-index/caring-without -sharing-final-report/ [accessed 29 July 2021].

Council of Europe. (2021). The COVID-19 pandemic and children: Challenges, responses, and policy implications – Updated 12 March 2021. Retrieved [online] at: https://rm.coe .int/covid-19-factsheet-revised-eng/1680a188f2

Craig, L. (2020). *COVID-19 has Laid Bare How Much We Value Women's Work & How Little We Pay For It*. Retrieved [online] at: https://womensagenda.com.au/latest/covid -19-has-laid-bare-how-much-we-value-womens-work-how-little-we-pay-for-it/

Cruse, L.R., Contreras Mendez, S. and Holtzman, T. (2020). Student parents in the COVID-19 pandemic: Heightened need & the imperative for strengthened support. # C492. Institute for Women's Policy Research.

Daniels, D. (2020). Reimagining parents' educational involvement during the COVID-19 lockdown. *Southern African Review of Education with Education with Production*, *26*(1), pp. 134–147.

Diaz-Serrano, L. and Flamand, S. (2020). Schools' attitudes towards single parents: Experimental evidence, IZA Discussion Paper No. 13699. Retrieved [online] at: https:// ssrn.com/abstract53695400

Febrianto, P.T. (2021). Single mothers' survival strategies of university students during COVID-19 pandemic. *Society*, *9*(1), pp. 19–36.

Fisher, J., Languilaire, J.C., Lawthom, R., Nieuwenhuis, R., Petts, R.J., Runswick-Cole, K. and Yerkes, M.A. (2020). Community, work, and family in times of COVID-19. *Community, Work & Family*, *23*(3), pp. 247–252.

Garthwaite, K. and Patrick, R. eds. (2022). *COVID-19 Collaborations: Researching Poverty and Low-Income Family Life during the Pandemic*. Great Britain: Policy Press.

Ghosh, M.R.C. (2020). Single mothers, the magically powered unicorns of their kids! Retrieved   [online]   at: https://moumitarcghosh.medium.com/single-mothers-the -magically-powered-unicorns-of-their-kids-c68bb1f30b36

Graham, L. (2020). Pandemic underscores gross inequalities in South Africa, and the need to fix them. *The Conversation*. Retrieved [online] at: https://theconversation.com /pandemic-underscores-gross-inequalities-in-southafrica-and-the-need-to-fix-them -135070

Grawe, N.D. (2018). *Demographics and the Demand for Higher Education*. Baltimore: JHU Press.

Gromada, A., Richardson, D. and Rees, G. (2020). Childcare in a global crisis: The impact of COVID-19 on work and family life. UNICEF Office of Research. Retrieved [online] at: http://www.cokmed.net/ps-sistem/dosyalar/kutuphane/Childcare%20in%20Global %20Crisis%20-%20Impact%20of%20Covid-19%20on%20Work%20and%20Family %20Life.pdf

Hall, K. and Sambu, W. (2019). Demography of South Africa's children. *South African Child Gauge*, pp. 216–220 http://www.childrencount.uct.ac.za/uploads/publications/ South%20African%20Child%20Gauge%202018_Children%20Families%20and%20the %20State.pdf#page=134.

Hertz, R., Mattes, J. and Shook, A. (2021). When paid work invades the family: Single mothers in the COVID-19 pandemic. *Journal of Family Issues, 42*(9), pp. 2019–2045.

Hillis, S.D., Unwin, H.J.T., Chen, Y., Cluver, L., Sherr, L., Goldman, P.S., Ratmann, O., Donnelly, C.A., Bhatt, S., Villaveces, A. and Butchart, A. (2021). Global minimum estimates of children affected by COVID-19-associated orphanhood and deaths of caregivers: A modelling study. *The Lancet, 398*(10298), pp. 391–402.

Kallitsoglou, A. and Topalli, P.Z. (2021). Coping with home-schooling and caring for children during the UK COVID-19 lockdown: Voices of working mothers. pp.1–17. https://doi.org/10.21203/rs.3.rs-333649/v1

Knottnerus, J.A. and Tugwell, P. (2020). Methodological challenges in studying the COVID-19 pandemic crisis. *Journal of Clinical Epidemiology, 121*, pp. A5–A7.

Lancet, T. (2020). Redefining vulnerability in the era of COVID-19. *Lancet (London, England), 395*(10230), p. 1089.

Langmeyer, A.N., Guglhör-Rudan, A., Winklhofer, U., Chabursky, S., Naab, T. and Pötter, U. (2022). Resources of families adapting the COVID-19 pandemic in Germany: A mixed-method study of coping strategies and family and child outcomes. *Journal of Family Research, 34*(1), pp. 333–366.

Leavy, P. and Shabel, P.N. (2022). Childcare and participation in the Global South: An anthropological study from squatter houses in Buenos Aires. *Third World Thematics: A TWQ Journal*, pp. 1–16. https://doi.org/10.1080/23802014.2021.2008268

Lian, B. and Yoon, S.Y. (2020). Burdens, resilience, and mutual support: A comparative study of families in China and South Korea amid the COVID-19 pandemic. *Journal of Comparative Family Studies, 51*(3–4), pp. 337–346.

Lu, Y.C., Walker, R., Richard, P. and Younis, M. (2020). Inequalities in poverty and income between single mothers and fathers. *International Journal of Environmental Research and Public Health, 17*(1), p.135.

Martínez, L., Valencia, I. and Trofimoff, V. (2020). Subjective wellbeing and mental health during the COVID-19 pandemic: Data from three population groups in Colombia. *Data in Brief, 32*, p. 106287.

Stats SA. (2018). Mbalo Brief the missing piece of the puzzle.). Pretoria. Retrieved [online] at: http://www.statssa.gov.za/wp-content/uploads/2018/03/Mbalo-Brief-March-2018 .pdf

Meng, X. and Yamauchi, C. (2017). Children of migrants: The cumulative impact of parental migration on children's education and health outcomes in China. *Demography, 54*(5), pp. 1677–1714.

Munje, P.N. and Mncube, V. (2018). The lack of parent involvement at the hindrance in selected public primary schools in South Africa: Educators' voices.

Ndebele, L. (2022). Rate of school dropouts tripled in SA due to Covid-19 – Unicef report. Retrieved [online] at: https://www.news24.com/news24/africa/news/rate-of-school -dropouts-tripled-in-sa-due-to-covid-19-unicef-report-20220331

Olaseni, V.M. and Olaseni, A.O. (2020). Covid-19 pandemic: Impact of socio-demographic factors and parent's life orientation on enforced learning in pupils during lock-down in Nigeria. *Cape Comorin, 2*(4), pp. 34–39.

Parry, B.R. and Gordon, E. (2021). The shadow pandemic: Inequitable gendered impacts of COVID-19 in South Africa. *Gender, Work & Organisation, 28*(2), pp. 795–806.

Sahu, P. (2020). Closure of universities due to coronavirus disease 2019 (COVID-19): Impact on education and mental health of students and academic staff. *Cureus, 12*(4) pp.2–6.

Schneider, B. and Coleman, J.S. eds. (2018). *Parents, their children, and schools.* New York: Routledge.

Seedat-Khan, M. and Ramnund-Mansingh, A. (2022). The sociology of a COVID-19 virtual university. Chapter 20. In Harsingh Gour, U.R. and Govender, J. *Exploring the Consequences of the COVID-19 Pandemic: Social, Cultural, Economic, and Psychological Insights and Perspective.* India: Taylor and Francis.

Silva, B.B., Sales, B., Lanza, A.C., Heller, L. and Rezende, S. (2020). Water and sanitation are not gender-neutral: Human rights in rural Brazilian communities. *Water Policy, 22*(1), pp. 102–120.

Taylor, Z.E., Bailey, K., Herrera, F., Nair, N. and Adams, A. (2021). Strengths of the heart: Stressors, gratitude, and mental health in single mothers during the COVID-19 pandemic. *Journal of Family Psychology*36(3), p 346.

Team, V. and Manderson, L. (2020). How COVID-19 reveals structures of vulnerability. *Medical Anthropology, 39*(8), pp. 671–674.

United Nations Women. (2020). Expert's take: By undercounting single mothers, we underserve families. Retrieved [online] at: https://www.unwomen.org/en/news/stories/2020/2/experts-take-antrabhatt-on-single-parent-households [accessed 27 September 2021].

Visagie, J. and Turok, I. (2021). Rural–urban inequalities amplified by COVID-19: Evidence from South Africa. *Area Development and Policy, 6*(1), pp. 50–62.

Williamson, E. (2020). What comes after COVID-19. *Somatosphere.* s/l: s/p. Disponível em http://somatosphere. net/forumpost/what-comes-after-covid-19.

Part V
Migration

14 Women's Memories in Brazilian Pandemic Times

Narratives of Migrants to Reframe Histories

*Fernanda Coelho Liberali, Viviane Letícia
Silva Carrijo, Daniela Aparecida Vieira,
Joyce Suellen Lopes Dias, and
Vanessa Cristina da Cunha Caires*

Introduction

The social scenario designed by the COVID-19 pandemic revealed the colours of inequalities and injustices committed against precarious workers, Black, indigenous people, immigrants, homeless people, women, and older people, groups pushed to the margins of society, 'left to live death in life' (Liberali, 2020). Santos (2020), when analysing this scenario, argues that 'every pandemic is always discriminatory,' mainly because 'it only exacerbates a crisis to which these groups have been subjected in the socio-historical-cultural and political-economic space-time of the South'. This concept is 'the metaphor of unjust human suffering caused by capitalist exploitation, besides racial and sexual discrimination' (Santos, 2020,p.16)[1]

Such a metaphor reveals the separation of humanity into two groups, i.e., a group of humans – worthy of rights and justice – and a group of sub-humans – historically inferior and disposable. A concrete example of these abyssal exclusions is the murder of Congolese Moïse Kabagambe in Rio de Janeiro on 24 January 2022 – a young man beaten to death for daring to request his employers for his late payment. This crime fuels the abyssal exclusion of the Global South in an analogy to slavery and the super-exploitation of work, in addition to reinforcing the elements of racism experienced by Black migrants in Brazilian lands. This scenario shows the abyssal line also hinders migration in Brazil. Haitians, for example, have been migrating to the country significantly since 2010, when an earthquake of catastrophic proportions hit Haiti. The population, which increased in number from 595, in 2010, to around 60,000 between 2010 and 2015 (Oliveira, 2017) in Brazil, and its 'forced migration' status – granted to those searching for survival – was not covered by the protection of refugees' law (Santos and Lima Júnior, 2018), as Haitians are not codified by the conventional refugee systems present in the 1951 Convention or the Convention from Cartagena. Due to the lack of jurisdiction to serve Haitian migrants and to reduce, or at least to circumvent

DOI: 10.4324/9781003267133-19

this problem, the National Immigration Council (CNI in Portuguese), through Normative Resolution nº. 97, on 12 January 2012, granted this group the humanitarian visa, issued by the international recognition of the post-earthquake severe situation (Baptistela, 2018).

Within such a complex migration situation, this chapter analyses the narratives of women, Haitian migrants, who are part of the Global South and, therefore, experience injustice, discrimination, social exclusion, racism, and sexism. Historically, these women were born into a world with stigmatised female roles in which social injustices culminate in stolen identities and lives. In the pandemic context, women became more susceptible to unemployment, informality, and domestic violence, as well as being even more involved in unpaid care work, and, when in transit, became more vulnerable to the actions and abuse of men (Annoni, 2020; Bergallo et al., 2021). When discussing the conditions of Haitian women, in addition to the aggravating factors described, there is the ethnic–racial/colour variable that corroborates the accentuation of inequality in Brazil – a country with ingrained racism in its social structure. According to Souza et al. (2020), Black Haitian immigrant women are generally poor and underemployed with competitive disadvantages due to cultural and linguistic adaptation, racism, and access to information, with little knowledge of their rights in Brazilian territory.

This chapter aims to discuss the narratives of women, two Haitian migrants, during the COVID-19 pandemic times. The chapter first presents the role of narratives in reframing histories, describing the context and methodological procedures for developing the research project from which this chapter derives in the sequence. Finally, it discusses the data and raises considerations about how these narratives support the development of new possibilities for survival for all.

Narratives to Reframe History

This section discusses the role of narratives in recovering memories as tools for the collective reconstruction of histories. Therefore, it discusses the concepts of counter-hegemonic narratives that dialogue with the concepts of memories and *perezhivanie* to reinforce the desire to leverage the voices of Haitian migrant women who seek, above all, to be heard within their social experiences. Being in this position gives these women, according to Collins (2016), a world perspective that goes beyond the orthodox; these Black women express their existence from experiences within the structures, from a non-place in a society shaped by the paradigms of white men, acting as tools for reframing history. The narratives enable the voices of others to be heard as they expose truths that have been denied, repressed, and kept as secrets (Kilomba, 2019).

It is noteworthy that this chapter brings narratives collected in interviews that cannot be seen only from the individual point of view. They are intertwined with the country's policies, ideologies, and cultures. It is within this process that it becomes possible to reframe our society regarding social justice, as pointed out by hooks (2020). In this sense, women's narratives enhance the subversive force of remembering suffering (Martín-Baró, 1998), possibly leading to the overcoming of presentism through access to the historical facts of their community since it allows minorities to understand the causes of their secular oppression.

Such a cathartic process involves 'an affective contradiction' that causes 'conflicting feelings and leads to the short-circuiting and destruction of these emotions' (Vygotsky, 1971, p. 213). In this context, Vygotsky (1994) uses the word *perezhivanie* to express the role of affect and drama in framing and interpreting human experience; that is, it expresses the transformational process in the struggle to live through a dramatic experience or trauma. In *perezhivanie*, environmental factors or experiences with others are refracted and help shape development. Understanding catharsis in 'the stage of life' then presumes people experiencing everyday drama as part of their engagement with society. So, in this chapter, we aim to reflect on narratives of memories of women as a cathartic stage of life that both created development and can become potent instruments for other people's development.

These memories, then, are viewed as models of anti-oppressive practice and intervention through stories of resistance and survival. Initially, they may be seen as vivid experiences of individuals. Gradually, they become a more collective vision of what happened to them. That is why, according to Moane (2009), historical memory, together with awareness, and radical social change, can play an essential role in addressing and transforming inequalities and social injustices.

Methodological Choices

This chapter is a partial discussion of the data collected for a Thematic Project 'Memories of migrants in the pandemic: narratives of resistance in confronting racism,' which aims to investigate, with young migrants from public schools in São Paulo, the possibilities of facing racism and social injustices they have experienced. The project involves producing interviews that are turned into narratives with the stories of migrants about their educational possibilities to face racism, social injustices, and the COVID pandemic. Regarding the methodological proposal, this project is grounded on Critical Collaboration Research (Magalhães, 2011), which is based on the intentional transformation of contexts with the involvement of all the participants. This methodology assumes that the process of transformation and collective engagement creates new shared and collaborative solutions that respond to the demands of subjects and their communities. Most of the interviews were conducted with students of CIEJA Perus I (Integrated Centre for Youth and Adults Education) which is Perus, a peripheral region of São Paulo. It is an institution of the municipal public education network and consists of one of the modalities of Youth and Adult Education (EJA) in this municipality. The target audience of EJA is formed by teenagers (from 15 years old onwards), young people, adults, and older people who could not start or finish their studies in the so-called 'right age' due to Brazil's marked history of social inequality.

At CIEJA Perus I, there are approximately 1,300 students, and almost all of them live in a situation of high social vulnerability. Between them, there are about 700 Haitian students. Brazilians believe and are believed to be welcoming towards migrants – a country that welcomes everyone. However, regarding migrants from impoverished countries, this receptivity is not the same, which is even more notice-able when the migrant is Black, as is the case with Haitian CIEJA students.

The interviews were mostly videotaped or audiotaped to compose the narra-tives and focus on a narrative structuring of migrants' memories. The narrativised interviews were analysed, interpreted, and transformed into collective accounts to denounce situations of racism and to propose didactic practices that can overcome them. For this chapter, two stories were the basis for discussing women, migration, racism, and education and how these accounts can create community histories of resistance based on collective memories to be used with critically and engaged students with a liberating quality. The interviews selected for this chapter were conducted by Daniela Vieira, one of the educators from CIEJA Perus I.

In this context, the two migrant women were selected for the first interviews of the project because of their close connection with Daniela. Flore (25 years) and Sergine (30 years) were born in Haiti, and they emigrated to São Paulo in 2019. At the time of the interview (2021), they were students at CIEJA. Their narratives were chosen since they materialised some of the main situations expressed by the groups of migrant women who have integrated the project. Besides, they were the two interviews that initially structured the narratives used by the researchers as initial triggers for many conversations and interviews with other migrants. The interviews with the students focused on the following guiding questions:

• How did you arrive, and what led you to move to Brazil?
• What was the period of the pandemic for you?
• What difficulties and possibilities did you experience?
• How did you get/create access to education?
• In the pandemic, did you feel changes in access to education, health, food, etc.? If yes, how was it?
• What financial support did you have during the pandemic?
• What was education like in Haiti?
• What was/is education like in Brazil before and during the pandemic?
• How did you survive all this?

Discussing Data

This section presents the stories of two migrant women whose histories were marked by Haiti's tragic ecological and historical problems, the need for migration movements, racism, gender discrimination, and the COVID-19 pandemic. Arne (2022), a Haitian graduate in International Relations who lives in Brazil and is a student at CIEJA Perus I, denounces social injustices with Haitian migrants liv-ing in Brazil and their struggles to deal with learning Portuguese as an additional language (AL). Like the study presented here and Arne's chapter, many other researchers discuss the role of schools, and learning Portuguese is seen as essential to the process of overcoming oppression (Vieira and Liberali, 2022).

Both socially and individually, these dramatic events can be seen as examples of *perezhivanie* once they were responsible for transforming the students' life histories, as expressed in the following discussion. These aspects were paramount for students' resistance, reframing histories from hegemonic paradigms which express diverse forms of living and existing in the world.

Two Haitian Women Students on the Move

The two migrant women presented their life histories, wishes, and desires. Both came alone to Brazil, looking for better living conditions.

Sergine

In the interview, Sergine described that, in Haiti, many children, teenagers, and adults could not read, which she associated with the increase in violence in the country: 'They stay on the streets, at home, without knowing how to read or write. They do not get a job (…), so they steal. They do not have a degree.' Education access remains a huge problem in Haiti since 20% of children up to 15 years are illiterate with the scarcity of public and unpaid schools. In many instances, educational access was not by merit but by political indication. The lack of job opportunities is characterised by a 15% unemployment rate in 2020, according to Trading Economics. Despite the 29% decline in 2018, the murder rate was 6.6 per 100,000 population, identical to Afghanistan. She explains that a few can enter Higher Education since there are more private, costly, charged-in-dollar schools than public ones. In her case, she could only start her undergraduate studies with the financial support of her relatives. Once an engineering student, she dropped out of the course after not finding job prospects in her future career.

To arrive in Brazil, she faced a move by bus, plane, and boat. At first, she had difficulties getting a job, but she worked as an administrative assistant in São Paulo at the time of the interview. She said it was very hard initially because she did not have any money to pay her rent, and she knew nobody who could help her. She knew that even with her diploma in hand, she would not be able to find work in her field, as she would have to master the local language: 'Finding a job was hard, extremely hard, because of racism. Sometimes you get to a place where people do not pay attention to other things. They look at your face everywhere you go, and they treat you badly. This is hard.' The way Sergine is treated in Brazil like 'the other' refers to what Kilomba (2019) discusses about white people who look at the migrant woman and see everything they create about the Black people histori-cally. She is seen as the different other – an enemy, this created racial enemy, an antagonist. Being new in the country and not knowing the language turned her life unbearable.

She was firm in saying that she wants to go back to Haiti to help families there: 'do something there for the other families and then return here.' However, to visit and help because, in her opinion, 'crime will not end there' because the children face too many problems and violence: 'People have expected crime to end for many years; however, it does not end, it only gets worse day by day.' This also happens in Brazil, not like in Haiti, but the oppressive historical treatment that Black people receive in Haiti and Brazil is structural, forged in the colonisation of the Americas and the modernisation of Europe. Moïse's case, referred to in the introduction of this chapter, epitomises such a history of brutality. Nevertheless, most of the time, these people and stories are neglected because the pain of the Black population is only considered when they politically affect the lives of white subjects, the ones who hold power (Kilomba, 2019).

Sergine repeatedly uses 'hard' to express her move to Brazil and her life in the country. However, she elucidated that all countries face difficulties, but she expresses the power of her resistance, explaining that one must always be positive and face problems using books and stories as instruments to keep fighting:

> Yes, there will be a problem, there is a problem with studying, speaking a language, or crime, but one must be positive. You must stay confident, but you also must continue reading and learning. A book can change your whole life until the end of your life. The first and greatest of all these books is the Bible, but there are other books that can also help a lot of people (…) because life is a struggle. (…) To grow, you must go through the fights, face the problems, and then there will be a light for you. You must be positive.

These dramatic movements can be seen as *perezhivanie* through voicing these hardships and resistance. Recovering these memories seems to suggest that she could look at her stories as ways to reconstruct her self-realisation and awareness (Martin-Baró, 1996), and her strength to survive. Such strength speaks to what Collins (2016) pictures as an outsider from within. Black women have always had this 'no place' in society – being inside the houses yet invisible. With this, they built paths to see themselves in this society and understand ways of dealing with and, possibly, transforming it.

During the pandemic, Sergine had little opportunity to work and could barely feed herself. She had no relatives in Brazil and received help from Haitian relatives. She explained that it was difficult because 'many things were closed, and the school was closed; we did not have access to the basic food basket.' According to her, 'It was difficult to eat and find a job.' Besides, the hospitals did not give the patients any help. Sergine says that if one immigrant got sick even before the pandemic, the hospital staff did not pay much attention. And to make things worse, the staff did not understand them because of language concerns and left them aside. So, when she needed help in the Emergency Room, they gave her little support and left her aside. She would eventually return home.

Flore

In similar circumstances, Flore interrupted the nursing course in the third year due to difficulties in paying her monthly fees. Encouraged by her stepfather, she searched for a new opportunity in another country. Flore was treated like 'a little princess' in her home country: 'In Haiti, I wouldn't do anything. My mother did everything for me.' In her memories, Flore would only sleep, eat, and take baths. However, she thinks it was unfair to her mother, who worked very hard for her and her siblings. According to the migrant student, her mother 'raised her children alone, without a father.' Although Flore loved her country, she said that one does not live well in Haiti, even with money, she had to move: 'Life in Haiti is very risky because there is a lot of insecurity.' As mentioned previously in Sergine's history, the criminality rates are very high in Haiti, despite the drop in the last report.

Since arriving in Brazil, Flore has suffered a lot because she can only find informal jobs where her condition as a Black migrant woman is despised. Initially, she lived with some girlfriends but was currently living with her boyfriend, an engineer who had arrived from Haiti in 2021. Her boyfriend was already working as a bricklayer's helper in Brazil and, although his present undervalued occupation was different from his qualifications, at least he could find a job. As expressed by Annoni (2020), Bergallo et al. (2021), and Tonhati and Macêdo (2021), it is possible to recognise that Flore's boyfriend had more opportunities in getting a job than her. Even having just arrived in Brazil, he already managed to get a job, an aspect that had escaped her possibilities so far.

Her life with Brazilians has not been easy at all. She has faced racism in its most brutal form. Her impressions and experiences as a Black migrant woman were refracted through *perezhivanie* and helped shape who she has turned into. Flore got a job delivering flyers at traffic lights. In Haiti, as a nursing student, she would never do it. As an immigrant, she saw no problem. However, many people did not take the leaflet, closed the window, and feared her. She cried and felt ashamed: 'The worst thing about street work is racism because many people close their car windows when we approach.'

She explained that she had cried a lot since arriving in Brazil:

Being a migrant is not something very easy. Getting in a different land, with a different culture, different language. Then you need to start to say … Being a migrant sincerely is not an easy thing. Maybe you can think: 'are they talking bad about me?' when I cannot understand something: 'Are they calling me names?'

The drama of taking a position considered inferior was not significant at first because she needed the money, and it was part of what she saw as possible for her. However, the reaction of the others, the way they despised her and were afraid of her, made her realise the story from a different perspective, which is stigmatised by social patterns. This account resonates with the danger of a single story, as Adichie (2019) pointed out regarding her experience as an African woman in the USA. Black people are villains of a story they did not write.

Despite these hardships, Flore would not return to her country. In her country, people think she is rich, which makes life more dangerous because some groups may kidnap her: 'If you're moving up in life, they'll hate you and kill you.' She intends to continue as an immigrant but aims to seek new opportunities in the USA: 'I love my country, but I don't want to go back. I love Brazil, but it's hard to make money here. If I go to the USA, I can send more money to my family.' The idea of the USA as the promised land seems to be reproduced in her speech when it is also well known how badly treated migrants and Black people are in that country. However, it also refers to her resistance and searches for better living conditions.

Besides, she also pointed out how much sorrow Haitian families have suffered and explained that she wanted to bring her whole family to Brazil or return there, but she understood that this is impossible right now. The student presents the awareness that the situation is not an individual problem but a social one that is part of everyone's life. Even though the situation is hard, Flore discussed picturesque Brazilian characteristics such as soccer and expressed how much she liked Brazil. Her tone of voice was happy, contrasting with all the sorrow and sad stories she reported and emphasising her strength to keep resisting and moving forward.

Flore had many projects when she arrived in Brazil, but they were postponed due to the pandemic. With emergency aid, a benefit granted by the federal government, she got the minimum necessary for her survival, such as paying rent and eating. She said:

> I can say that … the pandemic … I had a lot of projects, I wanted to take a course, I was working, and then the pandemic arrived … it stopped … I wanted to pay for my college, then it stopped … Then I just stayed at home, and I'm glad the government gave me emergency aid, which helped me a lot. I stayed at home; you must pay rent, you must eat, you must do everything.

The pandemic ended many of Flore's dreams and created a gap that was hard to fulfil. Besides, she feared becoming infected with COVID-19 in hospitals, and for this reason, she preferred to self-medicate and pray. She coped with her life issues the better she could:

> It was a challenging period, you know? I can say yes that I lost my right to study. Also, sometimes when I feel sick like I might get a headache, I want to go to the hospital, but I'm afraid. What if I go and I get the covid? So … I feel sick, but I pray and take dorflex medication to get rid of the pain … that's all.

Reflections on Narratives

The narratives of these migrant women describe a universe in that they may never have consciously reflected upon the need for racial justice and the elimination of prejudice against poor, Black migrant women. Their memories dialogue with Chimamanda's when she arrived in the USA. Due to the stereotypes created and different histories of colonisation, experiences of being Black in Brazil and the USA are quite different from Haiti and Nigeria. In countries such as Brazil and the USA, where there has been a long period of enslavement, being Black carries all the stereotypes that the word brings with it, making it difficult to recognise our humanity (Adichie, 2019).

Despite the economic difficulties presented in Haiti, Flore and Sergine lived the experience of being Black women in a primarily black country. In Brazil, Sergine feels these difficulties when looking for a job and because she still faces challenges in communicating in Portuguese: 'Having difficulty with the language closes doors.' On the other hand, Flore had a comfortable life, living with her mother and not having to dedicate herself to household chores. To survive in Brazil, she had to deliver pamphlets at traffic lights, which she would not do in her country. These experiences reflect social violence and lack of opportunity, a reality in large Brazilian capitals such as São Paulo and racism since Haitian immigrants are mostly Black.

Seeking social justice seems more difficult for poor Black migrant women as expressed by Tonhati and Macêdo (2021) about the role of women in migration movements and the complete invisibility they suffer. They represent the susceptibility of unemployment, race, and gender. The stories of their leaving their countries and the fears they face in the new society are part of the dramatic life they live and the ways they find to cope with a harsh reality. Their stories are intertwined with so many others and embody memories of dreams and sufferings that help visualise ways to cope with difficulties.

Their memories also represent the tragedy that faced the world during the most stressful moments of the pandemic which in Brazil was expanded by the lack of care for the vulnerable, so food insecurity, resulting from widespread social inequality, structural racism, and xenophobia became the main concern of their school. Students managed to find in their school a place of resistance and support. During the first six months of the pandemic, schools struggled and collectively worked to get food and support for their students and families since the government only implemented some actions after that, which lasted until the end of 2021.

In this chapter, migrant women's voices, as proposed by Collins (2016), create a counter-hegemonic construction of knowledge permeated by diversity and, simultaneously, similar situations because of its endemic and permanent connections with racism and ecological devastation. Their histories create potent means for constructing a different future (Martin-Baró, 1996, 1998).

Conclusion

This chapter aimed at analysing the narratives of women Haitian migrants, who experience injustice, discrimination, social exclusion, racism, and sexism, and as suggested by Martin-Baró (1996), transform their sufferings into subversive forces to overcome pain. The courage to seek better living conditions in a country with such a different culture is a virtue to be highlighted. The two interviewees left a country historically in civil conflict, aggravated by successive natural disasters, and arrived in Brazil alone, without someone who could support them. Both found in CIEJA a welcoming and resistant space, in addition to a learning environment. They, who had already started university education in Haiti, recognised the importance of seeking education in Brazil and understanding the importance of mastering the local language. The school contributed significantly so that the migrant women and so many other immigrant students could see that, even amid vulnerability, they are reversing the oppressive logic by continuing to study and helping to build the country where they chose to live.

Aware of secular oppression, society becomes responsible for designing processes of overcoming it through the search for ancestry, cultures, and experiences of diverse people and their memories. Despite the social injustice, inequalities, and racism faced during the Brazilian pandemic times, the courage expressed by these migrant women, from the Global South, in search of life, and life in expansion, can be connected to the scene from one of Evaristo's short story *We Agreed Not to Die* (2016): 'I don't know why the fear, thought Bica. If only fear made me retreat; on the contrary, I advance more and more in proportion to this fear. It's as if fear were courage in reverse: fear, courage, fear, courage–fear, and courage–fear of pain and panic'.

Note

1   In the original: 'a metáfora do sofrimento humano injusto causado pela exploração capitalista, pela discriminação social e sexual' (Santos, 2020, p. 16).

References

Adichie, C. N. (2019). *O perigo de uma história única*. São Paulo: Companhia das Letras.

Annoni, D. (2020). Mulheres migrantes e pandemia: vulnerabilidades sobrepostas diante da securitização internacional de fronteiras. In: Baeninger, Rosana et al. (Eds.). *Migrações internacionais e a pandemia de COVID-19*. Campinas: Núcleo de estudos de população "Elza Berquó" (Nepo/Unicamp).

Arne, C. (2022). Haiti, história e motivos que provocaram a migração do povo haitiano. In: Vieira, D. and Liberali, F. C. (Orgs.). *Português para imigrantes: denunciando injustiças sociais*. Campinas, SP: Pontes Editores, 29–40.

Baptistela, T. (2018). A problemática da tutela jurídica dos refugiados ambientais no Brasil: análise da concessão do visto humanitário concedido pelo Conselho Nacional de Imigração. *Revista Direito em Debate*, 27(49). doi: 10.21527/2176-6622.2018.49.156-176.

Bergallo, P., et al. (2021). The impacts of Covid-19 on women's economic autonomy in Latin America and the Caribbean. *UNDP LAC C19 PDS*, , 25.pp 1–32

Collins, P. H. (2016). Aprendendo com a outsider within: a significação sociológica do pensamento feminista negro. Tradução: Juliana de Castro Galvão. *Revista Sociedade e Estado*, 1(1), pp 99–127.

Evaristo, C. (2016). *Insubmissas Lágrimas de Mulheres*. 2. ed. Rio de Janeiro: Malê.

hooks, b. (2020). *Ensinando Pensamento Crítico: sabedoria prática*. São Paulo: Elefante.

Kilomba, G. (2019). *Memórias da plantação: episódios do racismo cotidiano*. Tradução: Jess Oliveira. 1. ed. Rio de Janeiro: Cobogó.

Liberali, F. C. (2020). Construir o inédito viável em meio a crise do coronavírus-lições que aprendemos, vivemos e propomos. In: Liberali, F. C., et al. (Eds.). *Educação em tempos de pandemia: brincando com um mundo possível*. Campinas, SP: Pontes Editores.

Magalhães, M. C. C. (2011). Pesquisa crítica de colaboração: escolhas epistemo-metodológicas na organização e condução de pesquisas de intervenção no contexto escolar. In: Magalhães, M. C. C. and Fidalgo, S. S. (Eds.). *Questões de método e de linguagem na formação docente*. Campinas, SP: Mercado de Letras.

Martín-Baró, I. (1998). *Psicología de la liberación*. Madrid: Trotta.

Martín-Baró, I. (1996). O papel do Psicólogo. *Estudos de Psicologia*, 2(1), pp. 7–27. Available in: https://www.scielo.br/j/epsic/a/T997nnKHfd3FwVQnWYYGdqj/?format =pdf&lang=pt. Access in: 06 February 2021.

Moane, G. (2009). Reflections on Liberation Psychology in Action in an Irish Context. In: Montero, M. and Soon, C. (Eds.). *Psychology of Liberation*. New York: Springer.

Oliveira, W. (2017). Haitianos no Brasil: Hipóteses sobre a distribuição espacial dos imigrantes pelo território brasileiro. *FGV DAPP*. Available in: http://dapp.fgv.br/ haitianos-no-brasil-hipoteses-sobre-distribuicao-espacial-dos-imigrantes-pelo-territorio -brasileiro. Access in: 01 February 2022.

Santos, B. (2020). *A cruel pedagogia do vírus*. São Paulo: Boitempo Editorial.

Santos, G. and Lima, Júnior, J. B. (2018). Refugiados no brasil: caracterizando as novas faces pelo país. In: Annoni, D. and Lysian, C. V. (Eds.). *O direito internacional dos refugiados e o Brasil*. Curitiba: Gedai/UFPR.

Souza, J., Heidemann, I.T.S.B., Pitilin, E.B., Bitencourt, J.V.O.V., Vendruscolo, C., Brum, CN. (2020). Determinantes sociais da saúde de mulheres imigrantes haitianas: repercussões no enfrentamento da Covid-19. *Revista Eletrônica Enfermagem*, 22. Available in: https://doi.org/10.5216/ree.v22.64362. Access in: 9 May 2021.

Tonhati, T. M. P. and Macêdo, M. (2021). Os impactos da pandemia de Covid-19 para as mulheres imigrantes no Brasil: mobilidade e mercado de trabalho. *Sociedade e Estado*, 36., pp 891–914.

Vieira, D. and Liberali, F. C. (Orgs.). (2022). *Português para imigrantes: denunciando injustiças sociais*. Campinas, SP: Pontes Editores.

Vygotsky, L. S. (1971). *The Psychology of Art*. Cambridge, MA: MIT Press.

Vygotsky, L. S. (1994). The problem of the environment. In: Van Der Veerand, R. and Valsiner, J. (Eds.). *The Vygotsky Reader*. Oxford: Blackwell.

15 Impact of COVID-19 on Policy and Support Services for Migrant Women Experiencing DV in Semi-Rural Areas of the UK

Loreen Chikwira and Alicja Blada Edgeley

Introduction

Gender and migration studies show that more women are migrating as international labour migrants on their terms, leading to a feminisation of migration (Kofman, 2020; Tittensor and Mansouri, 2017). Although the term migrant is contested (see the Migration Observatory), we use it to refer to first-generation migrant women who have settled in Britain for family, education, work, and leisure, and in Britain, they are often included in the category of ethnic minorities. The Migration Observatory data shows that in 2019, girls and women constituted 52% of international migrants in the UK. The migrant women are settling in an environment that is increasingly hostile because of political and social debates on immigration in the UK with certain narratives attributed to migrants and their contribution (or lack of) to the British economy (Thompson et al., 2013). These narratives position migrants and their cultures as counter and a threat to British values (Anthias, 2012). Within this context, the migrant women also face gendered specific challenges related to the labour market, immigration, integration, and access to support services.

Research on Domestic Violence and Abuse (DVA) against migrant women and their ability to access services has included a focus on social and cultural factors (Mahapatra, 2012), immigration policies and their impact (see Women's aid's report on the Migrant Victims of Domestic Abuse – Review Findings of July 2020, Domestic Abuse Bill 2020), and DVA policy design and implementation in different geographies (Mackenzie, Conway, Hastings, Munro, and O'Donnell, 2015). Findings and recommendations from the studies have led to third-sector support services, defined by The National Audit Office to include voluntary and community organisations, social enterprises, and co-operatives to make significant strides to demonstrate the diverse factors contributing to DVA (McKenzie et al., 2015). Understanding these factors has led to structural changes and multi-agency approaches to supporting families affected by DVA and acknowledging the women's complex needs (Frazer and Hutchings, 2020).

Recent studies during the pandemic show that an increasing number of migrant women experienced domestic abuse and the pandemic exacerbated existing issues

DOI: 10.4324/9781003267133-20

(Krishnadas and Taha, 2020). Both current and earlier research focused on specific geographical areas, i.e., urban areas, bringing the voices of women in these locations and the work being undertaken by services to address the specific needs of the women. We assert that within this research, there is a lack of critical analysis of the factors contributing to fewer migrant women accessing support from mainstream services within some rural areas of England where there is an increase in migrant settlements and dispersal of asylum seekers and refugees. Moreover, an examination of the impact of COVID-19 on policy and support services for migrant women experiencing domestic violence in semi-rural areas is important considering the current UK Domestic Abuse Act (2021), which has made significant changes to how victims are supported by the justice system in accessing protection orders, the prosecution of perpetrators, and a new statutory definition of DVA, which emphasises different types of abuse. These are only a few changes that the Act makes to offer more support to victims of DVA.

In this analysis, we aim to identify challenges that third-sector services faced supporting migrant women experiencing DVA during the pandemic in the semi-rural area of Cheshire East. We also discuss the impact of these challenges on service provision and make recommendations to improve policy and service provisions. The chapter starts with a discussion on migrant population settlements in rural/semi-rural areas of the UK over the last 10–15 years to provide context for the analysis. This will be followed by an examination of the effects of the pandemic on migrant women experiencing DVA. The discussion section and the conclusion will follow the methodological section.

Minority Ethnic and Migrant Populations in Rural England

Estimates of the migrant population, mainly from EU countries in rural areas of England, have increased over the last 20 years due to employment opportunities within the manufacturing, service industry, and agricultural sector (Neal, Gawlewicz, Heley and Jones, 2021; Storey, 2013). Data from the Migration Observatory shows that there are more than three million EU migrants who live in the UK. The figures have dropped due to Brexit and related consequences on migrants' lives. Non-EU migrants still form a majority of the UK migrant population with new settlements of asylum seekers and refugees dispersed in new areas (Alfano,Dustmann and Frattini, 2016; Office for National Statistics, 2021). The migrants often find themselves in low-paying jobs and may have to deal with poor living conditions, racism, and exclusions (Neal et al., 2021), which in turn affect their ability to access services if needed.

Figure 15.1, derived from the Statistical Digest of Rural England report (2021), provides an example of a detailed comparative analysis of minority populations between urban and rural areas in England between 2016 and 2020. Overall, Black African, Caribbean, or Black British groups are the smallest population within the rural areas. Conversely, the population of Chinese, Arabs, and other ethnic groups has increased over the same period.

It is important to note that population data on Eastern Europeans are not included in these statistics. Additionally, the categories used for the different ethnic groups

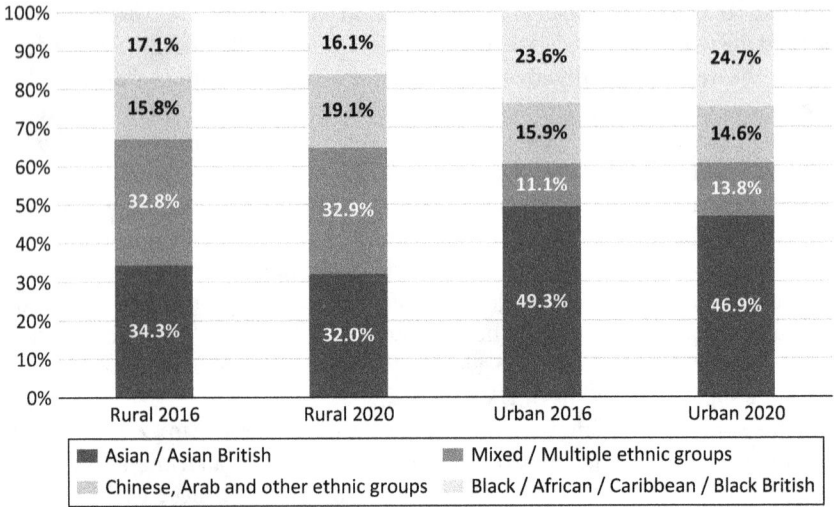

Figure 15.1 Detail for all minority ethnic group population in rural and urban areas, England, 2016 and 2020. Source: Department for Environment Food and Rural Affairs: The Statistical Digest of Rural England report (2021).

are too general and do not capture the nuances of identity and experiences for those categorised. Like the national rural migrant population statistics, Cheshire East is a rural county with a diverse migrant population with a higher population of Eastern Europeans, mainly Polish migrants. The strong economic situation in the UK, a plethora of jobs, and higher wages have always been a highly attractive push factor for EU migrants (Janta, 2011; Pemberton and Scullion, 2013; Harris et al., 2012). Some of the migrations are seasonal and temporary, which is important when one considers the intersectional factors concerning experiences of DVA and seeking support. For non-EU migrants, Cheshire East is a settlement region with migrants with diverse immigration statuses, refugees, and asylum seekers.

COVID-19, Migrant Women, and Domestic Abuse

A review of current literature shows that during COVID-19 and related lockdowns, there was an increase in the number of reported domestic violence cases against women in the UK (Safe Lives report, 2020-2021). In Cheshire, local news reports show that domestic abuse cases doubled during the pandemic, with local organisations like My CWA supporting more families than before (see Macclesfield news Hub, posted: 17.02.21 by James Kelly), job loss and related stress, and forced cohabitation contributed to these increased numbers (Vieira et al., 2020). Figure 15.2, published by the Office of National Statistics (ONS), summarises the percentages of adults (16–74) who experienced domestic abuse and violence by ethnicity and sex from April 2018 to March 2020. The data was collected from the Crime

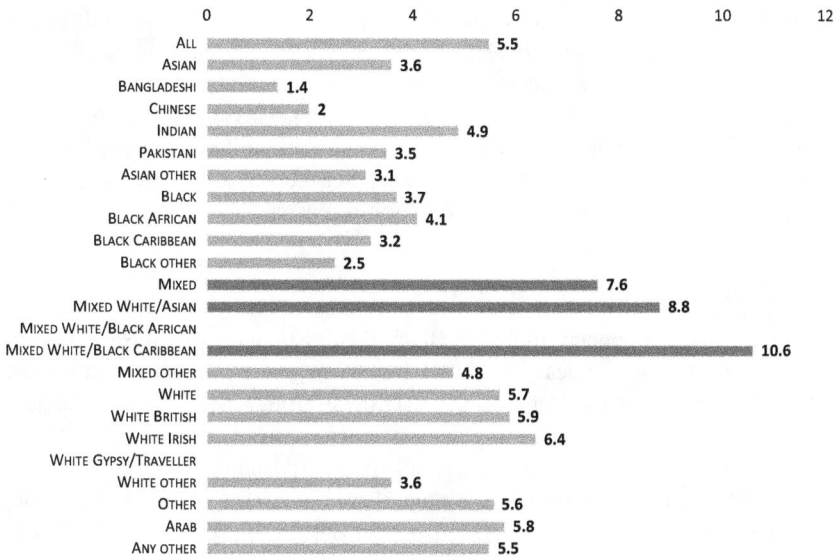

Figure 15.2 Percentage of 16–74 year-olds who reported being victims of domestic abuse.

Survey for England and Wales, which used questionnaires, and data from the criminal justice system across different police force areas of the UK. The reports show that in the year ending March 2020, 5.5% of people aged 16–74 years in England and Wales experienced domestic abuse with women being more likely than men to experience Domestic Violence and Abuse.

Overall, the data shows that relative to the populations of the different ethnic groups, the percentage of minority ethnic individuals who experienced DVA was more than their white counterparts. However, these figures are based on reported cases of DVA incidents, and the real numbers are unknown. It is also important to note that the sample sizes in the data were not consistent across the different groups. Additionally, the data does not further break down the different ethnicities within the broader categories and does not differentiate between those who are migrants and those who are British-born residents.

The UK Domestic Abuse Act enacted in 2021 has significantly changed the current legislation on how domestic abuse cases are dealt with and how victims are supported. Of significance are changes to what constitutes domestic abuse, the framework for how domestic abuse is addressed and the responsibilities of statutory organisations within each locality. Nevertheless, women's organisations, i.e., Sisters for Change, the Refugee Council, and the Step-Up Migrant Women (#SUMW), a coalition of more than 50 minority ethnic organisations, and human rights organisations have criticised the Act for not fully addressing specific issues related to the complexities of immigration and its effect on some of the migrant women's experiences of domestic abuse and the support available to them. For example, women who have No Recourse to Public Funds (NRPF) cannot access housing and some benefits when they flee domestic abuse. In Cheshire East, once a victim of domestic abuse reports the case to the police, it simultaneously goes through the local area's hotline where staff determine the case seriousness, and condition of the victims. The victims are then signposted to relevant support services. This single point of contact and ways of supporting and protecting victims and their children are only open to those who report or have the cases reported on their behalf. Although victims can, some victims may not report the cases for various reasons.

Intersectionality as Theory and Praxis

Intersectionality is a concept rooted in Black Feminism and Critical Race Theory (CRT) and provides a critical lens to analyse how gender, intersects with race, class, and other structural factors to reveal ways through which discrimination, exclusions, and oppression of marginalised communities occur within different contexts (Collins and Blige, 2016; Crenshaw, 1991; Lombardo and Rolandsen Agustin 2016; Rogers, 2020). For example, there are studies on DVA in lesbian, gay, and transgender relationships (Donovan and Barnes, 2020; Janice and Ristock, 2011), and gender-based violence and policy making (Gill, 2018). The studies show that women face complex challenges because of various sociocultural, political, and economic factors that position them in multiple complex ways resulting in challenges in reporting DVA and accessing support from services (Femi-Ajao, Kendal, and Lovell, (2018; Siddiqui, 2018). We employ intersectionality as an analytical framework to examine how third-sector support services recognise and have responded to the complex intersections of gender, ethnicity, immigration status, culture, religion, and other factors to support migrant women who are victims of DVA effectively.

Intersectionality also enables us as minority women (British Polish and British Zimbabwean) to write in ways that locate us as insiders and outsiders of the groups and services we are examining. Feminist scholars Hill Collins (2000) and Harding (2004) highlight the importance of women's vantage point of social reality and their locations within the interstices of the different spaces they occupy. As such, in this analysis we occupy spaces as migrant women and as professionals who have extensive experience working with organisations supporting migrant groups in Cheshire for 10+ years in various roles: one as a counsellor and clinical supervisor and another as a researcher and academic who has worked professionally with different organisations on addressing inequalities within policy and service delivery. The roles have given us insight into the challenges that migrant women face in semi-rural areas. We acknowledge that the concept of intersectionality is not a finished work; instead, it continually is shifting its boundaries.

Data Collection

Autoethnography is a data collection method which utilises researchers' experiences to examine a phenomenon within its sociocultural context (Ellis and Bochner,

2000). It challenges notions of objectivity, experience, and scientific knowledge production and emphasises 'subjectivity and researcher-participant intersubjectivity' (Foster, McAllister, and O'Brien, 2006, p. 47). Reflexivity is also central to autoethnography, and there are different ways of reflecting and writing the analysis. We employ collaborative autoethnography, which allows the researchers to examine their experiences and locations within the work from their standpoint. Collaborative autoethnography is about the collective interrogation and reflexive analysis of the researchers' experiences (Chang, Ngunjiri and Hernandez, 2016). The process of generating data and themes included the researchers meeting several times to reflect on our experiences and writing them up. This was followed by more reflection meetings, data collection, and generating themes. These themes were then grouped together into main themes and subthemes.

To further understand experiences of services during the pandemic, workshops were planned with two organisations, Women's Aid and My CWA that support families experiencing DVA in Cheshire. The two organisations were chosen because of the researchers' connections and understanding of their work. Unfortunately, due to the challenges of the pandemic and staff shortages, only one workshop was conducted with My CWA and only three staff members were able to attend, who included the service manager and two senior practitioners. My CWA is one of the main support services in the locality, working with the police, local authority, and other voluntary and national organisations to support families experiencing DVA and contribute to national policies. Ethical guidelines for conducting research were followed, including sharing information sheets highlighting the purpose of the workshop, issues of confidentiality, storage, and use of the data.

The workshop was divided into three themes including identifying the challenges that support services have faced during the pandemic in relation to supporting migrant women experiencing domestic violence, exploring how well-existing support services can address migrant women's needs and examining how services can develop evidence base to ensure that they are effective in targeting the needs of migrant victims. Due to the previous work with the organisations, we were aware of the challenges they faced engaging and working with minority communities pre-COVID-19 and we were able to have in depth discussions and reflections on the impact of the pandemic on their engagement. The discussions were recorded, analysed, and themes generated. Themes from the discussions were compared to the themes generated from autoethnographies to identify areas of similarity and differences because of the pandemic considering the recommendations from the Domestic Abuse Act (2021).

Discussion

A comparison of themes from the workshops and those generated by the authors highlighted two main challenges that underpinned some of the issues that the organisation faced during the pandemic. For example, their limited knowledge of where the migrant community groups were and lack of responses from the communities they contacted. We suggest that these issues are a result of lack of trust and communication with the long-standing communities. Themes generated were focused on:

i. Challenges of engagement and relationship building.
ii. A focus on national priorities that may not translate to local needs.

Challenges of Engagement and Building Relationships

On the question of the challenges that the organisation faced supporting migrant women experiencing domestic violence during the pandemic, conversations were preceded by a discussion on how the pandemic has intensified the disconnect between the service and migrant community groups. Unfortunately, the findings show that although the pandemic significantly affected families in various ways, discussions with My CWA demonstrate that COVID-19 has exacerbated already existing issues of engaging with minority and migrant groups in the locality. For example, organisations like My CWA relied on specific individuals (mainly from minority communities) to help them connect with communities. The heavy reliance on individuals meant that they did not build on the connections and establish their own relationships with communities. This has resulted in fewer self-referrals and a reliance on referrals through multi-agency work. At the time of the discussions, there were no clear plans on how to improve engagement post-pandemic.

One of the major issues in building relationships with minority and migrant communities is the lack of skills and knowledge on how to engage with the diverse, often termed 'hard to reach communities.' Community engagement is central to effective policy development and delivery of services. It includes participation and the ability of individuals to shape services (Smith, 2008). 'Hard to reach' communities are a contested term commonly used in the healthcare sector when discussing public participation in service design and delivery for the marginalised (Flanagan and Hancock, 2010). We assert that the notion of hard to reach is also based on narratives that define migrants in ways that problematise their cultural practises and based on the idea of their lack of integration. Furthermore, scholarship on the integration of migrants in rural areas is often framed within an idealised rurality and the place of the migrants within these spaces (Neal, 2013). The idea of being hard to reach has been challenged by both the communities and minority organisations that work with them, as it puts the onus on the groups to change and absolve the organisations from taking responsibility.

The lack of engagement with migrant groups is a long-standing issue within the area, as there are no visible community groups that the organisations can easily approach. Pre-COVID-19, some of the work we were involved in was around supporting both statutory and third-sector services to build better relationships with migrants and the importance of their inclusion in designing and delivering services. In the workshop, we once again had to share our knowledge of community groups and the migrant population in the area to help the staff in attendance.

Unlike the urban areas, where they have established community groups and voluntary organisations whose work is focused on supporting minority ethnics, for example, a good search on minority ethnic/migrant organisations groups in London, Manchester, or Liverpool show a plethora of organisations that work with minority women, similar google searches for rural areas like Cheshire East yield fewer numbers of organisations. There are advantages to providing specific support services to a community group; a report by Imkaan (2014), a UK-based Black feminist women's organisation dedicated to supporting Black and Minority Ethnic women experiencing DVA found that minority ethnic and migrant women prefer to seek specialist support from organisations run by minority women because they feel heard and safe. The organisations provide expertise to the specific groups they support and have more knowledge on the intersections of gender with culture, religion, and immigration policies on women's experiences.

We argue that building relationships with migrant communities creates a bio-dimensional communication channel where the organisations learn about the communities and how they can better support and work with them. There are cases where the service has successfully worked with a minority group, for example, through working with a Polish charity, the My CWA established a successful Polish DVA helpline to support those affected by domestic abuse. They further created social groups for Polish families experiencing domestic violence facilitated by the families themselves. Although such initiatives are important and a step in the right direction, the provision of such services is within the context of Brexit and the racialisation of Eastern Europeans and increased hate crime (Lumsden, Goode, and Black, 2019). These issues further create barriers to migrants seeking help. Moreover, there are 102 languages spoken in Cheshire East (Cohesion and Integration in Cheshire East Report, 2021). The question is, what happens to the other diverse migrant groups who may not have the resources to start a charity or a community group specifically for their nationality, especially if they do not speak English very well? This can lead to disparities in service provision across different migrant groups. It is worrisome when third-sector support services, like My CWA, continue to struggle to engage with marginalised communities and deprive them of opportunities to inform and shape policy and service design.

A Focus on National Priorities at the Expense of Local Contexts

In 2015, Cheshire East was part of the government's funded Syrian vulnerable person resettlement programme, the programme provided a multi-agency approach to supporting and settling the families across Cheshire. Part of the support provided by My CWA involved helping the families understand the different forms of DVA and how to access support if needed. A similar scheme was created for Afghan refugees. These national programmes drive the focus of local authorities and partners, who then must demonstrate how they are addressing them. One of the main challenges that organisations face is how to balance Government-led national priorities with local needs. Campbell (2021) conducted a qualitative study with 25 practitioners and professionals on their understanding of the drivers of DV and how they saw their own efforts impacting on DV; factors impacting multi-sectoral collaboration; and the relevance of feminism to their work/activism. The participants in the study included professionals who worked in the public sector (policymakers, police, social services, housing), the health sector (GP, psychiatrist, counsellors), the third sector (women's, men's, and children's charities), feminist organisations, and faith-based organisations. They found that one of the challenges of the effective delivery of services was the issue of top-down programmes, driven by government policies which they argue failed to consider local priorities. How can organisations, like My CWA, utilise the skills and learning from delivering on refugee and asylum seekers national programmes to better support existing migrant families and victims of domestic violence?

Other national priorities that have driven local activities are the issue of coercion and forced marriages amongst South Asian communities. These areas of focus do merit their prioritisation, we suggest that they may be at the cost of balancing national priorities with the local needs of migrant women, especially when one considers the lack of engagement with different migrant communities. We further note that the focus on specific migrant groups results in intersectional hypervisibility of one and invisibility of others. Ryland (2013) describes hypervisibility as where one is scrutinised based on perceived differences which may be interpreted as deviant and result in othering. The individual is then put under scrutiny and their failures are magnified and they have no control over how they are perceived. In this case, the South Asian women and their cultures are perceived as deviant, and they are viewed as victims needing to be saved. This has a significant impact in a context where the organisations do not have relationships with the communities where they can work with them to better understand their cultures and provide effective support.

One of the priorities of the new Domestic Abuse Act is the responsibility of local authorities and partners to create governing boards that develop and oversee implementation of DVA strategies locally. Each local partnership board has representation from different areas of health, policing, voluntary, and community sector. In Cheshire East, My CWA leads the domestic abuse partnership, and we suggest that the partnership provides an opportunity for support services to critically review their offer and address some of the issues they have faced supporting migrants during the pandemic. The reviews must focus on how they need to address barriers that make it challenging for victims to seek support, especially in cases of immigration and employment statuses that affect victims of domestic abuse. Findings and recommendations are then made central to the implementation of the Domestic Abuse Act (2021).

As migrant women ourselves, our starting point of discussion is the notion that the women are experts in their lives and use sociocultural and socio-economic resources available to them for resistance and survival. This is very important when discussions about DVA among migrant communities are shaped by fixed ideas on how their cultures and religions promote domestic abuse. Working with these communities from that approach helps services better understand how to use their cultural and religious resources to tackle domestic violence. We suggest that frontline workers should be equipped with cultural and social competency so that they are not afraid to reach out to communities and ask questions regarding the requirement for support for DVA in migrant households. Additionally, there needs to be an understanding of the intersections of gender, ethnicity, culture and religion, and immigration status, but also how these sites work to marginalise women, particularly, the way their locations as the 'other' is heightened in rural settings.

Conclusion

There is sparse research on migrant women's experiences of domestic abuse in rural areas, particularly, there are fewer studies on third-sector support services and some of the ways through which they create barriers to victims of domestic abuse accessing support. We demonstrated how a lack of engagement with migrant communities has a far-reaching impact on raising awareness of DVA and the ability of the women to trust the service and access support. We recognise that in Cheshire East, there is a lack of registered ethnic minority charities and active community groups that services can work with and increase their knowledge and understanding of the needs of diverse communities. This analysis is a starting point to ensuring that the issues are fully considered in the implementation of the Domestic Abuse Act (2021). Going forward third-sector organisations need to first find innovative ways of engaging with migrant communities, to build trust, and to provide support that is considerate of their social locations. Professionals working with migrant women can improve their knowledge by understanding how the migration process affects individuals' responses to engagement with DVA support. This can be achieved by listening to the women and working with minority ethnic voluntary organisations from other areas who have experience and expert knowledge engaging with migrant communities. Lastly, they need to recognise some of the narratives that are damaging to the effective delivery of services to migrant women in rural areas like Cheshire East. It is crucial to acknowledge these factors and the impact of migration on all people so that those affected by DVA can freely access the ongoing support they require

References

Anitha, S. (2022). Domestic violence during the pandemic: 'By and for' frontline practitioners' mediation of practice and policies to support racially minoritised women. *Organization Journal*29(3), 460–477. Doi.org/10.1177/13505084221074039.

Alfano, M., Dustmann, C. and Frattini, T. (2016). Immigration and the UK: Reflections after brexit. In *Refugees and Economics Migrants: Facts, Policies and Challenges*

Anthias, A. (2012). Transnational mobilities, migration research and intersectionality: Towards a translocational frame. *Nordic Journal of Migration Research*, 2(2), pp. 102–110. DOI: 10.2478/v10202-011-0032-y

Donovan, C. and Barnes, R. (2020). Help-seeking among lesbian, gay, bisexual and/or transgender victims/survivors of domestic violence and abuse: The impacts of cisgendered heteronormativity and invisibility. *Journal of Sociology*, 56(4), pp. 554–570.

Campbell, C. (2021). When the personal is not political: Experiences of collective agency amongst participants in the domestic violence response in London, UK. *Critical Public Health*, 31(3), pp. 280–292. DOI: 10.1080/09581596.2021.1874296.

Chang, H., Ngunjiri, F.W. and Hernandez, K.C. (2016). *Collaborative Autoethnography*. Oxon: Routledge.

Local Government Association. (2021). Report on Cohesion and Integration in Cheshire East. https://lginform.local.gov.uk/reports/view/lga-research/lga-research-cohesion-and -integration?mod-area=E06000049#Introduction. Accessed 17 May 2023.

Crenshaw, K. (1991). Mapping the margins: Intersectionality, identity politics, and violence against women of colour. *Stanford Law Review*, 43(6), pp. 1241–1299. DOI: 10.2307/1229039

Department for Environment Food and Rural Affairs: The Statistical Digest of Rural England Report. (2021). https://assets.publishing.service.gov.uk/government/uploads/ system/uploads/attachment_data/file/1043495/10_Statistical_Digest_of_Rural_England _2021_December_edition.pdf

Domestic Abuse. https://www.ethnicity-facts-figures.service.gov.uk/crime-justice-and-the -law/crime-and-reoffending/domestic-abuse/latest

Donovan, C. and Barnes, R. (2020). Help-seeking among lesbian, gay, bisexual and/ or transgender victims/survivors of domestic violence and abuse: The impacts of cisgendered heteronormativity and invisibility. *Journal of Sociology*, 56(4), pp. 554–570. DOI: 10.1177/1440783319882088.

Ellis, C. and Bochner, A. (2000). Autoethnography, personal narrative, reflexivity: researcher as subject. In Denzin, N.K. and Lincoln, Y.S. (eds.), *Handbook of Qualitative Research* (2nd ed.). London: Sage Publications, pp. 733–768.

Femi-Ajao, O., Kendal, S. and Lovell, K. (2018). A qualitative systematic review of published work on disclosure and help-seeking for domestic violence and abuse among women from ethnic minority populations in the UK. *Ethnicity & Health*. DOI: 10.1080/13557858.2018.1447652.

Foster, K., McAllister, M. and O'Brien, L. (2006). Making the personal, political—Using autoethnography as a method in mental health nursing research. *International Journal of Qualitative Methods*, 5(3), pp. 1–89. https://doi.org/10.1177/160940690600500303.

Frazer, E. and Hutchings, K. (2020). The feminist politics of naming violence. *Feminist Theory*, *21*(2), 199–216. https://doi.org/10.1177/1464700119859759.

Flanagan, S.M. and Hancock, B. (2010). 'Reaching the hard to reach' – Lessons learned from the VCS (voluntary and community Sector). A qualitative study. *BMC Health Services Research*, 10, p. 92. DOI: 10.1186/1472-6963-10-92.

Gill, A. (2018). Survivor-centered research: Towards an intersectional gender-based violence movement. *Journal of Family Violence*, 33, pp. 559–562. DOI: 10.1007/s10896-018-9993-0

Harding, S. (2004). *The Feminist Standpoint Theory Reader: Intellectual and Political Controversies*. 1st Edition. Routledge Publications.

Harris, C., Moran, D. and Bryson, J.R. (2012). EU accession migration: National insurance number allocations and the geographies of polish labour immigration to the UK. *Royal Dutch Geographical Society KNAG*, 103(2), pp. 209–221.

Hill Collins, P. and Blige, S. (2016). *Intersectionality (Key Concepts)*.Cambridge: Polity Press.

Hill Collins, P. (2000). *Black Feminist Thought: Knowledge, Consciousness, and the Politics of Empowerment* (2nd ed.). New York: Routledge.

Imkaan. (2014). *Supporting Black and Minority Ethnic Women and Girls: 10 Top Things for Commissioners of Ending Violence against Women and Girls' Services to Consider Summary*. London: Imkaan.

Janta, H. (2011). Polish migrant workers in the UK hospitality industry. *International Journal of Contemporary Hospitality Management*, 23(6), pp. 803–819.

Kofman, E. (2020). Unequal internationalisation and the emergence of a new epistemic community: Gender and migration. *CMS*, 8, p. 36. DOI: 10.1186/s40878-020-00194-1

Krishnadas, J. and Taha, S.H. (2020). Domestic violence through the window of the COVID-19 lockdown: A public crisis embodied/exposed in the private/domestic sphere. *Journal of Global Faultlines*, 7(1), pp. 46–58.

Lombardo, E. andAgustin, L. (2016). Intersectionality in European Union policymaking: The case of gender-based violence. *Politics*, 36(4), pp. 364–373. DOI: 10.1177/0263395716635184

Lumsden, K., Goode, J. and Black, A. (2019). 'I will not be thrown out of the country because I'm an immigrant': Eastern European migrants' responses to hate crime in a semi-rural context in the wake of Brexit. *Sociological Research Online*, 24(2), pp. 167–184. DOI: 10.1177/1360780418811967

Macclesfield news Hub. Posted: 17.02.21 by James Kelly. https://macclesfield.nub.news/n/domestic-violence-cases-double-in-cheshire-during-pandemic

Mackenzie, M., Conway, E., Hastings, A., Munro, M. and O'Donnell, C.A. (2015). Intersections and multiple 'candidacies': Exploring connections between two theoretical perspectives on domestic abuse and their implications for practicing policy. *Social Policy and Society*, 14(1), pp. 43–62. DOI: 10.1017/S1474746414000244

Mahapatra, N. (2012). South Asian women in the U.S. and their experience of domestic violence. *Journal of Family Violence*, 27, pp. 381–390.

Neal, S., Gawlewicz, A., Heley, J. and Jones, R.D. (2021). Rural Brexit? The ambivalent politics of rural community, migration and dependency. *Journal of Rural Studies*, 82, pp. 176–183.

Neal, S. (2013). Transition culture: Politics, localities and ruralities. *Journal of Rural Studies*, 32, pp. 60–69. https://doi.org/10.1016/j.jrurstud.2013.04.001.

Pemberton, S. and Scullion, L. (2013). The policies and politics of managed migration: Exploring mature labour migration from central and Eastern Europe into the UK. *Journal of Ethnic and Migration Studies*, 39(3), pp. 443–461.

Ristock, J.L. (Ed.). (2011). *Intimate Partner Violence in LGBTQ Lives.* 1st Edition. Routledge. DOI: 10.4324/9780203828977

RogersM. (2020). Domestic violence and abuse and hidden groups. In: Ali P., McGarry J. (eds) *Domestic Violence in Health Contexts: A Guide for Healthcare Professions.* Springer, Cham. DOI: 10.1007/978-3-030-29361-1_8.

Ryland, M. (2013, August 8). Hypervisibility: How scrutiny and surveillance makes you watched, but not seen [Tumblr blog]. Retrieved from http://thebodyisnotanapology.tumblr.com/post/57763238146/hypervisibility-how-scrutiny-and-surveillance.

Safe Lives Imapct Report. (2020–2021). https://safelives.org.uk/sites/default/files/resources/SafeLives_Impact%20Report%202020%E2%80%9321_Digital_A-compressed.pdf.

Siddiqui, H. (2018). Counting the cost: BME women and gender-based violence in the UK. *IPPR Progressive Review*, 24 (4), Special Issue: Forward March: The next destination for Feminism, p. 361–368. https://doi.org/10.1111/newe.12076.

Smith, A. (2008). Applying the lessons learnt: Community involvement in regeneration. *Public Policy and Administration*, 23(2), pp. 145–152. https://doi.org/10.1177/0952076707086252.

Storey, D. (2013). 'New' migrants in the British countryside. *Journal of Rural and Community Development*, 8(3), pp. 291–302.

Tittensor, D. and Mansouri, F. (2017). The feminisation of migration? A critical overview. In: Tittensor D., Mansouri F. (eds) *The Politics of Women and Migration in the Global South.* Palgrave Pivot, London. DOI: 10.1057/978-1-137-58799-2_2.

Thompson, P., Newsome, K. and Commander, J. (2013). 'Good when they want to be': Migrant workers in the supermarket supply chain. *Human Resource Management Journal*, 23, pp. 129–143.

Vieira, P.R., Garcia, L.P. and Maciel, E.L.N. (2020). The increase in domestic violence during the social isolation: What does it reveal? *Brazilian Journal of Epidemiology*, 23, e200033.

16 At Whose Cost? Vulnerable Female Migrants with No Recourse to Public Funds (NRPF) during the COVID-19 Crisis in England

Benedicte Brahic, Kim Heyes and Shoba Arun

Introduction

This chapter explores the experiences of vulnerable female migrants with No Recourse to Public Funds (NRPF) during the COVID-19 crisis in England. NRPF is a visa condition restricting specific migrant groups from accessing a range of support benefits. According to the Migration Observatory (2020a), there were around 1.376 million migrants with a NRPF condition attached to their visas in the UK. This number is presumed to have grown with the full implementation of the Brexit agreement in June 2021, which withdrew Britain from the European Union and changed the rights and entitlements for many European workers. Whilst migrants with the NRPF condition do not necessarily face hardship, many do (Smith, O'Reilly, Rumpel and White, 2021) and many of these are Black and minoritised women. Focusing on the gendered impact of the NRPF policy in the context of the COVID-19 crisis, this chapter explores the pervasive ramifications of this policy in vulnerable female migrants' lives including an increased risk of poverty, homelessness, illegal work, degradation in physical and mental health, and vulnerability to exploitation and violence. Locating the policy in its wider context of existence within the nexus of migration, race, and gender subordination, this chapter argues that the NRPF policy entraps female migrants into interlocking systems and structures of oppression and violence, reinforced, but also made more apparent by the pandemic. In other words, the current COVID-19 crisis did not create the hardship these women face, but it exacerbated their plight whilst exposing the patriarchal neoliberal ideology at the heart of the post-Brexit British migration system creating the so-called 'hostile environment.' This chapter is organised as follows: background and context are provided before relevant sociological theories are deployed to make sense of the evidence reviewed in the Findings and Discussion sections.

Background and Context

First introduced in Section 115 of the Immigration and Asylum Act 1999, the No Recourse to Public Funds (NRPF) policy prevents migrants subject to immigration

DOI: 10.4324/9781003267133-21

control (not having permanent residency) from accessing most state-funded benefits (such as welfare benefits and public housing benefits). The NRPF policy forms part of the regulatory arsenal designed to control and ultimately restrict incoming migrations. Developed by successive governments, these measures are deemed to protect public funds and, as such, be in the public interest. In 2012, the remit of the NRPF policy was widened to apply to a more diverse range of migrants as part of the UK Home Office 'hostile environment' strategy. In 2021, because of Britain leaving the European Union (and repelling free movement with EU member-states), the remit of the NRPF policy was extended to incoming EU migrants into the UK.

Many observers comment on the lack of data and transparency around NRPF (Project 17, 2019). According to the Institute for Public Policy Research (IPPR) based on the analysis of data published by the Home Office, in 2021, 1.31 million individuals residing in the UK had NRPF (IPPR, 2021). The Home Office describes the NRPF condition as a 'standard' condition applying to individuals subject to immigration control. For example, in 2015, the NRPF condition concerned 92% of migrants with Limited Leave To Remain (LLTR) (Wooley, 2019). Even though since its inception, the NRPF condition has been heavily criticised and challenged, the number of migrants with NRPF has grown and their percentage (out of the total UK migrant population) is expected to increase. Indeed, following the UK leaving the EU, incoming European migrants are now subjected to the NRPF condition – as are individuals entering the UK via the Hong Kong–British Nationals route. Furthermore, the 'Nationality and Borders' Act 2022 (royal assent received in April 2022) is also anticipated to tighten migration rules and increase the number of incoming migrants to the UK who have NRPF.

Incoming migrants to the UK with a NRPF condition are a heterogeneous group of individuals with a wide range of migratory statuses and migration trajectories. The IPPR estimates that three-quarters of migrants with a NRPF condition have work or study visas, and one-fifth have family visas (IPPR, 2021). Interestingly, according to the Policy Equality Statement (Home Office, 2020), in 2014, a larger proportion of males (96%, 4,944) were granted leave (under the 10-year settlement route) with NRPF than that of females (90%, 5,269). The lived experiences of migrants with a NRPF condition differ widely and, whilst the NRPF policy increased migrants' susceptibility to precarity (Wooley, 2019), many migrants with a NRPF condition are financially independent and presumably have their material needs met. Whilst the UK authorities and civil society organisations tend to refer to NRPF as a category to regulate, classify/describe incoming UK migration, migrants with NRPF only come to think about themselves in these terms in times of need and/or crisis.

Migrants at risk of extreme poverty or destitution can apply for a Change of Conditions (CoC) in a bid to overturn/lift the NRPF condition and gain access to public funds for the duration of the period of leave to remain. The Home Office reports on the CoC applications, it receives and adjudicates. Statistical data produced by the Home Office in relation to CoC applications is disaggregated by applicants' gender, age, and nationality. Exploring this data is illuminating and reveals how the

NRPF policy has a differentiated impact on individuals according to their personal characteristics. First and foremost, women are largely over-represented in CoC applications when there are slightly fewer female migrants with NRPF (see above). The number of female applicants for CoC on grounds of destitution has been more than double that of men since 2017 – except for 2020 during which, because of the COVID-19 pandemic, the number of applications has soared across genders, though the number of female applicants remains higher with 6,681 females, 4,735 males, and 16 unspecified (see Home Office, 2021). Various reports published by charitable organisations, practitioners, and researchers supporting migrants with NRPF in crisis (see also Wooley, 2019) supply further evidence ascertaining the detrimental impact of the NRPF policy on individuals/social groups experiencing systemic disadvantage and vulnerable to poverty and destitution; indeed the Unity Project supporting migrants to lift/remove the NRPF condition from their migratory status report that between 2017 and 2019, 90% of users were Black African or Caribbean, 87% were women, 96% had dependents, and 76% were single parents; 85% had a British child. Wooley (2019) makes similar observations and stresses that 30% of the sample of users (migrants with NRPF seeking support) surveyed reported a disability (as a point of comparison, 19% of working-age adults are disabled (The Department for Work and Pensions, 2021) with no data found for UK migrant population though the 'general' migrant population typically have better health outcomes than the general population – Migration Observatory, 2020b).

Statistical data produced to document the support and help sought by migrants with NRPF is illuminating and reveals how the NRPF policy has a differentiated impact on individuals according to their personal characteristics. For these reasons, restrictive migratory policies, such as the NRPF policy, have been brought into question as they have developed and become more stringent. Mediatised cases of British nationals and their non-British family members wronged by the NRPF policy have resulted in public outcry but no substantial change in policy. More recent legal challenges such as the lawsuit won by a five-year-old British boy to overturn his Zimbabwean mother's NRPF condition in April 2021 challenged the lawfulness of the NRPF policy strengthening the position of the growing number of advocates of its repeal.

Literature Review: Female Migrants in the Age of Crisis

As aptly captured in the title of the report published by Safety4Sisters in 2020 (Mort et al., 2020), migrant women with NRPF find themselves at risk of being locked out of safety and trapped in/by precarity and, for some, in/by abuse. The COVID-19 crisis has amplified the risks associated with the NRPF condition and, for many migrants, led to their materialisation – raising further questions on the tensions between migration control policies and human rights obligation. Locating the subject of this chapter in current theoretical debates, this section mobilises core theories, concepts, and ideas to make sense of the lived experiences of the female migrants with NRPF in times of crisis (and before it is considered in the concluding section how the present discussion of women migrant with a NRPF condition in the COVID-19 crisis contributes to these debates and extend them). Women migrants with NRPF caught in the COVID-19 crisis are trapped in a multi-layered web of discriminating systems – gender and migration status, among others, which oppressive outcomes have been amplified by the global health crisis. The notion of structural violence (Galtung, 1969 – discussed below) offers a fitting conceptual framework to make sense of the mutually reinforcing inequalities migrant women with NRPF face in times of crisis.

Gender Meets Migration or the Weight of Intersections in the Neoliberal Age

The neoliberal age of migration is shaped by two core trends: on the one hand, the increase and diversification of migratory flows (see the globalisation of migration in De Haas, Castles, and Miller, 2019), on the other hand, the politicisation of migration leading to the generalised drive to curtail (and criminalise) (certain) mobilities worldwide (often in breach with human rights commitment and in disregard of economic needs for workforce). In the neoliberal global age, migration remains globalisation's last frontier (Moses, 2006), the one arena of human activity where the neoliberal principles of laissez-faire do not apply. This section discusses gender and citizenship/migration status and their intersections as variables structuring migrant women's lived experiences in the neoliberal age of migration.

Gender is defined and understood as the identities constructed in relation to the perceived differences between sexes; the impact of gender differences has far-reaching material consequences in the social world. To this chapter and in relation to the social context at play for women migrants with NRPF in England, gender relations are herein described as patriarchal, forming a system of social structures and practices in which women are subordinated and at a disadvantage. Walby (1990) distinguishes six (independent but mutually reinforcing) structures through which patriarchy operates: relations in the household, paid work, the patriarchal state, male violence, relations in sexuality, and cultural institutions. As apparent in this chapter, these six structures inform and shape women migrants' lives and, for some, come to determine their life outcomes in times of crisis (particularly as access to public funds is conditional on citizenship or settled status).

The feminisation of migration (De Haas, Castles, and Miller, 2019) signals an increase in the number of women on the move since the 1960s (as workers and/or as family members). However, with many female migrants in low-paid (catering, cleaning) and/or care work (health and social care), this term also signals changes in the international division and reproductive labour (Naidu, 2010) as well as the precarity of migration (Arun, Brahic and Taylor, 2019; Chantler, 2012). Migration in the neoliberal global age is indeed articulated around two contradictions which lead to their precarious condition: (1) whilst the demand for (cheap and flexible) foreign labour – particularly in the Global North – is on the increase, restrictions on migration are mounting; (2) human rights and diversity are strong moral imperatives of the global age, yet migration policies and their operationalisation often contradict human rights and cannot be thought away from race and racism (Erel,

Murji and Nahaboo, 2016). As a result of these contradictions, female migrants' experiences are often marred by inequalities in the world of work, in the home, and in their relations with the host society. As suggested above, contemporary migrations ought to be understood beyond gender and migration status and in relation to race (Erel et al., 2017; Chantler, 2012), a social characteristic, identity, or division, which intersects with many variables such as class, religion, age, health, sexuality, and disability and result in shaping individuals' lives/life outcome.

African feminism creates a useful framework when linking together patriarchal societies, structural violence, gendered abuse, and migration. African feminist theories position migrant women within society, highlighting the inequalities and power struggles (Chikwira, 2021). Migration, like gender, shapes lives. Alongside neoliberal ideals, African feminist standpoint theory pulls apart the idea of intersectionality and allows for the 'calling out' of inherent epistemic privilege that has been allowed to continue through the guise of legislation and government control (Naidu, 2010; Oyekan, 2014). This adequately outlines the issues faced by migrants to the UK, whereby the political climate is using this epistemic privilege to exacerbate cultural differences, creating a 'them' and 'us' scenario of problematic othering that leads to a portion of the public viewing migrants as non-citizens.

Crisis Masking Structural Violence

Gendered inequalities are amplified in times of crisis (Walby, 2009, 2015). The financial crisis (2008) caused economies to shrink with depressed wages, soaring unemployment, and further precarisation of work, all of which disproportionately affected women (Fawcett Society, 2012). Following the bail-out of the financial system, austerity measures were introduced in response to the crisis and dramatically curtailed public expenditures, putting the most vulnerable members of society at further risk. Responses to the crisis amplified its gendered impact further (Walby, 2009). The gendered consequences of the COVID-19 crisis are still unravelling, yet a similar pattern is emerging whereby the responses to the crisis do not mitigate its gendered impact but instead have gendered consequences themselves (Power, 2020). These gender consequences intersect with other deep-seated inequalities – migratory status, race, class, age, health, and disability being some of them.

The inequalities are not caused by crises, they reach a heightened point and (re) surface with crises. In this chapter, we argue the lives of women migrants with a NRPF condition – given their gender, migratory status, and depending on their race and other intersecting characteristics shaping their lives – are constrained by structural violence. Developed by Galtung (1969), the term 'structural violence' refers to the constraints and limitations of one's potential brought by economic, political, legal, cultural, religious, and social structures. Unequal access to resources and marginalisation in these spheres of human activity constitute forms of structural violence. For Anglin (1998), structural violence refers to the violence produced by systems of domination and has a detrimental impact on mental and physical well-being. Furthermore, structural violence needs to be connected to physical violence. True (2012) indeed observes the heightened susceptibility to gender-based physical violence for women trapped in/by structural violence (see the sections 'Findings' and 'Discussion'). Chantler et al.'s (2022) study of domestic homicide in the UK shows how the perception of culture is a barrier to support. Those with NRPF are hidden further within those experiencing abuse in the home, with violence accepted as a cultural issue – clearly linked to the effect of the hostile environment (Chantler et al., 2022: tbc). Structural violence is therefore shown to be linked to the depletion of women's lives, of their physical and mental well-being, and the capabilities of those receiving their care (Elson, 2000, Rai et al., 2014). In this chapter, we argue that women migrants with NRPF (and needing RPF) experience structural violence linked to the neoliberal age of migration which the COVID-19 crisis amplifies but can also serve to recognise, a necessary step before it can be addressed.

Methodology

Using a narrative literature review approach, the present chapter is based on secondary and tertiary data analysis. Internet searches for academic and grey literature were conducted using Google and Google Scholar to gather relevant sources. Sources were initially identified by using combinations of the following keywords: migrant female/migrant women, NRPF, migration policy, COVID-19, coronavirus, health crisis, pandemic, England, the United Kingdom, put into Boolean search strings. The search dates were from March 2020 to December 2021 to coincide with the start of the COVID-19 pandemic lockdown in the UK, and the start of the analysis. As expected, very few publications were returned through the searches, and therefore the research team were able to quickly identify relevant papers. Titles were used to ascertain preliminary relevance before sources were scanned, reviewed, and analysed for the purpose of the paper. As a result, this chapter is based on a variety of sources from a range of disciplines, though the focus on sources using sociological epistemology is to be noted. The sources searched, reviewed, and in part included in this chapter include academic papers, reports, parliament-supporting evidence, legal documentation, grey literature, and newspaper articles. No quality review was conducted as most papers were not peer-reviewed and as there were so few, they were all to be included in the findings. We only included sources published in English. As this chapter focuses on the experiences of migrant women with NRPF during the COVID-19 crisis in England, the sources reviewed and cited in the findings and the concluding sections reflect the temporal and geographical remits of the paper.

Findings

The majority of the 13 papers included in the findings are reports published during the COVID-19 crisis and funded by charitable organisations working with women who have NRPF, with a noticeable lack of academic data at the time of writing. Most papers state that domestic abuse has risen since the onset of COVID-19, highlighting how migration policies can perpetuate gendered and racial inequalities. Indeed, because of their marginalised status in the UK, these women may not feel able to contact the Police, they are also unlikely to be able to leave the home that they share with the perpetrator due to a lack of financial support or access to services. The children witnessing this abuse are also at great risk, if not physically, then with long-term mental health trauma as a result. The voices of Black and minoritised women have not been heard within the wider response to COVID-19. They are also at a disadvantage as the pandemic has created an unfavourable environment for violence against women and girls with Black and minoritised women having access to fewer services, further enhancing inequalities and the likelihood of destitution.

The chapters reviewed shared several interconnected themes: fear and the continuum of violence, precarious employment and financial difficulties, health, and lack of access to help and support. The overarching theme of domestic abuse is woven through each of the other main themes.

Fear and the Continuum of Violence

As suggested previously, Black and minoritised women are impeded by an increasingly hostile environment in the UK forming a system of structural violence in which migrant women with NRPF are entrapped by policy and practice (Dawsey-Hewitt et al., 2021, Hobbs, 2021, McIlwaine, Granada, and Valenzuela-Oblitas, 2019). Mort et al.'s (2020) study found that migrant women with NRPF felt as though the Government were using their tenuous migration status as a tool to torment them, affecting their mental health. There is also significant evidence that perpetrators of domestic abuse use immigration status to exert control over the victim, weaponising immigration enforcement (Jacobs, 2021; The Children's Society, Project 17, and The Unity Project, 2020; Banga and Roy, 2020). Over 60% of women with NRPF stated that their partners had threatened them with deportation if they reported the violence, and over 50% thought that the Home Office or Police would believe the perpetrator over them (McIlwaine et al., 2019). This meant the women would not report the abuse for fear of deportation (The Children's Society, Project 17, and The Unity Project, 2020).

Dawsey-Hewitt et al. (2021) highlights the increased risk of domestic abuse to both children and migrant women. Forced lockdowns, fears associated with precarious migratory statuses, and economic pressures/uncertainties linked to the pandemic created an environment that was difficult to escape (Dawsey-Hewitt et al., 2021; Mort et al., 2020; The Children's Society, Project 17, and The Unity Project, 2020). For those women that managed to escape, the socio-economic issues they faced during the pandemic meant that they often felt under pressure to go back to their partners to avoid destitution and homelessness (Banga and Roy, 2020). Though this has been amplified by the conditions created by the response to the pandemic, the pressure to stay with the perpetrator needs to be understood as the by-product of migration policies designed with Western patriarchal definitions of the nuclear family which place the male 'head of household' at their core and, as a result, see migrant women and their children as mere dependents.

Precarious Employment and Financial Difficulties

Women migrant workers are the most vulnerable, but overall, contribute the most to global economies (UN Women, 2022). They are also more likely to be destitute, in poverty, and have jobs that have zero-hour contracts (Dawsey-Hewitt et al., 2021; Women's Budget Group, 2020, Dickson, 2021). The presence of COVID-19 has meant that frontline migrant women have been at most risk of losing their jobs, but even if they remain in employment, they generally have less disposable income and/or income to send home because of the general impact on living costs and extra childcare responsibilities during lockdowns (Dawsey-Hewitt et al., 2021; Gardner, 2021, Hobbs, 2021; UN Women, 2022). It is estimated that there are currently around 229,779 key workers among those with NRPF attached to their visa; however, they generally earn less than the general population, and 80% of those in work are earning less than they were at the start of the pandemic (Smith, O'Reilly, Rumpel and White, 2021).

Gardner (2021) found that many women with NRPF work in the industries that have been hit most by the pandemic hospitality and cleaning. Domestic workers face an increased risk of abuse; care workers are likely to contract COVID-19 and cleaners often must work harder without Personal Protective Equipment (PPE) and without extra pay (Hobbs, 2021; UN Women, 2022). They generally worked long hours with no guaranteed days off or any benefits such as paid sick leave. Care work also increased at home as schools closed, with the extra burden of unpaid work falling mostly on women (UN Women, 2022). Precarious employment puts these women at risk of destitution and homelessness with illegal and/or informal work (despite the risks associated with it) being one of the only forms of last recourse for these women. Although migrant women continue to contribute to UK society, there is no policy to include them as citizens or protect them as members of society.

Health

Around 53% of women surveyed by Safety for Sisters had a long-term health condition which is significantly higher than the 29% of people with long-term health conditions in the rest of the UK population (Mort et al., 2020). Smith, O'Reilly, Rumpel, and White (2021) found that around 83% of people with NRPFs felt that their mental health was suffering; however, 92% of Black women with NRPF felt that they were struggling with their mental health (Smith et al., 2021). Dawsey-Hewitt et al. (2021) stated that generally there has been an increase in domestic abuse throughout the pandemic, with perpetrators using the fear of COVID-19 to manipulate their partners. Domestic abuse has been worse due to forced co-existence and no escape, pressure around finances, and lack of access to services (Mort et al., 2020; UN Women, 2022; Smith et al., 2021). The cycle of abuse during such times as a pandemic is exacerbated by poverty and vulnerability (The Children's Society, Project 17, and The Unity Project, 2020). Psychological abuse and coercive control are the most experienced forms of domestic abuse, which makes it difficult to identify, but also to prove when seeking support (The Children's Society, Project 17, and The Unity Project, 2020; McIlwaine et al., 2019).

Women with NRPF are also generally at a higher risk of catching the COVID-19 virus. Their physical health may suffer further throughout the pandemic as they have a lack of understanding about the availability of COVID-19 testing and inoculation. The UK Government made the decision not to charge for COVID-19-related illness; however, this was not communicated well, particularly to women with NRPF (Mort et al., 2020). Gardner (2021) found that most people with NRPF were unlikely to be able to isolate at home, could be more at risk of catching the virus in their own homes, and more generally at risk in their frontline roles. Some people risked their health, and that of others, by going to work even if they felt unwell, as otherwise they would not get paid (Smith et al., 2021). Many people with NRPFs were unable to heat their homes, and around one in ten people with NRPF were unable to eat (Smith et al., 2021). Children with NRPF were also unable to access free school meals that were delivered to other children facing hardship in the UK during lockdown (Smith et al., 2021). Children's rights to education are therefore violated, and they are likely to be the victims of at least witnessing domestic abuse, if not abused themselves.

Lack of Access to Help and Support

Women with NRPF who are victims of domestic abuse face barriers to support are, with over half of Black and minoritised women stating they were not sure where to go (Women's Budget Group, 2020). Support has become harder to access since the pandemic (Dickson, 2021) and demand for domestic abuse support doubled between March 2020 (the beginning of the first lockdown in the UK) and September 2020 (Austin, 2020). All the women with NRPF trying to access refuge services through the Women's Aid 'No Woman Turned Away Project' had first been refused services elsewhere (Austin, 2020) which may be due to the lack of Government and local authority funding (Jacobs, 2021). Dawsey-Hewitt et al. (2021) found that women with NRPF are not always given the right advice from services that are trying to support them. Many support workers do not understand immigration rules, and a lack of understanding of culture can inhibit interactions. The report describes how this may lead to women not being referred to as refugees as they do not understand what they are (Dawsey-Hewitt et al., 2021). They may also fear having their data shared with immigration services (Jacobs, 2021).

There is an unwillingness from domestic abuse charities to support women with NRPF, unless they can secure funding in advance from other third-sector organisations (Dawsey-Hewitt et al., 2021). Safety for Sisters has also reported that other charities across the sector have refused women who are unable to speak English and have been excluding this vulnerable group from their services (Dawsey-Hewitt et al., 2021). The result of this lack of access to help and support means that many women are forced to reconcile with abusive partners (The Children's Society, Project 17, and The Unity Project, 2020). Forcing women to choose between going back to abusive partners or facing destitution is barbaric. Policies should include non-citizens, public health policies, and policies to tackle abuse ought to do so. A support system framed quasi-exclusively around citizenship as a condition of access inexorably casts migrants (particularly women and children) as outsiders and victims in need of help (rather than community members accessing support).

Discussion

The increasing rates of migrant populations in the UK pose challenges to the ways in which the welfare state is conceptualised and experienced, challenging notions of citizenship and residence-based territoriality. As Walzer (1983) notes, social policies based on citizenship benefit resident groups within closed systems who share these welfare entitlements (See Lafleur and Vintila, 2020). Without access to entitlements and rights such as work, housing, and legal aid, women identified as NRPF face multiple risks and insecurities posed due to their perceived legal status compared to men or other types of migrants. Despite residence rights, their inability to gain economic and social rights not only pushes them into poverty and insecurity, but also strips them of any agency to change the structural constraints of intersectional inequality. Female migrants with NRPF experiencing violence and abuse are trapped by abusers and the state, having no public institutions to turn to, their sole recourse being with friends and/or charitable organisations (or in some instances local authorities). They are indeed at the centre of intersecting systems of oppression – namely patriarchy, ethnic-based subordination, and the neoliberal migratory system. A support system framed quasi-exclusively around citizenship (or permanent leave to remain) as a condition of access inexorably casts migrants (particularly women and children) as outsiders and victims in need of help (rather than community members accessing support).

African feminist standpoint theory allows us to consider these intersecting systems and impugn the issues within the policy that allows women to be treated as non-citizens despite consistently contributing to society. The COVID-19 crisis has brought to the fore many injustices in our contemporary societies. Rather than causing them, the health crisis has been an exacerbating factor and an exposure of these injustices. As argued in this chapter, women migrants with a NRPF condition attached to their migration status find themselves at the centre of intersecting systems of oppression – namely patriarchy, ethnic-based subordination, and the neoliberal migratory system (known in the UK as 'hostile environment') – which puts them at risk. Although this is not always the case, the day-to-day experiences of these women are often shaped and constrained by structural violence, which entails marginalisation and a lack of access to resources and services. Within labour markets, we see they are represented in the lower rungs of labour market and subject to low wages, harsher working conditions, and prone to exploitation, with worse employment outcomes yet seemed to work in the frontline sector during times of crises such as the COVID-19 pandemic, and within exploitative and abusive conditions. Whilst the UK's Modern Slavery Act 2015 has been a step-change in tackling forms of exploitation at work in certain sectors as well as protecting victims of illegal migration, this legislation may not reach this group of NRPF migrants, even when they work in conditions akin to those discussed as forms of modern slavery. Thus, in the absence of an overall migrant integration policy at the national level, migrants will continue to be excluded from forms of social protection at both institutional and individual levels. Women migrants may face a double or triple jeopardy: being a woman, a migrant, and identified as Black or minoritised within the UK context, hence it is key to address the integration of migrant women in society as an important objective to advance social justice at large. This also helps address the gender and intersectional gaps, i.e., socio-economic gaps between men and women, and between groups of women in general and hence a strong driving force to promote the successful inclusion of children of migrants in the host society.

More importantly, the quality of life for children of NRPF categories goes against child rights and social justice advocated across Europe. Even though local authorities have a duty of care to all children under Section 17 of the Children's Act 1989 (and regardless of where these children are from), research shows that NRPF groups are either unaware of such provisions or afraid to seek assistance due to fear of being scrutinised (Jacobs, 2021; Erel et al., 2017). Thus, the overall context of gendered and social vulnerability requires a prompt and effective social protection response. The wider political context and negative media representation of migration fuel not only racism and xenophobia, which reproduce inequalities faced by ethnic minorities in the UK but reinforce stereotypes that stigmatise them. Changes to NRPF can not only guarantee social and economic rights for these groups, challenging stereotypes and addressing social and economic exploitation but also challenge the well-rehearsed trope of their victimhood as vulnerable, passive, and exploited in both economic and cultural/patriarchal contexts, and thus opening a space for instrumentalising change for gender equality through leveraging their agency and challenging patriarchal oppression. We see that migratory processes and systems reproduce and reinforce gendered systems through gender roles and their social outcomes, hence gender is a crucial variable within the contested policy area of migration in the UK. The lack of a gender perspective in migration, asylum, and integration policies has detrimental effects not only on the women themselves but for communities and society at large.

The hostile environment and its (in)human consequences are facing growing criticisms and the pandemic has brought the precarity of marginalised migrants into sharp relief. The public display of coalescence behind migrant essential workers (Broadhead and Ruiz, 2021) or the public sympathy attracted by high-profile court cases challenging the lawfulness of the NRPF condition show the level of interest these issues garner among the civic society. These public displays of support should however not obscure some of the damaging impact of the pandemic on migrations and transnational lives. The perception of the threat as coming from 'the outside' and strong public support for the quasi-closure of national borders at the height of the pandemic have participated in the demonisation of migrants and transnational lifestyles, and the further marginalisation of vulnerable migrants. These patterns of demonisation and criminalisation have in turn led to the silencing of migrants in relation to some of the specific challenges they faced during the COVID-19 pandemic and ranged from the impact of long-term separation from families and communities overseas, the impossibility to travel back to one's country of origin/former country of residence to uncertainties around visa renewal and remittances. The plight of female migrants seeking to overturn their NRPF condition during the pandemic discussed herein needs to be understood in this wider context of policies related to migration alongside the demonisation of specific migrant groups and behaviours. This has put female migrants with NRPF facing gender-based violence and their children at an increased risk of human rights abuses (Price, Viana and Ruiz (2021). The harm caused by these policies has been exacerbated by the crisis which has also served to reveal aspects of it. Many voices remain marginal, unheard (female migrants with NRPF living with a disability and/ or in areas not covered by charitable organisations), a shift towards a human rights-based approach to the relaxation of NRPF and migration regulations in general would provide the UK with a genuine opportunity to work towards its sustainable development goals pledge of 'leaving no one behind.'

Recommendations

This research shows the need to create fairer welfare policies that include supporting migrants. The support should not be provided because they are vulnerable or 'victims' and need help. If policy changes were put in place to address migrant needs, not only can they be supported to continue contributing to society, but the changes would be a start to tackling patriarchal and structural violence and eradicating gender inequalities. They would be viewed as community members rather than problematic 'others.'

Ad hoc responses (such as providing refuge and/or helping individuals with their request to overturn their NRPF condition) to the individual plight of female migrants with NRPF during the pandemic have been provided by charitable organisations working tirelessly and with limited financial support. Alongside their essential emergency work with women migrants, these organisations have also advocated for structural change and the repeal of the NRPF condition.

This call has been partially heard with a temporary relaxation of the NRPF condition on humanitarian grounds in the face of the pandemic. Whilst this is a welcome step, this should not be the last. Relaxation of the NRPF condition for women at risk of destitution should not be bound to emergencies (such as the health crisis) or locked in an essentialist reading of women's role as carer of a British child but afforded unilaterally on human rights grounds to reform neoliberal migratory policies rooted in post-colonial and patriarchal values.

Acknowledgements

The authors would like to thank Safety4Sisters for their participation in the Migration and Interdisciplinary Global Studies (MIGS, Manchester Metropolitan University) participatory workshop on the legacy of COVID-19 for migrant-background communities in Manchester. Their essential work with migrant women inspired this paper.

References

Anglin, M. K. (1998). Feminist perspectives on structural violence. *Identities*, 5(2), pp. 145–151.

Arun, S., Brahic, B. and Taylor, S. (2019). Global mobilities: United by dividing and accelerating precarities. *Migration and Development*, 9(1), pp. 1–7.

Austin, J. (2020). *Nowhere to Turn. Findings from the Fourth Year of the No Woman Turned Away Project, Women's Aid*. Retrieved from https://www.womensaid.org.uk/wp-content /uploads/2020/06/Nowhere-to-Turn-2020.pdf

Banga, B. and Roy, S. (2020). *The Impact of the Dual Pandemic's: Violence Against Women & Girls and COVID-19 on Black and Minoritised Women & Girls*. Retrieved from https://829ef90d-0745-49b2-b404-cbea85f15fda.filesusr.com/ugd/2f475d_6d6dea4 0b8bd42c8a917ba58ceec5793.pdf

Broadhead, J. and Ruiz, I. (2021). *Public Attitudes to Labour Migrants in the Pandemic: Health and Welfare*. Retrieved from https://migrationobservatory.ox.ac.uk/resources/ briefings/public-attitudes-to-labour-migrants-in-the-pandemic-health-and-welfare/

Chantler, K. (2012). Gender, Asylum Seekers, and mental distress: Challenges for mental health social work. *British Journal of Social Work*, 42(2), pp. 318–334.

Chantler, K., Bracewell, K., Baker, V., Heyes, K., Traynor, P. and Ward, M. (2022). An analysis of minoritisation in domestic homicide reviews in England and Wales. *Critical Social Policy*.https://doi.org/10.1177/02610183221133052.

Chikwira, L. (2021). Contested narratives of belonging: Zimbabwean women migrants in Britain. *Women's Studies International Forum*. https://doi.org/10.1016/j.wsif.2021 .102481

Dawsey-Hewitt, S., Jnagel, T., Kalia, S., Royal, K., Seshadri, S., Sutherland, L., Magić, J., McGivern, M. and Wilson Garwood, R. (2021). *Shadow Pandemic – Shining a Light on Domestic Abuse During Covid*. Retrieved from https://www.womensaid.org.uk/wp -content/uploads/2021/11/Shadow_Pandemic_Report_FINAL.pdf

De Haas, H., Castles, S. and Miller, M. (2019). *The Age of Migration, International Population Movements in the Modern World* (6th ed.). London: Bloomsbury.

Dickson, E. (2021). (No) recourse to lunch: A frontline view of free school meals and the immigration control during the COVID-19 pandemic. *Families, Relationships and Societies*. https://doi.org/10.1332/204674320X16076180418172

Elson, D. (2000). Empowerment and economics. In K. Judd (Ed.), *The Progress of the World's Women* (pp. 15–36). New York: United Nations.

Erel, U., Murji, K. and Nahaboo, Z. (2016) Understanding the contemporary race–migration nexus, Ethnic and Racial Studies, 39:8, 1339–1360. https://doi.org/10.1080/01419870 .2016.1161808.

Erel, U., O'Neill, M., Reynolds, T. and Kaptani, E. (2017). Crisis upon crisis: Migrant families with no recourse to public funds. *Discover Society*. Retrieved from https:// discoversociety.org/2017/05/02/crisis-upon-crisis-migrant-families-with-no-recourse-to -public-funds

Fawcett Society. (2012). *Policy Briefing: The Impact of Austerity on Women*. London: Fawcett Society. Retrieved from https://www.fawcettsociety.org.uk/the-impact-of -austerity-on-women

Galtung, J. (1969). Violence, peace, and peace research. *Journal of Peace Research*, 6(3), pp. 167–191.

Gardner, Z. (2021). *Migrants with No Recourse to Public Funds' Experiences During the COVID-19 Pandemic*. The Joint Council for The Welfare of Immigrants. Retrieved from https://www.jcwi.org.uk/Handlers/Download.ashx?IDMF=17805c35-d3bc-4251-9ada-6dfdae8dbca6

Hobbs, L. (2021). Opinion: Precarity, a pandemic and a 'hostile environment'. *Interdisciplinary Perspectives on Equality and Diversity*. Retrieved from http://journals.hw.ac.uk/index.php/IPED/article/view/106/76

Home Office. (2020). *Borders Immigration Citizenship Systems, Asylum & Family Policy Unit, Policy Equality Statement*. Retrieved from https://assets.publishing.service.gov.uk/government/uploads/system/uploads/attachment_data/file/880531/Policy_Equality_Statement__PES__21_April_2020.pdf

Home Office. (2021). Immigration and protection, UK Visa & Immigration transparency data Q4 2020. Retrieved from https://assets.publishing.service.gov.uk/government/uploads/system/uploads/attachment_data/file/965708/UKVI_IP_Q4_2020_Published.ods

Institute for Public Policy Research. (2021). *IPPR: 1.3 million People Living in the UK with No Access to Social Security are Sign of 'Broken System'*. Retrieved from https://www.ippr.org/news-and-media/press-releases/ippr-1-3-million-people-living-in-the-uk-with-no-access-to-social-security-are-sign-of-broken-system

Jacobs, N. (2021). *Safety Before Status. Improving Pathways to Support for Migrant Victims of Domestic Abuse*. London: Domestic Abuse Commissioner. Retrieved from https://domesticabusecommissioner.uk/wp-content/uploads/2021/10/Safety-Before-Status-Report-2021.pdf

Lafleur, J. M. and Vintila, D. (2020). *Migration and Social Protection in Europe and Beyond (Volume 1): Comparing Access to Welfare Entitlements*. Imiscoe Research Series: Springer Cham.

McIlwaine, C., Granada, L. and Valenzuela-Oblitas, I. (2019). *The Right to be Believed. Migrant Women Facing Violence Against Women and Girls (VAWG) in the 'Hostile Immigration Environment' in London*. London: Kings College. Retrieved from https://stepupmigrantwomenuk.files.wordpress.com/2019/05/the-right-to-be-believed-full-version-updated.pdf

Migration Observatory. (2020a). *Between a Rock and a Hard Place: The COVID-19 Crisis and Migrants with No Recourse to Public Funds (NRPF)*. Retrieved from https://migrationobservatory.ox.ac.uk/resources/commentaries/between-a-rock-and-a-hard-place-the-covid-19-crisis-and-migrants-with-no-recourse-to-public-funds-nrpf/

Migration Observatory. (2020b). *The Health of Migrants in the UK*. Retrieved from https://migrationobservatory.ox.ac.uk/resources/briefings/the-health-of-migrants-in-the-uk/

Mort, L., Sharma, S., Marsh, V. and Clarke, B. (2020). *Locked in Abuse, Locked Out of Safety. The Pandemic Experiences of Migrant Women*. Manchester: Safety 4 Sisters. Retrieved from https://static1.squarespace.com/static/5af498dd3c3a53848b8530b6/t/5f8d43da5688f32ed1347aaa/1603093480213/Locked_in_abuse_locked_out_of_safety_S4Sreport.pdf

Moses, J. (2006). *International Migration: Globalization's Last Frontier*. London: Bloomsbury.

Naidu, M. (2010). Wrestling with standpoint theory…some thoughts on standpoint and African feminism. *Agenda*, *24*(83), pp. 24–35. https://doi.org/10.1080/10130950.2010.9676289

Oyekan, A. O. (2014). African feminism: Some critical considerations. *Philosophia*, *15*(1), pp. 1–10.

Power, K. (2020). The COVID-19 pandemic has increased the care burden of women and families. *Sustainability: Science, Practice and Policy*, *16*(1), pp. 67–73.

Price, M. C., Viana, M. and Ruiz, M. (2021). *The Criminalization of a Pandemic*. Retrieved from https://resurj.org/wp-content/uploads/2021/03/ENG-The-Criminalization-of-a-Pandemic.pdf

Project 17. (2019). *No Data, No Recourse: How a Lack of Information Limits Access to Support for Vulnerable Families*. Retrieved from https://www.opengovernment.org.uk/2019/02/19/no-data-no-recourse-how-a-lack-of-information-limits-access-to-support-for-vulnerable-families/

Rai, S., Hoskyns, C. and Thomas, D. (2014). Depletion: The social cost of reproduction. *International Feminist Journal of Politics, 16*(1), pp. 86–105.

Smith, C., O'Reilly, P., Rumpel, R. and White, R. (2021). *How Do I Survive Now? The Impact of Living with No Recourse to Public Funds*. Citizen's Advice. Retrieved from https://www.citizensadvice.org.uk/Global/CitizensAdvice/welfare%20publications/How%20do%20I%20survive%20now_%20November%202021.pdf

The Children's Society, Project 17 and The Unity Project. (2020). *Domestic Abuse in Families with No Recourse to Public Funds (NRPF). Briefing for the Domestic Abuse Bill 2020*. Retrieved from https://www.project17.org.uk/media/101935/Domestic-Abuse-in-Families-with-No-Recourse-to-Public-Funds-Briefing.pdf

The Department for Work and Pensions. (2021). *National Statistics: Family Resources Survey: Financial Year 2019 to 2020*. Retrieved from https://www.gov.uk/government/statistics/family-resources-survey-financial-year-2019-to-2020/family-resources-survey-financial-year-2019-to-2020#disability-1

True, J. (2012). *The Political Economy of Violence against Women*. New York: Oxford University Press.

UN Women. (2022). *Addressing the Impacts of the COVID-19 Pandemic on Women Migrant Workers*. UN Women Headquarters. Retrieved from https://www.unwomen.org/sites/default/files/Headquarters/Attachments/Sections/Library/Publications/2020/Guidance-note-Impacts-of-the-COVID-19-pandemic-on-women-migrant-workers-en.pdf

Walby, S. (1990). Theorising patriarchy. *Sociology, 23*(2), pp. 213–234.

Walby, S. (2009). *Gender and the Financial Crisis, Paper for UNESCO Project on 'Gender and the Financial Crisis'*. Retrieved from https://www.lancaster.ac.uk/fass/doc_library/sociology/Gender_and_financial_crisis_Sylvia_Walby.pdf

Walby, S. (2015). *Crisis*. Cambridge: Polity.

Walzer, M. (1983). States and minorities. In *Minorities: Community and Identity* (pp. 219–227). Berlin, Heidelberg: Springer.

Women's Budget Group. (2020). *BAME Women and Covid-19 – Research Evidence*. Retrieved from https://wbg.org.uk/wp-content/uploads/2020/06/BAME-women-and-Covid-FINAL.pdf

Woolley, A. (2019). *Access Denied: The Cost of the 'No Recourse to Public Funds' Policy*. Retrieved from https://static1.squarespace.com/static/590060b0893fc01f949b1c8a/t/5d021ada54e8ee00013fe5b9/1560419116745/Access+Denied+-+V12+%281%29.pdf

Part VI
Adversity and Resilience

17 Women behind Bars in the United States

A Hidden and Vulnerable Population in Pandemic Times

Daniela Jauk-Ajamie

Introduction

The United States of America is the largest incarcerator in the world. The US incarceration rate of 698 per 100,000 people is 1.07% of all working adults in the country (Wagner and Bertram, 2020). While male incarceration is in a slight downturn, female incarceration has risen by 700% over the last few decades (Sentencing Project, 2020). As of 2019, 231,000 women and girls are behind bars in the USA. Over one million women are under criminal justice system supervision including probation and parole (see Kajstura, 2019; Sentencing Project, 2020).

This chapter sheds light on the hidden and vulnerable population of women and girls incarcerated in the USA and the impact of the COVID-19 pandemic. The research report comes from reports on women in American correctional institutions and a study of a clinical sociological gardening programme for women in a residential community correction setting in the American Midwest. Clinical sociology as a rights-based and liberatory approach to sociological practice calls for a sociology that reflects the needs of all humans (Brunsma et al., 2013; Fritz and Rheaume, 2014). Along these lines, the gardening programme uncovers voices hidden behind barbed wire fences, while growing more nutritious food and providing meaningful leisure time behind prison walls.

While I use the term 'woman/women' to refer to individuals held in correctional facilities for individuals assigned female at birth, it should not be forgotten that at least 4,890 transgender individuals are held in prisons in the USA, the vast majority not accommodated based on their lived gender identity (Lacoste et al., 2021). Transwomen of colour (who are overrepresented in prison) are particularly vulnerable to mistreatment behind bars from staff and fellow residents and are ten times more likely to experience sexual assault (National Centre for Transgender Equality, 2018). For the USA, there is no published research on COVID-19 and the transgender incarcerated population currently.

The American corrections system is broadly divided into institutional and community-based supervision. Institutional corrections facilities encompass prisons and jails. Typically, prisons are state or federal facilities that hold people convicted of felonies with sentences longer than a year. Jails are facilities of local

DOI: 10.4324/9781003267133-23

law enforcement and usually hold individuals with sentences of one year or less and those awaiting trial. Community supervision includes probation, parole, and residential community corrections programmes. Residential community corrections are housing facilities that count as re-entry or prison diversion programmes. Residents are entirely confined for a defined period and then gradually gain access to the community based on their treatment progress. However, during their stay in a community corrections facility, residents technically count as 'incarcerated' and lose state-sponsored health benefits.

In the next section, I give a brief overview of the problem of mass incarceration of women and girls in the USA, followed by a review of the research on COVID-19 behind bars in the USA with a focus on women. I then turn to the clinical sociological Garden Project, explaining the methodological approach and data analysis. The analysis draws from data collected during the COVID pandemic and speaks to women's perceptions of the lack of protection, inconsistent institutional responses, limited access to treatment and social support, and deteriorating food quality in the facility. The chapter concludes with a call to embrace a feminist clinical sociology that can be of service to incarcerated women and girls and their communities and for gardening to be used as a therapeutic intervention that can bring respite and a sense of agency to incarcerated women.

Literature Review

How Does Mass Incarceration Impact Women and Girls in the USA?

Over the past quarter-century, women have been significantly more involved with the criminal justice system in the USA because of more expansive law enforcement efforts, stiffer drug sentencing laws, and post-conviction barriers to re-entry that uniquely affect women (Kajstura, 2019; Swavola, Riley, and Subramanian, 2016). In recent decades, the female incarcerated population has grown at twice the pace of men's incarceration and is now eight times higher than in 1980. Wacquant (2001) argued that 'hyper-incarceration' describes the phenomenon because the risk of imprisonment is heavily weighted towards sub-communities. Hyper-incarceration of women is gender-based but also reveals a racialised dynamic (Richie, 2012; Kaba, 2018). For example, while the rate of imprisonment for African American women has been declining since 2000, in 2019, the imprisonment rate for African American women (83 per 100,000) was still over 1.7 times the rate of imprisonment for white women (48 per 100,000). Additionally, Latinx women were imprisoned at 1.3 times the rate of white women (63 vs. 48 per 100,000; Sentencing Project, 2020).

It is critical to understand women's criminalisation and incarceration in the larger context of the patriarchal gender order that permeates the socialisation and life chances of women and girls (including gender diverse identities). Ranking 30 of 156 in the latest Global Gender Gap report, American society is characterised by systematic gender violence (36% of women experience violence in their lifetime) and low political participation of women (World Economic Forum, 2021). Substance abuse, mental illness, and severe physical, sexual, and mental abuse often predates women's convictions; a pattern that has been captured in feminist criminology literature, particularly by the 'Pathways Perspective' (Chesney-Lind and Pasko, 2013; Daly, 1992; Kruttschnitt et al., 2019). This perspective accounts for five gendered pathways to crime in response to traumatisation and victimisation (Daly, 1992) and calls for a gender-responsive approach in correctional treatment (Covington and Bloom, 2007; Wright et al., 2012). Empirical evidence shows that more incarcerated women than men struggle with severe psychological distress (Bronson and Berzofsky, 2017) and substance use challenges (Swavola et al., 2016). Class also matters, and economic marginalisation may play a more significant role than originally theorised (Kruttschnitt et al., 2019). Criminal justice-involved women face greater economic marginalisation and poverty than their male counterparts. Additionally, incarcerated women are also often financially responsible for dependents. The vast majority (80%) of women in jails are mothers and frequently the primary caretakers of their children and families (Sawyer and Bertram, 2018). Over half (58%) of women in state and federal prisons reported having at least one minor child (Maruschak et al., 2015).

Women's bodies pose a unique challenge not adequately addressed in the American criminal justice system. More than half of women in jails have a current medical problem (compared to 35% of men). About two-thirds of jailed women report a chronic condition – compared to half of the men in jails and 27% of people in the general population (Swavola et al., 2016). Gynaecological, obstetric, and pregnancy care are often unavailable, especially in jails where women have shorter stays (Swavola et al., 2016). As of 2021, 29 states shackle women during childbirth, and the practice of immediate postpartum separation is still widely used (Swavola et al., 2016). As of 2019, only prisons in eight states (Illinois, Indiana, Nebraska, New York, Ohio, South Dakota, Washington, and West Virginia) hosted nursery programmes that allow women to care for their infants for varying periods of time (Arregi et al., 2020).

What Do We Know about COVID-19 behind Bars in the USA?

Mass incarceration and prison overcrowding have been a structural driver of health inequities, amplifying COVID-19 and health disparities in already disproportionately policed communities (Novisky et al., 2021; Reinhart and Chen, 2021). Prisons and jails continue to be hotbeds of COVID-19 infection and source of spread in the USA (Macmadu et al., 2020; Marquez et al., 2021; Saloner et al., 2020). Information on the extent of the pandemic crisis has been lagging and deliberately omitted by some states. While for much of the pandemic, at least data on COVID infections and deaths of residents and staff in state and federal prisons were available on individual State Departments of Corrections (DOC) websites, some states have ceased publication of data; others have decreased the frequency of reports and the variety of data provided (Lao and Behne, 2021). Generally, there is no concerted effort from the Department of Justice in the USA to report on COVID-19, and data is being collected from independent research teams.[1] As a result, data on the vaccination status of incarcerated people and staff across all states remain vague.[2]

Bearing in mind that we face under-reporting, as of 14 June, 590,757 COVID-19 infections and 2,896 related deaths of incarcerated people have been reported (data derived 15 June 2022 from https://covidprisonproject.com/). Marquez et al. (2021) compared these rates with the overall USA population for the first 52 weeks of the pandemic and found that the incidence rate of COVID-19 in incarcerated settings was more than three times higher than in the general populations (30,780 cases of incarcerated people versus 9,350 cases in 100,000), and the mortality rate more than double the community death rate (80.9 deaths per 100,000 in the general population versus 199.6 among incarcerated individuals). Data are primarily collected from the federal and state prison system, and no conclusions can be made about the pandemic within jails. Jails currently host some 650,000 detainees every day with a 55% weekly turnover rate and involve approximately 220,000 full-time jail staff who commute from their communities each day (Reinhart and Chen, 2021). The 'jail churn' thus poses a threat not only to those incarcerated but to the community exposed to elevated infection risks outside the jail walls.

What Do We Know about the Impact of COVID-19 on Incarcerated Women?

There is a lack of official reporting on COVID in sex-aggregated form. However, a few independent studies have been published about women and girls during the pandemic (Arregi et al., 2020; Lacoste et al., 2021; Welch and Deitch, 2021). Lacoste et al. (2021) compiled the most comprehensive report on gender-specific data on COVID-19. They identified at least 54 women's prisons that have reported more than 100 infections and 56 with cumulative infection rates above 15% (as of November 2021), showing at least 20,125 documented COVID-19 infections among incarcerated women during the pandemic. These data are drawn from 107 state and federal prisons; many more prisons and jails do not report this information. It is thus impossible to know how many cases occurred in women's facilities (Lacoste et al., 2021). Even in systems that report facility-level data, data are not disaggregated by sex within mixed facilities. Lacoste et al. (2021) complement available quantitative data with narratives from California women's prisons that demonstrate how systematic transparency failures have hidden the impacts on women.

Welch and Deitch (2021) describe a 'pandemic gender gap' with faltering services for women in prisons that are still predominantly designed for males. They suggest that releasing women with nonviolent charges would be the best mitigation strategy in the pandemic, yet androcentric risk assessments result in women's 'over classification' and overly restrictive eligibility criteria for release (Welch and Deitch, 2021). In addition, pregnant women have not been prioritised for release, even though they are especially vulnerable to complications from COVID (Arregi et al., 2020; Ellis, 2020; Welch and Deitch, 2021).

Andrea High Bear was the first woman to die in an American prison from the novel virus. She had been transferred to a federal prison in Texas on a nonviolent drug-related charge in North Dakota when she was seven and a half months pregnant; she contracted COVID-19 shortly after her arrival. After being put on a ventilator, she delivered a premature baby on 1 April 2020 by caesarean section and passed away on 28 April 2020 (Ellis, 2020; LeBeau, 2020). Andrea High Bear's grandmother, who is caring for the infant, called for accountability, saying she never received any information. The first communication from the prison was a letter stating that Andrea had died (LeBeau, 2020). This is symptomatic of the separation women and their families suffer, exacerbated in the pandemic through lockdowns and the non-transparency of decisions by prison officials.

Arregi et al. (2020) compiled a snapshot of data available in September 2020 on COVID infections in women's prisons, including an interactive map. They offered profiles of the hardest hit prisons (for which data were available) located in Louisiana, Florida, Texas, Massachusetts, California, and Michigan (Arregi et al., 2020). However, nearly half of incarcerated women are held in jails (Kajstura, 2019) which act as pandemic super spreader sites (Reinhart and Chen, 2021).

The Garden Project

In this chapter, I draw from available reports on women in the American prison system during the pandemic, as well as my research in a residential community corrections facility for women with the goal of diverting clients from prison and facilitating their re-entry into the wider community (give the place a name so you can reference it throughout). The field site for this clinical sociological intervention is a residential community facility in which female clients are incarcerated on a full-time basis for a minimum of 30 days; they gradually receive access to the community. The length of stay depends on progress towards treatment goals and compliance in the programme and averages approximately 4.5 months. The facility had an average of 215 intakes/year from 2015 to 2018, with a 76% programme completion rate. Clients in this time had a median age range of 26–35, and 40% did not have a high school degree. In terms of race, about 75% of clients identified as white, and about 12% identified as African American. The racial identity of the remaining 13% was undetermined.

My research interest emerged when I worked as a full-time applied sociologist for the large community corrections agency (hereafter called 'the agency') that operates the field site. As an applied sociologist for the agency, I analysed 'exit evaluations' of residential clients. Clients complained with the highest frequency about the low quality of the food and the extensive 'downtime' between treatment classes. To address these needs by taking women's voices seriously and seeking to empower them (Mancini, Billson, and Disch, 1990), I helped to develop a therapeutic garden programme (Jauk and Blackwood, 2022; Jauk and Blackwood, 2020) inspired by the need for gender-responsive programming (Covington and Bloom, 2007; Fleming et al., 2021) and research evidence of the benefits of gardening in correctional settings (Ascencio, 2018; van der Linden, 2015; Toews et al., 2018).

The curriculum was adapted from a prison garden project developed by fellow clinical sociologists in Alabama, with the goal of comparative research (Jauk, et al., 2022; Jauk and Everhardt, 2018).

Two crucial community partners supported the garden project: *Sunflower Gardens*,[3] a local food justice initiative that supports 100 community gardens in the urban area where the facility is located, and the local Extension Office.[4] As such, the garden intervention is an example of a clinical sociological community intervention (Fritz and Rheaume, 2014) that connects incarcerated women with community resources. Thanks to the hands-on help and material donations of *Sunflower Gardens*, a garden of approx. 400 square feet was established in May 2019 and doubled in fall 2019 to 800 square feet. A horticultural curriculum was administered to clients weekly from May to November 2019 with the goal of creating a nurturing space of agency for the women inside the facility, addressing the problem of idle time, supplementing healthy snacks, and equipping women with re-entry skills.

Data Collection

I used multiple qualitative methods to answer the research question '(How) Can an educational horticultural programme in a community correction setting benefit female clients?' The larger data pool I derived from the clinical sociological garden

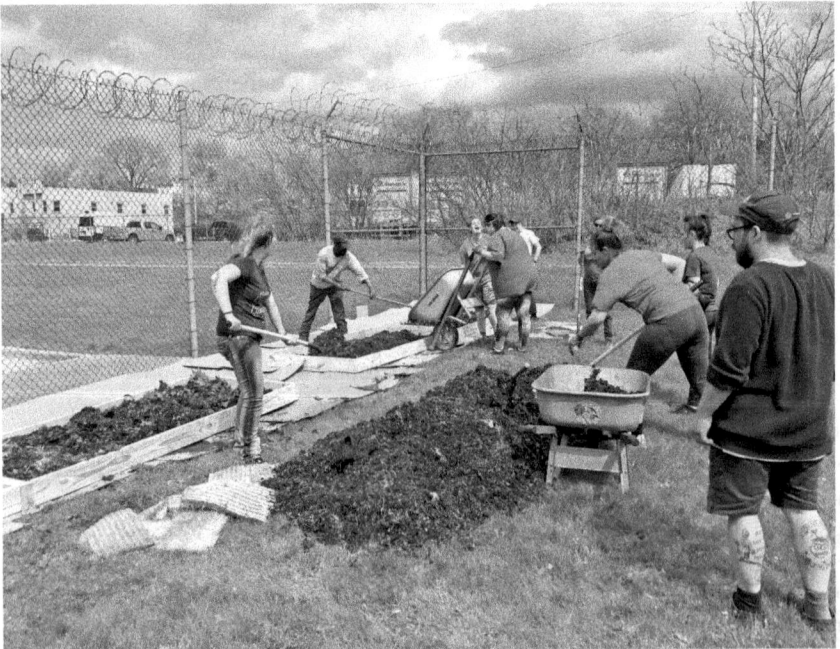

Figure 17.1 Establishing the garden in 2019 (image by author)

intervention includes participatory observation of gardening lessons, a focus group with clients discussing food and facility experiences and expectations of the garden programme, and a focus group with all stakeholders including facility management and community partners. Participatory observation meant that I was actively participating in the garden, working alongside the women, engaging in deep and natural field conversation, and observing social interactions closely. I wrote copious fieldnotes and additionally conducted interviews with community partners (n = 5) and staff members (n = 2) involved in the garden programme. The data set also includes written anonymous reflection narratives (n = 120) from female clients after the completion of individual gardening lessons.

With the onset of the COVID-19 pandemic in early Spring 2020, facility management terminated the garden programme, and the field site was on complete lockdown until August 2020. The garden operated for four weeks in August 2020 before shutting down again. During the pandemic, the garden programme director and I met for five weeks with an average of five women weekly in the garden. We were supported by a Social Work intern who helped develop the women's programme in prior months. From these five weeks of gardening in the women's corrections facility during the pandemic, I have rich fieldnotes I draw on for this chapter.

Research Results

Perceived Lack of Protection from COVID

Prisons and jails in the USA are overcrowded and social distancing is impossible. At the beginning of the pandemic, incarcerated people faced inadequate healthcare and lacked access to supplies like soap and masks (Ellis, 2020; Scott, 2021; Reinhart and Chen, 2021). Jennifer, imprisoned for life at a Florida Reception Centre, reports in April 2020 that 'they told us we must remain six feet apart. But I sleep in an open dorm with 78 beds, eight showers, 12 toilets, and eight sinks. Our bunks are only two feet apart, side by side' (quoted in Lewis, 2021). The women I worked with in the agency were not affected by overcrowding, as the facility was not at maximum capacity during this time. Yet, they did not feel adequately protected from COVID-19. The participants reported that they had not received any COVID-19 testing and that 'someone is always sick in there,' and when they report sick, they are told 'not to spread panic' (Fieldnotes, 1 August 2020).

In contrast to women's reports, the garden program director of the agency cautioned that COVID-19 rapid tests were widely available in the agency (Fieldnotes, 3 August 2020). In addition, masks seemed available, as all women who came out to the garden were in possession of masks (some wore them below their chin). Other problems women noted related to water quality. One participant shared, 'The water is brown and yellow. We must take our medications with brown water' (Fieldnotes, 3 August 2020). Given the cancellation of in-person visits and lockdown restrictions, the correctional staff was likely the leading factor in introducing the virus into facilities (Lacoste et al., 2021). While I did not observe staff members disregarding safety precautions at my field site, incarcerated women across the USA reported that correctional staff had not complied with safety protocols. Women were concerned about retaliation if they voiced their concerns (Scott, 2021; Welch and Deitch, 2021).

Inconsistent Responses from the Criminal Justice System

Reinhard and Chen (2021) estimate that non-carceral management of nonviolent alleged offences would have been associated with a 2.0% reduction in daily COVID-19 case growth rates. This would have amounted to more than ten million cases that could have been avoided. At the beginning of the pandemic, significant policy changes were enacted to depopulate crowded prisons and jails by reducing admissions and increasing releases. Most policy changes were late and insufficient, and states and counties abandoned their efforts as the pandemic wore on (Prison Policy Initiative, 2021).

The court in the county where my field site is located shut down for a year, with most trials delayed and handled via telephone and video conferencing. That also meant that the court reduced intake numbers for the facility because fewer women were sentenced in the first year of the pandemic. While this was a positive development, detained women in our research revealed dynamics that created strain. A few women consistently reported attempts to keep them in the facility longer. Entering the garden for the first time after the shutdown, I noted that the facility, which holds approximately 60 beds, was only filled to a third, according to staff and participant reports. I documented in my field notes:

> The unit for medication-assisted drug treatment is currently closed, and two of the three garden volunteers today reported that there were attempts to keep them in the facility for a lot longer than their original sentencing. Both had to contact their lawyers to confirm that they could be released because there were. (Fieldnotes, 1 August 2020)

Natalie, a frail young white woman, eagerly participated in every gardening lesson we offered during the pandemic. She was new to the facility, having been incarcerated because she failed to show up for three drug tests due to a lack of childcare and transportation, typical barriers for women's re-entry (Michalsen, 2019). Missing the drug tests was a violation of her probation, but Natalie said she had been sober and clean and had not relapsed.

Overall, one-third of incarcerated girls are held for status offences or for violating the terms of their probation (Sentencing Project, 2020). For example, Natalie 'believed she would be in there for three months, but she did not know.' It is concerning that there is a lack of transparency about the length of her confinement that can be reduced or extended depending on a client's treatment completion and compliance violations. Facility management decides release dates together with treatment and counselling staff. Given the fact that the agency receives day rates for each client, a financial motive for the practice of sentence extensions is plausible. Kouri and Lemoine (2021) find a similar dynamic in their analysis of a roundtable with representatives of eight community-based residential facilities in Canada. Participants highlighted that the use of de-carceration measures can conflict with maintaining the financial stability and capacity of agencies and described challenges to advocating for the release of lower-risk individuals.

Limited Access to Social Support, Treatment, and Programming

Overall, women reported that access to treatment was limited in pandemic times due to the cessation of movement between inside and outside. We were invited back to the garden for a short period in August 2020 because it was the safest leisure time activity the facility could offer at the time. It was outdoors, which allowed for social distancing, and we made sure to bring gloves, surgical masks, and sanitiser to every session. However, other programming had been entirely cut. External contractors and volunteers provide much of prison programming (12-step programmes, faith groups, educational classes, etc.), and family and friend visits are essential for social support. Unfortunately, these opportunities for outside contact had been halted as part of the agency's COVID-19 policies.

One of the garden evaluation outcomes was how much the women appreciated that people came in from the outside and took the time to work with the women (Jauk and Blackwood, 2021; Jauk, Blackwood, and Boros, 2020). Unfortunately, this outlet was wholly erased for them during COVID-19. All programming had ceased because the facility was on lockdown, and the women were deprived of social contacts that had been minimised as a protection measure. Maintaining contact with family members during incarceration significantly lowers concerns about re-entry (Baker et al., 2021) and is crucial for women's desistance from crime (Michalsen, 2019).

Consider the case of Lillith, a Black woman in her mid-20s, who missed her five-year-old son's birthday. She reported that she was allowed one meeting a week, but her counsellor said that the meeting must be in the treatment plan, and seeing her son is not part of the treatment. She was furious and stated she didn't get any treatment. She said that she saw a crisis counsellor for two weeks but never again (Fieldnotes, 3 August 2020). Brenda, a young white woman nearing her release date, said she kept requesting appointments with her caseworker that were then postponed (Fieldnotes, 20 August 2020). Our observations confirmed analyses of other researchers. In-person counselling has been suspended in most facilities and available activities did not substitute for professional treatment. Compounding this gap, the COVID crisis required correctional health care staff to focus on the needs of people with the virus, reducing their ability to provide critical preventive care for women in custody. Without access to care, stress can exacerbate mental health challenges and cause the immune system to deteriorate, leading to worse outcomes for those infected with COVID (Arregi et al., 2020; Ellis, 2020; Welch and Deitch, 2021).

Deteriorating Food Quality and Quantity

Access to healthy food at my field site had been a problem before the pandemic. 'This food is not for human consumption' was one of many complaints in the

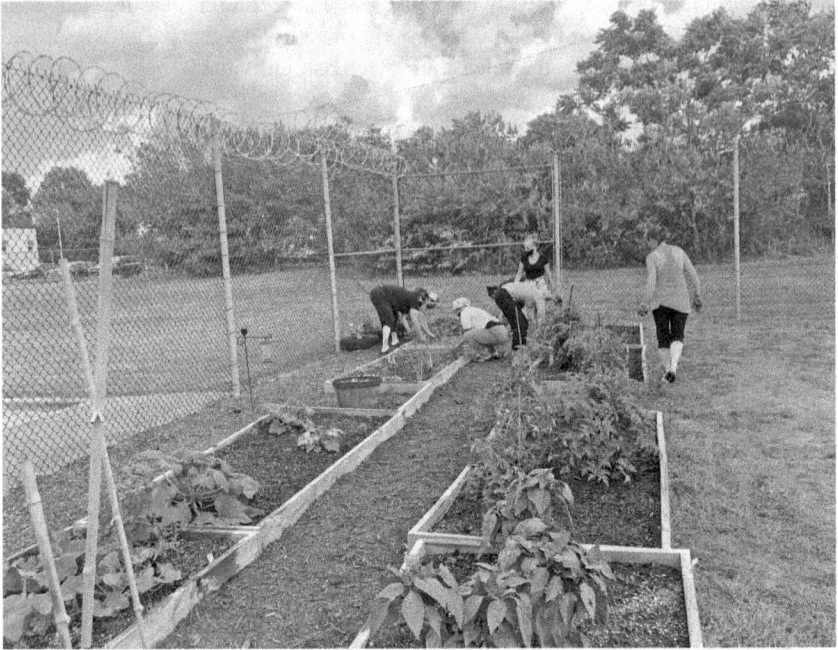

Figure 17.2 Pandemic gardening (image by author)

anonymous exit evaluations. 'It's not good enough for humans, not good enough for dogs like that's how bad it is … it's like punishment in itself,' said Etta in a focus group I conducted shortly before the pandemic (Focus Group, 18 February 2020). The food for my field site is supplied by the largest of the three major corporations that share the 4.1-billion-dollar prison food industry in the USA. Still, incarcerated people and their loved ones must spend an additional 1.4 billion dollars a year to supplement the inadequate and often spoiled food (Camplin, 2017; Worth Rises, 2020). On average, just over $2 per day is spent on food for an incarcerated person (Soble et al., 2020) for a diet typically composed of low-cost carbohydrates and processed meat. In the most comprehensive report on prison food to date, carceral institutions are conceptualised as 'out-of-sight food deserts' (Soble et al., 2020), perpetuating patterns of ill health amongst marginalised populations that already experience profound inequalities and food insecurity in their home communities (Testa and Jackson, 2019).

While the high-carb diet that often leads to weight gain and obesity is more common among incarcerated women (37%–43%) compared to incarcerated men (20%–27%) (Maruschak et al., 2015), data from our research indicate that meal skipping is a strategy women use, especially if they lack funds to supplement their diet. Amber reported that 'I lost weight when I couldn't eat the food anymore. I didn't want to eat it anymore. I didn't have money to buy vending machines stuff.'

Instead, Amber would just eat one piece of bread a day, a practice she kept up for an entire month (Focus Group, February 18.2020). This finding is in line with Soble et al. (2020) who found that 94% of survey respondents reported never being full in prison, and 93% being hungry between meals.

The pandemic has exacerbated the dire food situation behind bars. According to Blakinger (2021), prisoners said the food had become largely 'inedible and sometimes unidentifiable.' Many facilities reduced from three meals to two meals a day. In several instances, 'lockdown meals' or 'emergency menus' were served, and these tended to leave residents hungry and without a warm meal for weeks. The Marshall Project published pictures of 'food' served in American jails and prisons since the onset of the pandemic in early Spring 2020. The pictures reveal dry milk powder as a meal, green-grey meat patties, mould spots on bread, and a food diary revealing that many meals were skipped altogether (Blakinger, 2021). During the first visit and the preparation for the short pandemic gardening season, I noted:

> They also said they have been eating baloney sandwiches ninety days in a row every night and that the 'food is garbage.' And they also said that they call it 'mystery meat' because they never know what kind of meat they get to eat or if it is even real meat. (Fieldnotes, 1 August 2020)

The garden programme was attractive to the women because it offered access to alternative food sources. After the first gardening session, we decided we would bring some snacks. We brought celery sticks in individual plastic snack bags, portioned peanut butter in containers, and flavoured water, which the participants eagerly ate. Even if only briefly, the garden provided respite from a harsh environment that had become a danger zone in a global pandemic. The engagement of women and the opportunities for nurturing interactions with humans and plants demonstrate the potential for clinical sociology to permeate total institutions and bring hope to hidden and vulnerable populations.

Conclusion

This chapter focused on the effects of COVID-19 on the hidden and vulnerable population of women and girls behind bars in the USA during the pandemic through the lens of a clinical sociological garden project in a women's community corrections facility. Data speak to the perceived lack of protection from COVID-19, inconsistent and opaque responses from the criminal justice system, limited access to social support, and deteriorating food quality during the pandemic. As clinical sociologists, we find creative and research-based interventions to improve human lives. With this line of work, I seek to develop and apply a feminist rights-based approach in clinical sociology that focuses on healing and strengthening the voices of incarcerated women and girls (Brunsma et al., 2013; Fritz and Rheaume, 2014; Mancini Billson and Disch, 1990). Gardening can be designed as a gender-responsive treatment (Covington and Bloom, 2007; Fleming et al., 2021) that empowers women and in the spirit of clinical sociology, gardening in correctional settings can help to strengthen human rights for the female prison population in the USA (Barberet and Jackson, 2017).

In the truncated growing season during the pandemic, I saw the garden in the women's community corrections facility as a respite and sociological intervention that was able to bring positive interaction, extra healthy outside time, and validation for the women's voices we were able to capture. This applied not only to the women residents but also to the staff member who had been assigned to supervise the gardening lessons. I noted in my field notes:

Andria did a lesson on soil today and brought a jar filled with soil and water to explain the different layers of sediment. Women were eagerly listening and sitting around her in a half-circle. She brought a compost tumbler set that had to be put together for the practical part. It was remarkable how staff member Misty was really into gardening and actively participated throughout the entire session. This has never happened before. When asked how she feels

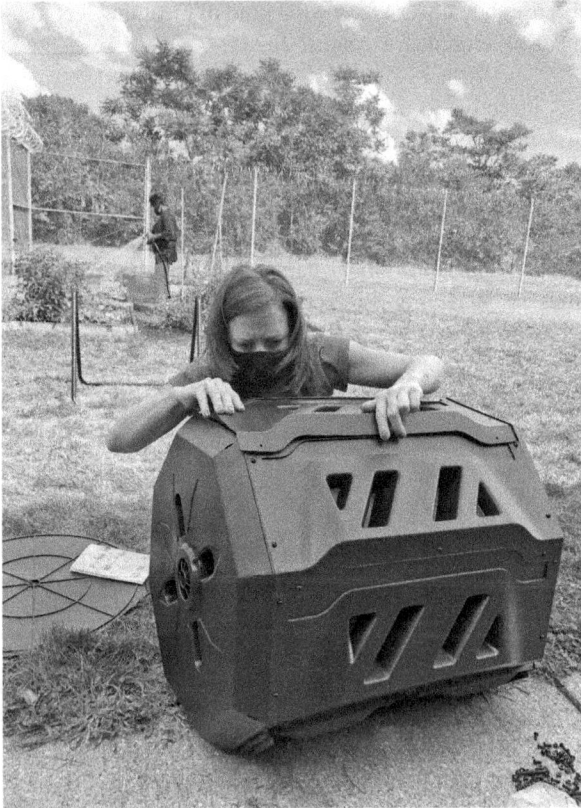

Figure 17.3 Building a tumbler and staff member watering in the background (image by author)

about the garden, she said, 'wonderful.' She feels 'wonderful and excited about the garden and eager to see the fruits.' Misty and Natalie jumped at the opportunity to put the tumbler together, and it took a good half hour to 40 minutes to put all the parts in the right places. It was so fulfilling to see how Misty and Natalie collaborated as equals, and hierarchical boundaries were transgressed as they struggled with the black plastic and the vague instructions. It made clear to me that collaborative gardening is not only good for the rapport between staff and clients but also empowers women to be active and 'create' something as well as strengthens skills (in this case, following instructions, persevering through challenges, communicating), and finally, is also an outlet for staff members to break through routines and get some extra outside time.

(Fieldnotes, 13 August 2020)

In terms of the larger context of COVID-19 in American penal institutions, there is an urgent need for de-carceration, i.e., the release of incarcerated populations, especially women serving time for nonviolent offences (Arregi et al., 2020; Lacoste et al., 2021; Reinhart and Chen, 2021; Welch and Deitch, 2021). We need to move away from hyper-imprisonment and adopt a healthier approach that will simultaneously strengthen public health and improve safety for women in custody and their children, families, and communities. We must view women in prison and jails as a priority group with unique needs in our responses to the COVID-19 crisis (Ellis, 2020), and urge institutions to better implement the UN Rules for the Treatment of Women Prisoners (Bangkok Rules) as human rights framework that recognises that female incarcerated individuals have different needs respecting their diverse backgrounds (Barberet and Jackson, 2017; Welch and Deitch, 2021).

The strategies that correctional systems have implemented to mitigate the spread of the virus within prisons and jails (i.e., additional separation and isolation) exacerbate harm for women (Welch and Deitch, 2021). Additionally, DOCs and the Department of Justice need to be held accountable to report COVID-19 metrics disaggregated by facility and sex-disaggregated for mixed facilities to help researchers and the public better understand the COVID-19 situation in carceral institutions (Lacoste et al., 2021; Welch and Deitch, 2021). While these are more significant big-picture issues and need a radical restructuring of the penal complex, we can take actions today to support incarcerated women and girls in the USA.

Arregi et al. (2020) suggest supporting organisations led by formerly incarcerated women, such as the National Council for Incarcerated and Formerly Incarcerated Women (https://www.nationalcouncil.us/). Another option is contributing to bail-out funds for incarcerated mothers such as The National Bail Out Collective (https://www.nationalbailout.org/) which is a Black-led initiative coordinating the #FreeBlackMamas campaign. We can also promote the planting of more prison gardens for women who remain in custody. Researchers of the pandemic in women's penal institutions in the USA have loudly called to expand and enhance the programmes and services available for women and particularly expand wellness programmes that promote women's health, including better food options (Arregi et al., 2020; Ellis, 2020; Lacoste et al., 2021; Welch and Deitch, 2021). Educational gardening is a restorative practice and a safe outdoor activity with the potential to enhance health and well-being and supply additional nutrition. Gardening as a clinical sociological intervention should challenge dominant discourses of personal responsibility and employ a gender-sensitive and trauma-informed approach that can account for structural violence and injustice shaping re-entry experiences for women. It is a space for women's agency and resistance in pandemic times. It is a space to envision a better future and create a better Now.

Acknowledgements

I want to warmly thank Dr Andria Blackwood for her brainwork and hands-on work in the garden, the garden is her legacy as she served as the director of the garden programme in 2019 and 2020, and her comments have greatly improved this chapter. I am indebted to *Let's Grow Akron*, particularly Lisa Nunn and Sam Phillips, for their generous support of the project and Jacqueline Kowalksi from the *OSU Extension Office* for many hours spent as co-conspirator and guest lecturer. I also thank Dr Alec Boros, a champion for the garden programme in the agency. I thank Dr Kathryn Feltey and the anonymous reviewers for valuable comments on the chapter, and finally, I thank the editors for their excellent support despite pandemic times.

Notes

1 The two major data hubs are *The UCLA Law COVID Behind Bars Data Project* (https://uclacovidbehindbars.org) and The Covid Prison Project (https://covidprisonproject.com/) collecting and combining available data published by individual DOCs.
2 Data on vaccination frequency and status is tracked and updated based on media reports and DOC websites and shows gaping holes; see_https://covidprisonproject.com/covid-19-vaccinations-system-report/, accessed 18 November 2021.
3 All names in this chapter are altered for confidentiality; geographic data is de-identified.
4 Extension Offices are sponsored by the United States Department of Agriculture in collaboration with land-grant universities and state and local governments. They provide research-based information and education to the public on subjects relating to agriculture and food, home, the environment, community economic development, and youth.

References

Arregi, A., Bridget C., Siegel, M., and Herzig, A. (2020). Forgotten victims? Women and COVID-19 behind bars. Retrieved from https://sites.tufts.edu/wpf/files/2020/11/Forgotten-Victims-Women-and-COVID-19-Behind-Bars-Final.pdf.

Ascencio, J. (2018). Offenders, work, and rehabilitation: Horticultural therapy as a social cognitive career theory intervention for offenders. *Journal of Therapeutic Horticulture* 28(1), pp. 21–28.

Baker, T., Mitchell, M., and Gordon, J. (2021). Prison visitation and concerns about reentry: Variations in frequency and quality of visits are associated with reentry concerns among people incarcerated in prison. *International Journal of Offender Therapy and Comparative Criminology*. doi: 10.1177/0306624X211013516.

Barberet, R., and Jackson, C. (2017). UN rules for the treatment of women prisoners and non-custodial sanctions for women offenders (the Bangkok Rules): A gendered critique. *Revista de Sociologia 102*(2), pp. 215230. doi: 10.5565/rev/papers.2336.

Blakinger, K. (2021). *Inside Frigid Texas Prisons: Broken Toilets, Disgusting Food, Few Blankets*. Retrieved from https://www.themarshallproject.org/2021/02/19/inside-frigid -texas-prisons-broken-toilets-disgusting-food-few-blankets.

Bronson, J., and Berzofsky, M. (2017). *Indicators of Mental Health Problems Reported by Prisoners and Jail Inmates, 2011–12*. U.S. Department of Justice. Retrieved from https:// bjs.ojp.gov/content/pub/pdf/imhprpji1112.pdf.

Brunsma, D., Iyall Smith, K., and Gran, B. (Eds.). (2013). *The Handbook of Sociology and Human Rights*. Boulder, London: Paradigm Publishers.

Camplin, E. (2017). *Prison Food in America*. Lanham, MD: Rowman and Littlefield.

Chesney-Lind, M., and Pasko, L. (2013). *Girls, Women, and Crime: Selected Readings*. 2nd ed. London: SAGE.

Covington, S., and Bloom, B. (2007). Gender responsive treatment and services in correctional settings. *Women and Therapy 29*(3–4), pp. 9–33. doi: 10.1300/ J015v29n03_02.

Daly, K. (1992). Women's pathways to felony court: Feminist theories of lawbreaking and problems of representation. *Southern California Review of Law and Women's Studies 2*(11), pp. 11–52.

Ellis, R. (2020). *In Prison in a Pandemic: Gender behind Bars*. The Gender Policy Report. Retrieved from https://genderpolicyreport.umn.edu/in-prison-in-a-pandemic-gender -behind-bars/.

Fleming, E., Lopez Wright, F., Wurzburg, S., and Nevi, B. (2021). *Adopting a Gender-responsive Approach for Women in the Justice System: A Resource Guide*. New York: The Council of State Governments Justice Center. Retrieved from https://csgjusticecenter .org/publications/adopting-a-gender-responsive-approach-for-women-in-the-justice -system-a-resource-guide/.

Fritz, J., and Rheaume, J. (Eds.). (2014). *Community Intervention: Clinical Sociology Perspectives*. New York: Springer.

Jauk, D., and Blackwood, A. (2021). The Serenity in the Garden project. Virtual presentation conducted for Social and Ecological Infrastructure for Recidivism Reduction Conference. Virtual. Retrieved from https://www.youtube.com/watch?v=db4irl-dvwoandt=2530s.

Jauk, D., Blackwood, A., and Boros, A. (2020). 'We are a creation just like these are creations and we deserve that chance.' Gardening as clinical sociology for women in community corrections. Virtual presentation for *Association for Applied and Clinical Sociology Annual Meeting*. Retrieved from https://www.youtube.com/watch?v =j2Ym3HOfnRkandt=7s.

Jauk, D., and Everhardt, S. (2018). Veggies against barriers: Feminist methodologies of gardens for women in correctional settings. *Presented at the Sociologists for Women in Society Winter Meetings*, February 7, Denver, CO.

Jauk, D., Gill, B., Everhardt, S., and Caruana, C. (2022). Systemic inequality, sustainability, and covid-19 in US prisons: A sociological exploration of women's prison gardens in pandemic times. In *Research in Political Sociology, Vol. 29*, edited by S. Aladuwaka, B. Weijnert, and A. Alagan. Bingley, West Yorkshire: Emerald Group Publishing Ltd.

Kaba, M. (2018). *Criminalizing Survival: A Resource of Curricula and Activities*. Retrieved from https://survivedandpunished.org/2018/10/16/criminalizing-survival-a-resource-of -curricula-and-activities/.

Kajstura, A. (2019). Women's mass incarceration: The whole pie 2018. *Prison Policy Initiative*. Retrieved from https://www.prisonpolicy.org/reports/pie2019women.html.

Kouri, D., and Lemoine, J. (2021). Challenges and promising practices in correctional healthcare during the Covid-19 pandemic: A perspective from community-based residential facility operators in Canada. *Advancing Corrections Journal 12*, pp. 30–52.

Kruttschnitt, C., Joosen, K., and Bijleveld, C. (2019). Research note: Re-examining the gender responsive approach to female offending and its basis in the pathway's literature. *Journal of Offender Rehabilitation 58*(6), pp. 485–499. doi: 10.1080/10509674.2019.1621415.

Lacoste, A., Paliwal, S., Tyagi, E., and Johnson, H. (2021). *'Horrible Here': How Systemic Failures of Transparency have Hidden the Impacts of Covid-19 on Incarcerated Women.* UCLA Covid Behind Bars Project. Retrieved from https://uclacovidbehindbars.org/horrible-here-covid-impacts-incarcerated-women.

Lao, J., and Behne, F. (2021). States halt COVID data publication. *COVID Prison Project*. Retrieved from https://covidprisonproject.com/blog/data/states-halt-covid-data-publication/.

LeBeau, C. (2020). Opinion | The Federal Bureau of Prisons must be held accountable for the death of my granddaughter. *The Washington Post*. 22 May 2020. Retrieved from https://www.washingtonpost.com/opinions/2020/05/22/federal-bureau-prisons-must-be-held-accountable-death-my-grandaughter/.

Lewis, N. (2021). How we survived COVID-19 in prison. *The Marshall Project*. Retrieved from   https://www.themarshallproject.org/2021/04/23/how-we-survived-covid-19-in-prison.

Macmadu, A., Berk, J., Kaplowitz, E., Mercedes, M., Rich, J., and Brinkley-Rubinstein, L. (2020). COVID-19 and mass incarceration: A call for urgent action. *The Lancet Public Health 5*(11), pp. e571–572. doi: 10.1016/S2468-2667(20)30231-0.

Mancini Billson, J., and Disch, E. (1990). Empowering women: A clinical sociology model for working with women in groups. In *Handbook of Clinical Sociology*, edited by J. G. Bruhn and H. M. Rebach (pp. 323–342). Berlin: Springer Science and Business Media.

Marquez, N., Ward, J., Parish, K., Saloner, B., and Dolovich, S. (2021). COVID-19 incidence and mortality in federal and state prisons compared with the US population, April 5, 2020, to April 3, 2021. *JAMA 326*(18), pp. 1865–1867. doi: 10.1001/jama.2021.17575.

Maruschak, L., Berzofsky, M., and Unangst, J. (2015). *Medical Problems of State and Federal Prisoners and Jail Inmates, 2011–12*. NCJ 248491. U.S. Department of Justice. Retrieved from https://bjs.ojp.gov/content/pub/pdf/mpsfpji1112.pdf.

Michalsen, V. (2019). *Mothering and Desistance in Reentry*. Milton Park: Routledge.

National Center of Transgender Equality. (2018). LGBTQ people behind bars. A guide to understanding the issues facing transgender prisoners and their legal rights. *National Center for Transgender Equality*. Retrieved from https://transequality.org/sites/default/files/docs/resources/TransgenderPeopleBehindBars.pdf.

Novisky, M., Nowotny, K., Jackson, D., Testa, A., and Vaughn, M. (2021). Incarceration as a fundamental social cause of health inequalities: Jails, prisons, and vulnerability to COVID-19. *The British Journal of Criminology 61*(6), pp. 1630–1646. doi: 10.1093/bjc/azab023.

Prison Policy Initiative. (2021). Criminal justice responses to the coronavirus pandemic. Retrieved from https://www.prisonpolicy.org/virus/virusresponse.html.

Reinhart, E., and Chen, D. (2021). Association of jail decarceration and anticontagion policies with COVID-19 case growth rates in US counties. *JAMA Network Open 4*(9), p. e2123405. doi: 10.1001/jamanetworkopen.2021.23405.

Richie, B. (2012). *Arrested Justice: Black Women, Violence, and America's Prison Nation.* New York, NY: NYU Press.

Saloner, B., Parish, K., Ward, J., DiLaura, G., and Dolovich, S. (2020). COVID-19 cases and deaths in federal and state prisons. *JAMA 324*(6), pp. 602–603. doi: 10.1001/jama.2020.12528.

Sawyer, W., and Bertram, W. (2018). Jail will separate 2.3 million mothers from their children this year. *Prison Policy Initiative.* Retrieved from https://www.prisonpolicy.org/blog/2018/05/13/mothers-day-2018/.

Scott, M. (2021, March 15). I'm trapped in a women's prison during a pandemic. *Elle.* Retrieved from https://www.elle.com/culture/career-politics/a35766530/prison-pandemic-story-michele-scott/.

Sentencing Project. (2020). Incarcerated women and girls. *The Sentencing Project.* Retrieved from https://www.sentencingproject.org/publications/incarcerated-women-and-girls/.

Soble, L., Stroud, K., and Weinstein, M. (2020). Ending the hidden punishment of food in prison. *Impact Justice.* Retrieved from https://impactjustice.org/impact/food-in-prison/#report.

Swavola, E., Riley, K., and Subramanian, R. (2016). *Overlooked: Women and Jails in an Era of Reform.* New York, NY: VERA Institute of Justice. Retrieved from https://www.vera.org/publications/overlooked-women-and-jails-report.

Testa, A., and Jackson, D. (2019). Food insecurity among formerly incarcerated adults. *Criminal Justice and Behavior 46*(10), pp. 1493–1511. doi: 10.1177/0093854819856920.

Toews, B., Wagenfeld, A., and Stevens, J. (2018). Impact of a nature-based intervention on incarcerated women. *International Journal of Prisoner Health 14*(4), pp. 232–243.

Van der Linden, S. (2015). Green prison programmes, recidivism, and mental health: A primer. *Criminal Behaviour and Mental Health 25*(5), pp. 338–342.

Wacquant, L. (2001). Deadly symbiosis: When Ghetto and prison meet and mesh. *Punishment & Society 3*(1), pp. 95–133. doi: 10.1177/14624740122228276.

Wagner, P., and Bertram, W. (2020). What percent of the USA is incarcerated? (And other ways to measure mass incarceration). *Prison Policy Initiative.* Retrieved from https://www.prisonpolicy.org/blog/2020/01/16/percent-incarcerated/.

Welch, A., and Deitch, M. (2021). *The Pandemic Gender Gap Behind Bars: Meeting the Needs of Women in Custody during COVID-19 and Planning for the Future.* May. Austin: The Lyndon B. Johnson School of Public Affairs at the University of Texas at Austin. Retrieved from https://repositories.lib.utexas.edu/handle/2152/85440.

World Economic Forum. (2021). *Global Gender Gap Report 2021.* Retrieved from https://www.weforum.org/reports/global-gender-gap-report-2021.

Worth Rises. (2020). The prison industry: The curriculum. *Worth Rises.* Retrieved from https://worthrises.org/wk8-telecom.

Wright, E., Van Voorhis, P., and Salisbury, E. (2012). Gender-responsive lessons learned and policy implications for women in prison. *Criminal Justice and Behavior 39*(12), pp. 1612–1632. doi: 10.1177/0093854812451088.

18 Food or Data

The Realities of the Online Teaching Transition during COVID-19 in South Africa

Mariam Seedat-Khan, Quraisha Dawood and Aradhana Ramnund-Mansingh

Introduction

The extent of COVID-19 and the subsequent worldwide lockdowns have metamorphosed a histrionic shift in the education sector. The age-old tradition of a conventional contact teaching model at universities has never experienced such profound amendments. Suddenly, academics and students were hurtled into an unaccustomed technological domain of electronic learning. This has emerged as the archetype for education amid a pandemic. The appeal for social distancing, self-isolation, travel limitations, and computer-based virtual instruction has become the leading new interface for academics and learners. Naturally, the consequences are both advantageous and disadvantageous. This is exceptionally diverse in the context of South Africa (SA), where the pandemic and inequality have laid bare the conspicuous gap between the rich and poor. The original founding of an insular university archetype remains a momentous, ubiquitous component of 21st-century institutions worldwide. Universities act as catalysts regulating each country's universal pecuniary standings amidst the worldwide novel COVID-19 pandemic. The earliest tradition of specialised degree programmes and rigorous scientific research has continued unremittingly. Academics have efficaciously sustained conscientious scientific research necessitated by COVID-19 hazards. The mandate foisted on academics has seen the university archetype experience an unprecedented transfiguration. The directive implored academics to intellectualise pedagogic prototypes realising the delivery of professional degree specifications (Dwivedi et al., 2020; García-Morales, Garrido-Moreno & Martín-Rojas, 2021). Once upon a time, university classes necessitated a class occupied by students and an academic dispensing the discourse. Scholars worldwide responded to the call for the meteoric revolutionisation of a COVID-19 academy.

The timely, pioneering inventiveness of academics recognised the significance of treatises grounded in socially constructed realities (Seedat-Khan, Ramnund-Mansingh & Johnson, 2020). The new normal necessitates the formation of a university archetype contemplating new measures indicated by synchronous and asynchronous pedagogies. Incongruities with staff and students' ownership of

DOI: 10.4324/9781003267133-24

technological hardware, software, and access to the world wide web have uncovered the actualities of the digital divide. Scrutiny of complexities includes several unrestricted virtual platforms offering multiple subscribers uncomplicated access via innumerable personal electronic devices, with substantial hardware dissimilarity for users. The lengthened teaching and preparation hours necessitate participation in elementary training for specialised proficiencies burdens required for a possibly plausible titanic amendment to every aspect of teaching and learning. The augmented workload imposed on academics fails to cogitate the impact on the merit of discourse delivery distinction. This novel virtual didactic design impacts unsympathetically on students and academics. The cutting-edge new socially constructed normal calls for swift clarifications from academics to safeguard the strategic online instruction, erudition, and evaluation archetype. Vanguard instruction and erudition approaches are steeped in existing theoretical models and pedagogies on the social construction of knowledge. The import of COVID-19 dictates progressive technological acquaintance. Auxiliary fiscal resources are necessitated to support augmented administrative responsibility, software and hardware costs, access to technical support and merchandise vital to maintaining virtual classrooms. This study examines the substantial body of brand-new 2019–2020 erudition toward an online pedagogical teaching and learning enhancement. It takes into account the delivery of sociological intelligence and clinical intermediations, cogitating the shock of COVID-19, complexities, challenges, and possibilities that lie ahead when teaching online. As sociologists, we have positioned our study to concentrate on the causative components of a fragmented society that favours the rich and neglects the poor. It considers the legacy of apartheid and the pressure put on the socio-economic context by the fourth Industrial Revolution (4IR) and then leads the reader to a risk assessment and suggested recommendations.

Methodology

A qualitative desktop methodological approach has been selected, which reconnoitres the bearing of online teaching and learning on academics and students at universities in South Africa and worldwide. The analysis of secondary scholarship and the use of theory around the social construction of knowledge facilitates the presentation of virtual education in an unjust society. This study originates with recognising technological, social, and economic impediments that commence with cognising academic limitations in realising optimum online instruction. The complexities amidst COVID-19 are compounded by the remnants of the apartheid education system and the unscathed racial and economic divide immortalised in South Africa. Secondary methods or desktop research was used to conduct the study. This method was elected to react cursorily to the requirements of the pandemic. The suitability of budgetary concessions and the complexities of primary research amid COVID-19 reinforced the cogency of selection.

The purpose of primary research generally should be to fill in gaps in existing knowledge. These gaps cannot be identified without an understanding of the existing knowledge base. The term does not imply anything about the importance of the information, only that it is being used for research beyond the specific informational need that prompted the original gathering of the data. All primary research may ultimately become someone else's secondary source.

(Stewart & Kamins, 1994, p. 4)

The integrity of the research is, however, maintained. Academics and authors at both public and private institutions facilitated reflective acumens. They are aligned to recent COVID-19 scholarship; scrutiny of current literature sanctioned researchers to postulate first-hand perceptiveness into a clinical model for the application. The model integrates the inimitably South African perspective that higher education institutions should consider as a risk mitigation perspective.

The Social Construction of Knowledge

The social construction of reality advanced by Berger and Luckmann (1979) is grounded on pre-existing knowledge from individuals and their environments. Entrenched in knowledge and social education theories, the unambiguous application is established in an analogous paradigm by Vygotsky in Cole et al. (1978) and Freire (1972). Collectively acquiesced knowledge that interaction between academics and students was mandatory. Whilst the assessment advanced by Freire (1972) in the Pedagogy of the Oppressed on banking theory indicates how an academic might use their position of authority to 'force' socially constructed philosophies, it is noted as one of the detrimental outcomes of the social construction of reality. Though Vygotsky cogitates this power when he affirms,

important learning by the child occurs through social interaction with a skilful tutor. The tutor may model behaviours and provide verbal instructions for the child. Vygotsky refers to this as a cooperative or collaborative dialogue. The child seeks to understand the actions or instructions provided by the tutor (often the parent or teacher), then internalises the information, using it to guide or regulate their performance.

(Mangal & Mangal, 2019, p. 209)

Organised theoretical frameworks accentuate the significance of the educator is palpable concerning both constructive and ineffectual inferences. Vygotsky discerned that a constructive academic could have a proportionately reformist bearing. Irrefutably, these philosophies can be expanded to substantiate the assertions of controlled virtual learning, notwithstanding its physical or virtual staging. This theoretical lens is further shaped by the intricacies of the unequal context of education, the pressure of 4IR, and the distinction between public and private universities.

The South African Context

Education underpins economic, political, and social advancement in a contemporary globalised capitalist economy. It has been used as an instrument for subjugation in the once apartheid state. Conversely, it was utilised as a liberation tool to construct indispensable tools required to destabilise the apartheid state. In COVID-19, the digital aperture is the sine qua non of the solution; it is a significant concern and requires prioritisation if we can guarantee to learn through the lockdown. This chapter is a fragment of sociological reconnaissance into the existing condition of higher education in South Africa amid a global pandemic. We have initiated eminent sociological questions that have been relegated for too long. If education is to realise a learning model, we must begin cognising and contextualising the multifarious provisos and proficiencies for academics and students. We cannot ignore the decisive intersections of class, race, gender, access, privilege, and unequal resources when pondering innovative learning pedagogies in an inimitable global epoch. The veracity of these factors is multifaceted and translates adversely into unemployment, poverty, and employability in society. South Africans have an incomparable socially constructed reality based on a series of social and political encounters in their lives. This South African actuality is differentiated and established on race, class, gender, religion, ethnicity, and political and socio-economic intensified by COVID-19. The splinters in post-apartheid education are a precise cause for panic when repositioning curricula to a virtual platform. In addition to these, higher education institutions continue to adapt and endure challenges from the 2004 post-apartheid reorganisation, where the merger of racially distinct universities unlocked institutions for all students. Academics continue to feel the burden of the corporatisation of universities, and female academics are encumbered by gender-specific challenges that impact their classroom roles and lives as academics (Ramnund, 2019).

The Remnants of Apartheid Education

The legacy of apartheid cannot be negated amidst COVID-19 for some indispensable explanations. South African universities were founded on racial separateness. The significance of infrastructure and allotment of treasuries to apartheid universities occurred relative to race. The University of Fort Hare was founded for African students; Indian students attended the University of Durban Westville while Coloured students obtained a qualification from the University of Western Cape; these apartheid universities were referred to as bush colleges (Ramnund, 2019). Privileged white students read for degrees at small universities equipped with exceptional infrastructure; these included the erstwhile University of Natal, Stellenbosch University, Rhodes University, and the University of Cape Town. Post-2004, the merged institutions were ineffectually equipped for students' demand and exponential growth and subsequently failed to expedite analogous academic staff development. Lecture venues and academics struggled to cope with the need for access to higher education, and the academic, administrative, and teaching workload multiplied rapidly, placing pressure on academics to maintain academic excellence without additional support and resources (Seedat-Khan, Ramnund-Mansingh & Johnson, 2020). Institutions across the country had reached the breaking point regarding capacity to accommodate students in residences and the classroom. The repercussions of apartheid education are unceasing, with poverty bolstering low levels of education. Formal schooling statistics are signifiers functioning on a continuum to higher education and employment indicators.

South African 2019 statistics (Education.gov.za) indicate the existence of 1,966 independent- private schools and 23,796 public schools, of which 11,000 of all public schools are mainly located in the rural districts of the Eastern Cape KwaZulu Natal and Limpopo province. Inadequate infrastructure, under-qualified educators, and partial resources indispensable to facilitate prescribed learning are absent. The previously widespread inequality gap is compounded by poor access to adequate education at a primary level impacting higher education successes. Public universities in South Africa are oversubscribed with extraordinarily large student bodies. In 2015, 25% of White matriculants had completed a bachelor's degree as opposed to 15% of Indians and 5% of Black and Coloured students (Maluleke, 2019). This oversubscription was supervened by private higher education institutions responding to student needs for access. This context incentivised private international higher education institutions to establish campuses in South Africa. Public universities have been slow to follow the lead of private universities, primarily due to the digital divide. The news of universities proceeding with the resumption of the academic programme was exceedingly hostile to student representative councils nationally. The lack of access, resources, and capabilities by a large contingent of the student body was cited as the critical reason for objection.

The Fourth Industrial Revolution

The past decade has prepared the world for the fourth Industrial Revolution (4IR). South Africa only initiated preparation for 4IR in 2017 (Xing, Marwala & Marwala, 2018). Smart technology has been embraced in various industries such as manufacturing, medicine, aeronautics, and global businesses such as Amazon, which has embraced drone technology to deliver goods to customers. Higher education ministries have promptly recognised the significance of their binary role in expeditiously bringing into line 4IR advancements. This certainty prompted the alignment of academic discourse to capabilities offered by 4IR. The different Industrial Revolutions have all impacted education and employment in histrionic and ubiquitous ways of their time. The fourth Industrial Revolution is often orientated with technology; however,

> within the Third Industrial Revolution, the expansion of access to higher education rose to even greater prominence with significantly increased diversity on campuses and globalisation of academic research accelerated by online technologies. An intensified commitment to large-scale higher education worldwide has increased participation rates in higher education.
>
> (Penprase, 2018, pp. 211–212)

In a South African context, we have not reached the advanced stages of robotics and AI in learning. Due to historical inequalities, we continue to equalise and align with the Third Industrial Revolution benchmarks. Higher education globally has long embraced a fully functional blended approach. Reference to an adaptive model by Xing, Marwala, and Marwala (2018) lends frameworks to the accessibility and acceleration to environmental contexts. This successful implementation is challenging from a South African perspective due to several gaps, including but not exclusive to digital literacy and accessibility to resources.

South Africa Playing Catch Up

The delayed response to 4IR and the rapid onset of COVID-19 has required universities to adopt virtual education prototypes. The South African education ministry previously envisioned a three to five-year plan to remodel academic discourse, teaching pedagogies, research, and assessment frameworks in line with 4IR trends (Gleason, 2018). Priorities within South African education have been relatively complex. The past decade has left us with insurmountable challenges within academia. Aligning with global higher education trends, South Africa had to play catch up in the operationalisation of institutions. At the same time, the traditional, cultural, and academic challenges such as the 'old boys' network' continue to ravage and destabilise female academics (Ramnund-Mansingh & Seedat-Khan, 2020). This is covertly executed whilst concurrently undertaking the mammoth task of decolonising a racially based apartheid-designed curriculum. The timing of a global pandemic could not have been worse. The distress of the COVID-19 pandemic has expedited the apportioning of these undertakings by forcing the higher education ministry to formulate an effective model guaranteeing the execution of the prescribed academic schedule.

Teaching and Employability

The meteoric reconfiguration of teaching pedagogies has been propelled by graduate employability in contradiction to the apartheid framework. Theoretically, employability has been transmuted with unconventional recruitment and interview practices such as gamification, which embraces technology to involve and inspire individuals to accomplish career objectives. Graduates leave universities with a collection of imperative skills and abilities, acknowledging their competence to contend in a universal employment market (Suleman, 2016; Al-Karaki et al., 2021). Failure to equip students with imperative proficiencies impacts the workplace and the economy. Learning begins the moment we are born and continues until our death. South Africa is only just becoming acquainted with changes in workplace trends and the impact of millennials in the workplace. This is yet another complexity, as workplaces must configure their workspace to accommodate a blend of 4IR intricacies with the millennial and growing digital native workforce. The traditional higher education structures have been instrumental in preparing different generations, and cognisance needs to be given to the conventional approach of sitting in a lecture hall and taking in academic theory. One is drawn to the educational pedagogies Freire (1972) designed, which denigrates these traditional approaches based on his theory of the banking approach. He was not in favour of the constant power educators had over students and the fact that they would impart their ideologies, values, and perceptions to students. This impacted the students' constructions of reality. Light (2001) concurs that learning difficulties that have not been treated appropriately and remedied facilitate extensive social problems of crime, deviance, and violence.

Private and Public Universities

The requisite for private higher education escalated dramatically, prompting international universities to establish roots in South Africa. The associated extraordinary cost of private higher education has triggered the admission of students from reasonably affluent backgrounds. These students are equipped with advanced technology and adequate financial resources to increase opportunities for success amid the pandemic. Private universities intensified the already wide socio-economic rift. While the digital divide has impacted private institutions on a smaller scale, it has not arrested, nor delayed, the delivery of curricula virtually (Lebelo, Moloi & Jaffer, 2020). The primary distinction between private and public universities is access; government-funded National Student Financial Aid Scheme (NSFAS) students cannot access entry to private institutions using the funding. Private higher education institutions MANCOSA, Regent Business School, Rosebank, Milpark Business School or Varsity College and universities that fall under the authority of the Independent Education Institute have since inception integrated various absentee configurations to facilitate distance learning. They were among the first institutions to migrate to online teaching and assessment models. The measured response to COVID-19 resulted in a seamless, prompt transition to online teaching, learning, and assessment. Students were offered multiple virtual platforms, which integrated content formulation, academic enhancement, and assessment evaluation webinars to fortify academic content delivery. These resources were further enhanced with discussion assemblies, instant communication services, audio-supported PowerPoint lectures, supplementary videos, prescribed and additional academic readings, and a learning journey with module-specific learning outcomes. Students unable to partake in live sessions are offered recorded sessions where the information is available.

The entanglement of COVID-19 lies in the deferment of 4IR, decolonisation and employability, instigating a paradigm shift to the urgency of an indispensable strategic focus on virtual education. Whilst researchers devise scientific studies which address up-to-date discourse for South Africa's gradual transition, and the higher education public sector is working feverishly to facilitate the immediate implementation of viable prototypes. During this time of uncertainty, a better solution for students would have been a private-public partnership. Public institutions can glean on experiences and infrastructure of private institutions where their online learning experience seems to be faring well with the student community. Private institutions have expeditiously transitioned during COVID-19 and have offered students an online summative assessment replacing the traditional sit-down examination, in line with the South African presidency's public gathering and social distancing requirements. Timely planning on the part of private universities has contributed to the swift transition to virtual classes on existing institutional portals. This is not without its unique challenges, with various categories of students centred on their access, mental health, and students who need to suspend, defer, or abandon the academic programme. There are substantial concerns with in-person and online exams. Access to data impacts largely on students who have only re-entered the province under stage three protocol after spending lockdown in rural familial homes. Students registered for professional degrees and engaged in ethnographic research require access to laboratories (Lebelo, Moloi & Jaffer, 2020). These factors characterise students who have only re-entered the province after spending lockdown in rural areas with their families. Working, scholarship, and self-funded students have by no means escaped the financial wrath of the pandemic. Job losses and modifications to privately funded agreements have compromised the ability of some students to make the requisite payments (Armoed, 2021).

Technological Transformation and Threats

Online platforms, such as Blackboard, Google classroom, Zoom, Microsoft Teams, and Skype have swiftly become familiar; universally, these are signifiers of a new socially constructed normal. Negotiations with data service providers have resulted in the availability of a limited number of zero-rated data tools, one of which is the commonly adopted online platform Moodle (Tamrat & Teferra, 2020). These concessions are only available to public university students. However, downloading videos, pre-recorded lessons, or presentations and attending virtual classes are not currently recognised as zero-rated. The implications for students at public universities are colossal. Downloading pre-recorded webinars or participating in virtual Zoom, Skype, or Microsoft Teams classes will require between 500 megabytes to 1.2 gigabytes of data. The current rate of 100 megabytes of data is R 15.00, an expense that students cannot incur. During this time, even students at private institutions find difficulty accessing online content due to data restrictions. Students' exclusive reliance on NSFAS funding and institutional infrastructure, computer facilities, library resources, printing, and internet services has been disconnected by COVID-19. This disengagement from essential physical university resources has further abated the students' prospect for academic success.

The Digital Divide

The alienation caused by the protracted lockdown since the 24th of March 2020 has required families to live in isolation, creating either an exclusion or an increase in professional and social engagement. The restrictions thwart socialisation, family gatherings, and in-person celebrations to avert the proliferation of the virus. Congruently families with limited internet access are excluded from involvement in virtual religious, social, and professional responsibilities, fostering social isolation. Pecuniary means and geographic location further constrain accessibility to connectivity. Virtual platforms are extraordinarily exorbitant, necessitating substantial bandwidth for a single computer per household. These South African contexts magnify the digital divide between the affluent and the underprivileged, impacting university students (Xing, Marwala & Marwala, 2018). A technological intervention has become vital to preserve a positive level of normalcy amid

COVID-19. It is precisely this access to technology that is revealing the veracity of inequality. The digital divide amplifies the space between rich and poor in an already fractured society, differentiating citizens by race and social class (Mhlanga & Moloi, 2020).

Donnelly and Kyriazopoulou (2014) delineate comprehensive education as an exercise of strengthening the capability of education structures to extend to every student. Comprehensive education necessitates educational institutions to deliver adequate resources to facilitate learning and teaching. Technological learning models have been fast-tracked, and academics and students have been mandated to become savoir-faire technologically instantaneously. However, notwithstanding the exponential expansion of technology in the 21st century, with the 4IR, the disproportionality between individuals with unencumbered access to the internet and individuals with no access is impenetrable. Ownership or access to a personal processor, laptop, or mobile device is forsaken on account of the expense; the accessibility to a dependable and secure internet connection and the capability of individuals to exploit devices optimally to obtain instructive resources is the fundamental impairment that South African academics and students face. Failure to acknowledge the prejudice, buttressing systematic inequity for the poor, threatens the success of a virtual learning model (Matli & Ngoepe, 2020; Van Wyk et al., 2020; Tamrat & Teferra, 2020).

The South African statistics present a picture consistent with the aftermath and remnants of apartheid. 10.4% of urban homes had access to the internet. Other homes relied on public access, including work and higher education institutions. 1.7% of rural households had internet connectivity. Internet access using mobile devices was 60.1%, while access at home was 10.4%, at work 16.2%, and elsewhere 10.1%. Mobile internet access devices in rural areas were 45.0% as opposed to 67.5% in metropolitan areas. Household access to the internet at home was highest in Western Cape (25.8%) and Gauteng (16.7%) and lowest in Limpopo (1.7%) (Maluleke, 2018). This is a part of the challenges students in public universities face. Other peripheral struggles include the lack of a device. The risk in these instances is significant during the global pandemic. In rural communities and informal settlements, the shared use of all commodities is due to necessity. The compulsion for online learning is likely to cause pandemonium in these areas. The two most severe consequences are that several students will be sharing a laptop, personal computer, tablet, or smart device (Mhlanga & Moloi, 2020; Van Wyk et al., 2020; Tamrat & Teferra, 2020). This increases the risk of COVID-19 contamination among the students. In addition, there is an opportunity for the exploitation of students. An individual with one of the above devices can hire it at a nominal cost. It is unlikely the sanitation protocols will be observed, thus increasing the risk of infection. It must also be noted that many rural parts do not accommodate internet access.

No Computers – No Data

Notwithstanding the emboldening prospect and gains that virtual learning depicts, online modalities have concurrently laid bare the inequalities around access to the requisite technologies, devices, and resources required to activate access to academic content. Although learning software has been zero-rated, asynchronous lessons deliver expediency for academics and learners. OECD data accentuates access to a computer workstation as a significant challenge (Li & Lalani, 2020). Li and Lalani (2020) report that 95% of learners in Switzerland and Austria have access to computer workstations to facilitate learning. In an unambiguous contrast, only 34% of learners in Indonesia, India, and Africa have access to a computer workstation. This is compounded by COVID-19, which has mandated parents to import their workday into the familial domain. This unfamiliar territory has compromised extended households in developing countries that do not necessarily possess the veracious and requisite quantity of computer workstations vital for multiple family members simultaneously. A computer workstation is a fundamental necessity for academics and learners; the auxiliary expenditure of internet access must congruently be measured. This disproportionate access marks indiscriminate participation in virtual classes. The unexploited opportunities are associated with reduced connectivity and inadequate pecuniary means. The rapid migration to virtual platforms bared technological drawbacks with academics and students, recognising the mandatory need for expert skills training, facilitating the seamless use of online media, book repositories, educational, research software, and associated portals. Access is more than acquiring a computer workstation or downloading virtual curricula; it is contingent on contextual factors, such as geographic location and data access. The lockdown resulted in thousands of students and academics returning to familial homes in remote rural areas. These outlying areas are commonly situated outside the internet and mobile network connectivity zones. The remote geographic location disturbs the ability of academics and learners to connect and participate virtually Mhlanga & Moloi, 2020; Matli & Ngoepe, 2020; Van Wyk et al., 2020; Tamrat & Teferra, 2020).

The Complexities of Online Teaching

Without a definite return date to a pre-COVID-19 existence, the higher education ministry has quickly recognised that academics and students must embrace electronic learning methodologies as the 'new normal.' Virtual learning in South Africa embraces both synchronous and asynchronous curricula. Synchronous curricula occur in real-time via digital platforms, which support audio and visuals for academics and learners to interact virtually. Asynchronous curricula include recorded lectures stored on a shared online platform accessible for learners to download and view at a convenient time. Empirical evidence of virtual methods demonstrates that learners retain added academic content because they can stop and repeat virtual lessons at leisure. Predominantly, emphasising the time redeeming component for the academic exercise depends on age, connectivity, and auxiliary circumstantial factors (Li & Lalani, 2020). Technology use has increased, with several virtual platforms offering free access to online meetings, resources, and educational software. Cogitating the merits of online teaching and learning, Li and Lalani (2020) proclaim that e-learning is 'here to stay.' 'There is no doubt that teaching and learning with technology make the learning exciting, effective, and efficient. There is a revolution in how teachers/lecturers are expected to teach the students and learners in the classroom' (Kwinana & Mohau, 2019, p. 18). The expeditious transference to a virtual platform has flouted the different skill sets academics require to circumnavigate synchronous online curricula (Moorhouse, 2020) and guarantee assessments emulate models of instruction to produce a quality experience for both academics and learners. Li and Lalani (2020) contend that perhaps a hybrid model which amalgamates face-to-face and virtual lessons necessitates priority and development as this express transference to virtual learning cannot be sustained indefinitely. The assessments have turned out to be stimulating and with the sole rationale of assessing to make sure that learning has occurred. Through the online formative and corrective evaluations, students can test their knowledge of the subjects taught repeatedly until an understanding is attained (Mashifana in Kwinana & Mohau, 2019, p. 18). Overall, teaching in the phase of COVID-19 increases mental health concerns and challenges for academics, learners, and parents. The 'uncertainty' identified by Sahu (2020) revolves around financial security, job security, and physical health. Families from all socio-economic strata have been affected in one way by the loss of income, job losses, and job insecurity. Yet, they are still held accountable for their financial commitments to educational institutions. Craig (2020) asserts that this is even more stressful for single mothers studying further and students who work to pay their university tuition. Sahu (2020) identifies the need for a social scientific study to quantify the value of online instruction and assessments designed for traditional face-to-face instruction. This primarily includes difficulties in delivering applied and clinical curricula where laboratory work is a substantial portion of the assessment.

Leaving the Children Behind

The inequalities of a South African society have developed progressively, becoming increasingly apparent in the COVID-19 context. The possibility of a bungled academic year has distressing pecuniary repercussions for South African students and their families. Unemployment in South Africa is presently at 29% and is conjectured to reach 36% in December 2020.

> Among those supported by the national financial aid scheme, two-thirds of undergraduate students have become dropouts five years after entering. Most drop out after the first year, many because the financial support is insufficient, and accommodation and transport are too expensive. Still, mostly because they fail to pass exams.
>
> (Tionneland, 2017, p. 4)

Data published by the South African Department of Higher Education and Training (DHET) indicates that 72% of all public university students are African, many of whom are the first in their families and communities to access higher education. The incalculable burden placed on students to graduate and secure suitable employment is impelled by their families' entrapment in the poverty cycle. They face several historic challenges elucidated by Tionneland (2017, p. 4):

> While there has been an impressive increase in the number of black students, from very poor households, the proportion of poor black students at South

African universities is limited. Less than five per cent of black secondary students with parents earning less than 120 000 qualify for entry into universities while the percentage of students with parents earning more than 600 000 is 70 per cent.

The South African government announced incentive schemes to alleviate citizens' limited financial burdens, but the system has been peppered with technical malfunctions and payment deferments. The dissemination and allocation of funds are guided by Black economic empowerment policy guidelines and have initiated prodigious discontent amongst South Africans. The manacles of the race once again force post-apartheid South Africa amid the devastating pandemic. This decision's repercussions have seen intense unemployment growth, impacting the poorest. The tenuous South African economy has witnessed 'the means to survive,' and others will 'struggle just to survive'; thus, du Plessis (2020) expounds that 'we live in two South Africas.'

COVID-19 has accentuated disproportions, particularly among higher education students. The resources for students to facilitate the completion of assigned academic workload via online curricula have left those with few options compromising the completion of their studies. Mathiba (2020) develops this take, enquiring how universities plan to accommodate stranded international students, with Mzileni (2020) querying the status of university residences. Poor students from rural areas rely on the proximity to campus and its infrastructure (computers, printers, books) to engage in academic work; the lockdown has denied students' access. The displacement has prompted pervasive insecurity resulting in mental health concerns (Sahu, 2020). An urgent plea for resources appears to eclipse government attempts at monetary relief. The converse of residences is problematic, with institutional accountability for sanitation protocols and social distancing.

COVID-19 Risks in the Academy

Identifying threat categories that consider inimitable dynamics intersecting on multifarious levels has been recognised in creating a clinical risk paradigm. We have proposed a distinctive phased three-pronged South African COVID-19 clinical approach to teaching pedagogies and academic content delivery. The model considers the role of all academics, teaching assistants, administrators, technical support, library services, risk management services, and health services in identifying a viable COVID-19 teaching model. The model offers three threat levels, with COVID-19 guidelines and accountability. These include Table , which is no threat-no risk; Table , which is intermediate threat medium-high risk; and Table which is utmost threat high risk. Each of these levels measures the role of academics, tutors, administrators, technical support, library services, and COVID-19 screening services to maintain and advance the intellectual project during a global pandemic. The interventions, Tables 18.1, 18.2 and 18.3 were designed by chapter author and clinical sociologist Prof Mariam Seedat-Khan.

Table 18.1 No threat-no risk in the academy

Threat Level *Covid-19 Guidelines* *Accountability*	*Teaching*	*Covid-19* *Class Configuration*	*Summative And Formative Assessments*
No Threat-No Risk *No physical submissions.* *No physical contact.* *No in-office consultations.* *Data provided to students.* *Data provided to staff.* *Data provided to tutors.* *Data provided to contract lecturers.* *Data provided to administrators* *Data provided to the disability office.* *No physical presence on campus.*	**Academic**	**Academic**	**Academic**

(Continued)

Table 18.1 (Continued)

Threat Level Covid-19 Guidelines Accountability	Teaching	Covid-19 Class Configuration	Summative And Formative Assessments
Dean of School **Office Administrators** **Head of Department** **Academic** **Contract Staff** **ICS**	Online teaching only. Email communication. Online consults. Specified consultation times. Moodle for slides. Moodle for video clips. Moodle forum discussions. Moodle announcements. Moodle online assessments. No physical contact. WhatsApp student support. Weekly tutor meetings. Liaison with the disability office. Separate support group. Mental health resources guidelines.	Virtual classes. Individual remote locations. Use of Zoom. Use of Skype. Use of Microsoft Teams. Use of Facebook. No restrictions on size. Length of class not exceeding 1 hour. Cost of class considered. Reconcile data-time and access. Recorded classes. WhatsApp student support. Tutors manage WhatsApp.	All online assessments and preparation of examinations. Moderation of exam papers, password protected. Electronic communication external examiners. We have specified time allowances. Minimum usage of data. Students download assessment and template. Work offline until ready to submit. Multiple choice questions for undergraduates. Microsoft Forms assessments. Administered on MS Teams. Administered on Moodle and Blackboard. No paper submissions. Electronic feedback assignments. tests Exams and tutorial activities.

(Continued)

Table 18.1 (Continued)

Threat Level Covid-19 Guidelines Accountability	Teaching	Covid-19 Class Configuration	Summative And Formative Assessments
Programme co-ordinator **Academic** **Contract Staff** **Head of Department** **Administrator**	**Tutors** Online tutorials only, email communication. Online consults specified times. Moodle for slides, video clips, forum discussions, announcements, and online assessments. No physical contact. WhatsApp student support, tutors managed. Weekly tutor meetings. Liaison with the disability office, access team, and contract staff. Separate support group. Mental health resources guidelines. **Administrators** Online queries and email communication. Online forms submission. Online requests specified times. No physical contact. Weekly team meeting.	**Tutors** Virtual tutorials. Individual remote locations. Use of Zoom, Skype, Microsoft Teams, Facebook, and Moodle. No restrictions on size. Length of class not exceeding 1 hour. Cost of class considered. Reconcile data-time and access. Recorded classes. No physical contact. WhatsApp student support. Tutors manage WhatsApp. **Administrators** Online queries and email communication. Online academic, tutor support. Technical bookings, meeting requests, timetables. No physical contact.	**Tutors** Consolidate content online. Examination revision, past papers. Electronic communication specified time. Minimum usage of data. Download past assessment, work offline. Provide model answers. Multiple choice questions. Essay questions and definitions. No paper submissions, no physical contact. Electronic feedback assignments, tests, exams Tutorial activities. Processing online exams. WhatsApp student support. Tutors manage WhatsApp. **Administrators** Online exam queries via Email Medical certificates and academic support. Submission to examiners. Processing results, class lists. Technical bookings and timetables. No paper submissions, no physical contact. Electronic feedback marks DP, assignments, tests, exams, and tutorial activities. Processing online exams.
Office Manager **Dean** **Head of Department** **Programme Co-ordinator**			

(Continued)

Table 18.1 (Continued)

Threat Level Covid-19 Guidelines Accountability	Teaching	Covid-19 Class Configuration	Summative And Formative Assessments
Technical Manager **Technical Hotline** **Technical Email** **Technical Contact**	**Technical Support** Online telephone queries. Email communication. Facilitate seamless classes. No physical contact.	**Technical Support** Rapid response to queries. Facilitate seamless online classes. No physical contact.	**Technical Support** Monitor online assessments, technical support. Standby for examinations. No paper submissions, no physical contact. Processing online exams.
Subject Librarian	**Library Services** Online email and telephone queries. Textbook availability. No physical contact, no library access.	**Library Services** Online training no physical contact. Telephone, email communication. E-textbook available.	**Library Services** Sufficient licences for texts. Virtual workshops. No exchanges of paper, no physical contact.
RMS **Clinic–Campus Health**	**Screening** Permits from RMS online. Pre-screening at home. Temperature check at university. Follow department of health protocol.	**Screening** Permits from RMS online. Pre-screening at home. Temperature check at university. Follow department of health protocol.	**Screening** Permits from RMS online. Pre-screening at home. Temperature check at university. Follow department of health protocol.

Table 18.2 Intermediate threat medium-high risk in the academy

Intermediate Threat Medium–High Risk	Academics	Academics	Academics
Social distancing rules applied. *No physical submissions.* *No physical contact.* *No in-office consultations.* *Data provided to students.* *Data provided to staff.* *Data provided to tutors.* *Data provided to contract lecturers.* *Data provided to administrators* *Data provided to disability office.* *No physical presence on campus.* **Dean of School** **Office Administrators** **Head of Department** **Academic** **Contract Staff** **ICS**	Electronic feedback on assessments. Online teaching 75%, In-person classes 25%. Email communication, online consults. Specified times. Moodle for slides, video clips, forum discussions, announcements, and online assessments. No physical contact. Weekly tutor meetings. Liaison with the disability office. Separate support group. Mental health resources guidelines.	25% of students attend class on a weekly rotational basis.75% of access recorded lectures. Virtual classes. Individual remote locations. Use of Zoom, Skype, Microsoft Teams, and Facebook. 25% restriction on class size. Online class not exceeding 1 hour. Reconcile data-time and access. Recorded classes. WhatsApp tutor managed.	All assessments continue online Specified time frame. Minimum usage of data Students download assessment and booklet. Work offline until they submission. MCQs administered for undergraduates. Microsoft Forms assessments administered on MS Teams, Moodle, and Blackboard.

(Continued)

Table 18.2 (Continued)

Intermediate Threat Medium-High Risk	Academics	Academics	Academics
Programme co-ordinator **Academic** **Contract Staff** **Head of Department** **Administrator**	**Tutors** Electronic feedback on assessments. Online 75%, in-person tutorials 25%. Email communication, online consults. Specified times. Moodle for slides, video clips, forum discussions, announcements, and assessments. No physical contact. Weekly tutor meetings. Liaison with the disability office. Separate support group. Mental health resources guidelines. **Administrators** Online queries and email continue. Online forms submission continue. Online requests specified times. No physical contact continues. Weekly virtual team meetings continue.	**Tutors** Virtual tutorials 75%. In-person tutorials 25%. Individual remote locations. Use of Zoom, Skype, Microsoft Teams, Facebook, and Moodle. No restrictions on size. Length of class not exceeding 1 hour. Cost of class considered. Reconcile data-time and access. Recorded classes. 25% physical contact. WhatsApp student support. Tutors manage WhatsApp. **Administrators** Online queries and email continue. Online academic and tutor support continue. Technical bookings, meeting requests, timetables. 25% physical contact.	**Tutors** Consolidate content online. Examination revision, past papers. Electronic communication specified time. Minimum usage of data. Download past assessment, work offline. Provide model answers. Multiple choice questions. Essay questions and definitions. No paper submissions, 25% physical contact. Electronic feedback Assignments, Tests, Processing online exams. WhatsApp student support tutor managed. **Administrators** Online exam queries via email. Medical certificates and academic support. Submission to examiners. Processing results, class lists. Technical bookings and timetables. No paper submissions, no physical contact. Electronic feedback marks DP, assignments, tests, exams, and tutorial activities.
Office Manager **Dean** **Head of Department** **Programme Co-ordinator**			

(Continued)

Table 18.2 (Continued)

Intermediate Threat Medium–High Risk	Academics	Academics	Academics
Technical Manager **Technical Hotline** **Technical Email** **Technical Contact**	**Technical Support** Online telephone and email communication continues. Facilitate seamless online classes 75%. Facilitate seamless in-person classes 25%. Physical contact 25%.	**Technical Support** Rapid response to queries. Facilitate seamless online classes. No physical contact.	**Technical Support** Monitor online assessments, technical support. Standby for examinations. No paper submissions, no physical contact. Processing online exams.
Subject Librarian	**Library Services** Online, telephone, and email communications continue. Textbook availability electronic. Sufficient licences for texts. Physical contact at 25%. Library access 25%. Virtual workshops 75%. In-person workshops at 25% Limited physical contact. Social distancing protocol.	**Library Services** Textbook availability electronic. No physical contact at 25%. Sufficient licences for texts. Virtual workshops 75%. In-person workshops 25%. No paper resources. Limited physical contact. Social distancing protocol.	**Library Services** Textbook availability electronic. Increased in library electronic access. Physical contact at 25%. Sufficient licences for texts. Access to library 25%. In-person workshops 25%. No paper resources limited physical contact. Social distancing protocol.
RMS **Clinic–Campus Health**	**Screening** Permits from RMS online, 25% access. Pre-screening at home. Temperature check at university. Follow department of health protocol.	**Screening** Permits from RMS online, 25% access. Pre-screening at home. Temperature check at university. Follow department of health protocol.	**Screening** Permits from RMS online, 25% access. Pre-screening at home. Temperature check at university. Follow department of health protocol.

Table 18.3 Utmost threat high risk in the academy

Utmost Threat High Risk	Academic	Academic	Academic	Academic
Social distancing rules applied. *No physical submissions.* *No physical contact.* *No in-office consultations.* *Data provided to students.* *Data provided to staff.* *Data provided to tutors.* *Data provided to contract lecturers.* *Data provided to administrators* *Data provided to disability office.* *No physical presence on campus.* **Dean of School** **Office Administrators** **Head of Department** **Academic** **Contract Staff** **ICS**	Online classes – 50–75% (depending on class sizes and venues regarding social distancing regulations). In-person classes – 50% In-person consults – specified times Online consults – specified times. Electronic feedback on all assignments and tests. WhatsApp groups for student support managed by teaching assistants. Discussion groups on online platforms such as Moodle and Blackboard.	Virtual classis's remote locations residences. 50–75% of students attend class on a weekly rotational basis. 50–75% access recorded lectures.		Smaller postgraduate 100% exam. Assessments based on venue configuration Social distancing protocol. Online assessment with a specified time frame. Minimum usage of data. Students download assessment and booklet. Work offline until they ready to submit. MCQs can be administered for undergraduates. Microsoft Forms assessments. Administered MS Teams, Moodle, and Blackboard

(*Continued*)

Table 18.3 (Continued)

Utmost Threat High Risk	Academic	Academic	Academic
Programme co-ordinator **Academic** **Head of Department** **Administrator**	**Tutors** Electronic feedback on assessments. Discussion groups Moodle and Blackboard. Online tutorials 75%, In-person tutorials 25%. Email communication, online consults. Specified times. Moodle for slides, video clips, forum discussions, announcements, and online assessments. No physical contact. Weekly tutor meetings. Liaison with the disability office. Separate support group. Mental health resources guidelines. **Administrators** Online queries and email continue. Online forms submission continue. Online requests specified times. No physical contact continues. Weekly virtual team meetings continue.	**Tutors** Virtual tutorials. Individual remote locations. Use of Zoom, Skype, Microsoft Teams, Facebook, and Moodle. No restrictions on size. Length of class not exceeding 1 hour. Cost of class considered. Reconcile data-time and access. Recorded classes. No physical contact. WhatsApp student support. Tutors manage WhatsApp. **Administrators** Online queries and email continue. Online academic and tutor support continue. Technical bookings, meeting requests, timetables. 50% physical contact.	**Tutors** Consolidate content online. Examination revision, past papers. Electronic communication specified time. Minimum usage of data. Download past assessment, work offline. Provide model answers. Multiple choice questions. Essay questions and definitions. No paper submissions, no physical contact. Electronic feedback assignments, tests, exams. Tutorial activities. Processing online exams. Whatsapp student support. Tutors manage WhatsApp. **Administrators** Online exam queries via email Medical certificates and academic support. Submission to examiners. Processing results, class lists. Technical bookings and timetables. No paper submissions, no physical contact. Electronic feedback marks DP, assignments, tests, exams, and tutorial activities.
Office Manager **Dean** **Head of Department** **Programme Co-ordinator**			

(Continued)

Table 18.3 (Continued)

Utmost Threat High Risk	Academic	Academic	Academic
Technical Manager **Technical Hotline** **Technical Email** **Technical Contact**	**Technical Support** Online telephone and email continue. Facilitate seamless online classes 50%. Computers in-person classes 50%. Access to computers 50%.	**Technical Support** Rapid response to queries. Facilitate seamless online classes. 50% physical contact.	**Technical Support** Monitor online assessments, technical support. Standby for examinations. No paper submissions, 50% physical contact. Processing online exams.
Subject Librarian **Head of Department**	**Library Services** Online telephone, email continue. Textbook availability electronic. Physical contact at 50%. Virtual workshops, no paper resources. Social distancing protocol. Library access 50%. Electronic forms.	**Library Services** Textbook availability electronically. Physical contact at 50%. Sufficient licences for texts. Virtual workshops. In-person workshops 50%. Social distancing protocol.	**Library Services** Textbook availability electronic. Increase in library electronic access. Increase computers 50%. Open study carrels. Physical contact at 50%. Access to library 50% occupancy. In-person workshops 50% occupancy. Social distancing protocol.
RMS **Clinic-Campus Health**	**Screening** Permits RMS online, 50% access Pre-screening at home. Temperature check at university. Follow department of health protocol.	**Screening** Permits RMS online, 50% access Pre-screening at home. Temperature check at university. Follow department of health protocol.	**Screening** Permits from RMS online. Pre-screening at home. Temperature check at university. Follow department of health protocol.

Conclusion

Established on the findings of this all-encompassing social scientific erudition, the ensuing mandatory clinical interventions need to be affected proximately. If universities in South Africa and worldwide intend to realise ground-breaking teaching pedagogies advanced by leading scholars, three fundamental extents compel instantaneous precedence. The precondition for a successful practicable virtual curriculum that is anticipated to be the principal model espoused by South Africa's 26 public universities has been identified. These include three key areas; the primary areas that require the attention of key South African government departments include but are not limited to the ministry of communication and higher education. They ought to be liable for the facilitation of infrastructure required by students and academics for the successful completion of the 2020 academic year. By way of a solution, partnerships between the private and public sectors must be fortified and compensated by tax concessions. The private information and technology sector should be integrated into a government strategy that addresses the inadequate software and hardware for students and academics. The objective is to ensure that every academic and student has a personal electronic device that facilitates virtual education. South Africa has a protracted history of inequality, resulting in well-resourced affluent residential areas and under-resourced townships. This geographical diversity is a representation of South Africa's inequality. Students and academics dwell in these different suburbs and townships, differentiating access. The lack of internet coverage prevents users from connecting to a network in specific locations.

By way of a solution, initiatives between the telecommunication and engineering sectors must be facilitated and compensated via amendments to the regulatory guidelines of both sectors. The objective is to secure access to reliable, affordable uninterrupted data that permits participation and facilitation of virtual learning. Specialised training for advanced technological proficiencies when teaching virtually. The deficiency of these proficiencies is common among academics who have previously not been required to possess such intricate knowledge. Online classes' recording, transmission, and delivery will fail if academics are not precisely competent therein. By way of a solution, initiatives between the software developers, information technology companies and academics in the field need to be accelerated and recompensed via a reconsideration of licence agreements and taxation. The objective is to equip academics with the requisite technical skills to prepare and deliver virtual lectures

References

Al-Karaki, J.N., Ababneh, N., Hamid, Y. and Gawanmeh, A. (2021). Evaluating the effectiveness of distance learning in higher education during COVID-19 global crisis: UAE educators' perspectives. *Contemporary Educational Technology*, 13(3) . pp.1–16

Armoed, Z. (2021, February). The Covid-19 pandemic: Online teaching and learning at higher education institutes. In *IOP Conference Series: Earth and Environmental Science* (Vol. 654, No. 1, p. 012026). IOP Publishing.

Berger, P.L. and Luckmann, T. (1979). *The Social Construction of Reality: A Treatise.* Wahlström and Widstrand, Penguin.

Cole, M., John-Steiner, V., Scribner, S. and Souberman, E. [eds]. (1978). *L.S. Vygotsky Mind in Society – The Development of Higher Psychological Processes.* United Kingdom:Harvard University Press.

Craig, L. (2020). *COVID-19 has Laid Bare How Much We Value Women's Work & How Little We Pay For It.* Retrieved from: https://womensagenda.com.au/latest/covid-19-has -laid-bare-how-much-we-value-womens-work-how-little-we-pay-for-it/

Dwivedi, Y., Hughes, L., Coombs, C., Constantiou, I., Duan, Y., Edwards, J., et al. (2020). Impact of COVID-19 pandemic on information management research and practice: Transforming education, work, and life. *International. Journal Information Management,* 55, 102211. https://doi.org/10.1016/j.ijinfomgt.2020.102211

Donnelly, V. and Kyriazopoulou, M. [eds]. (2014). *Organisation of Provision to Support Inclusive Education – Summary Report.* Denmark: The European Agency for Special Needs and Inclusive Education.

Du Plessis, E.A. (2020). *Out-of-Field Teaching and Education Policy.* Singapore: Springer.

Freire, P. (1972). *Pedagogy of the Oppressed.* New York: Herder and Herder.

García-Morales, V.J., Garrido-Moreno, A. and Martín-Rojas, R. (2021). The transformation of higher education after the COVID disruption: Emerging challenges in an online learning scenario. *Frontiers in Psychology,* 12, 196. https://doi.org/10.3389/fpsyg.2021 .616059

Gleason, N.W. (2018). *Higher Education in the Era of the Fourth Industrial Revolution.* Springer Nature.

Kwinana, A. and Mohau, P. [eds]. (2019). *Education Conversations' Occasional Publication Series.* Johannesburg: Kagiso Trust and the University of Johannesburg.

Lebelo, R.S., Moloi, K.C. and Jaffer, S. (2020). Corona virus pandemic and change to online learning in one South African private higher education institution: An action research. *Loyola Journal of Social Sciences,* 34(2).

Li, C. and Lalani, F. (2020). *The COVID-19 Pandemic has Changed Education Forever. This is How.* World Economic Forum. Retrieved From: https://www.weforum.org/ agenda/2020/04/coronavirus-education-global-covid19-online-digital-learning/

Light, J.S. (2001). Rethinking the digital divide. *Harvard Educational Review,* 71(4), 709–774.

Maluleke, R. (2018). *General Household Survey 2018.* Pretoria: Statistics South Africa.

Maluleke, R. (2019). *Education Series Volume V: Higher Education and Skills in South Africa, 2017.* Pretoria: Statistics South Africa.

Mangal, S.K. and Mangal, S. (2019). *Childhood and Growing Up.* India: PHI Learning Private Limited.

Mathiba, G. (2020). COVID-19 and South African Universities: A raft of problems to ponder. Retrieved from: https://www.dailymaverick.co.za/opinionista/2020-04-09-covid -19-and-south-african-universities-a-raft-of-problems-to-ponder/#gsc.tab=0

Matli, W. and Ngoepe, M. (2020). Capitalising on digital literacy skills for capacity development of people who are not in education, employment or training in South Africa. *African Journal of Science, Technology, Innovation and Development,* 12(2), 129–139.

Mhlanga, D. and Moloi, T. (2020). COVID-19 and the digital transformation of education: What are we learning on 4IR in South Africa? *Education Sciences,* 10(7), 180.

Moorhouse, B.L. (2020). Adaptations to a face-to-face initial teacher education course 'forced' online due to the COVID-19 pandemic. *Journal of Education for Teaching,* 46 (4) pp. 609–611

Mzileni, P. (2020). *How COVID-19 Will Affect Students*. Retrieved from: https://mg.co.za/education/2020-04-23-how-covid-19-will-affect-students/

Penprase, B.E. (2018). *Higher Education in the Era of the Fourth Industrial Revolution*. In N. W. Gleason [ed]. Singapore: Palgrave Macmillan.

Ramnund, A. (2019). *Exploring the Link between Institutional Culture and the Career Advancement of Female Academics in Higher Education: A Case Study of the University of Kwazulu-Natal, South Africa*. PhD thesis. Durban: UKZN.

Ramnund-Mansingh, A. and Seedat-Khan, M. (2020). Move over Ms. Professor! A review of the challenge's women experiences in academia. *Journal of Higher Education Service Science and Management*, 3(1), 1–14.

Sahu, P. (2020). Closure of universities due to Coronavirus Disease 2019 (COVID-19): Impact on education and mental health of students and academic staff. *Cureus*, 12(4), p. e7541.

Seedat-Khan, M., Ramnund-Mansingh, A. and Johnson, B. (2020) Welcome to university: Have a seat please! *Journal of Higher Education Service Science and Management (JoHESSM)*, 3(2) pp. 1–15.

Stewart, D.W. and Kamins, M.A. (1994). *Secondary Research – Information Sources and Methods*. California: Sage Publications.

Suleman, F. (2016). Employability skills of higher education graduates: Little consensus on a much-discussed subject. *Procedia-Social and Behavioral Sciences*, 228, 169–174.

Tamrat, W. and Teferra, D. (2020). COVID-19 threat to higher education. *International Higher Education*, (102), 28–30.

Tionneland, E.N. (2017). Crisis at South Africa's universities – What are the implications for future cooperation with Norway? *CMI Brief*, (16), 3–4.

Van Wyk, B., Mooney, G., Duma, M. and Faloye, S. (2020, October). Emergency remote learning in the times of COVID: A higher education innovation strategy. In *Proceedings of the European Conference on e-Learning, ECEL, Berlin, Germany* (pp. 28–30).

Xing, B., Marwala, L. and Marwala, T. (2018). Adopt fast, adapt quick: Adaptive approaches in the South African context. In N. W. Gleason [ed]. *Higher Education in the Era of the Fourth Industrial Revolution*. Singapore: Palgrave Macmillan.

Part VII

Conclusion

Interventions and Change

19 New Clinical Sociology for a Post-COVID World

Jayanathan Govender and Usha Rana

Introduction

As the world prepares for the lifting of the COVID-19 lockdown, new and stimulating opportunities are presented to the discipline of clinical sociology. These opportunities come in the form of new knowledge, methodology, and theory. As a discipline of the social sciences and humanities, clinical sociology possesses both intellectual and scientific capabilities to view society differently, allowing for a post-COVID-19 evaluation of social relations globally. Crucially, the discipline of clinical sociology could lead a way forward at viewing afresh the relationship between science and society.

This chapter examines the nature of pandemic crises and the global response to the pandemic. The focus is on two aspects: the first is people's responses to the authoritarian protocols imposed by government to the point of intolerable isolation fatigue and violent resistance; the imperative of returning the world economy to functionality; as well as the pressure to restart social systems. The question arising from this aspect is: *Because of the nascent revelations made possible by unravelling the pandemic, will there be a return to the status quo, and if not, what possibilities may be expected for a more equal and just global society.* The second aspect to be pursued is: *Is a new clinical sociological discipline possible that is better placed at understanding a post-COVID-19 world?*

The External Face of the COVID-19 Crises

This epoch that experienced the pandemic led to sharpening focus on global and local inequality, injustice, political malice, climate change, and the perennial struggles of children, women, migrants, and those on society's fringes. The pandemic revealed the cleavages, unevenness, and hopelessness wedged within society during wealth, comfort, and power. The strongest, that is, those possessing historical and accumulated capacities, having access to opportunity and unrestricted freedoms, were not only the safest and best protected under the pandemic, but also determined the debates, political economy of the pandemic, as well the scientific interventions. The vaccines that emerged from the most organised scientific communities and private companies are earning profits that would never have been possible under non-pandemic conditions. This is notwithstanding that the drug

DOI: 10.4324/9781003267133-26

industry's average net profit margins show that it has long been the most profitable sector, exceedingly even the energy and financial industries globally (Hawksbee, McKee et al. 2022). The huge government subsidies for vaccine production benefitted only ten companies across the world (WHO 2022; (Le, Andreadakis et al. 2020). Along with massive profits, the COVID-19 vaccines saga has introduced new controversies, including health before profits debate, vaccine nationalism, vaccinophobia, vaccine passports, conspiracy theories, personal liberty, and a gamut of ethical issues.

The COVID-19 pandemic has had effects on employment, distributive practices, living standards, gender relations, and institutional relations. However, the differential effects on societies in respect of political systems, markets, inequalities, and so on require a consensus for an empirical framework. These different sociological categories must be framed within a qualitative matrix to both understand and respond to the COVID-19 crisis. The respective histories, contradictions, and freedom struggles of societies place them on divergent capability platforms, such as in respect of public health policies. The current approach to the science of the COVID-19 pandemic is fragmented and not contiguous from government to government. Some are conflicted by philosophy, political will, and standard of scientific capability. There are also a set of new contests among societies, including vaccine hegemony and nationalism; medical capitalism; scientific popularism; and universal public health policy.

The analytical framework is therefore compelled to hone into global debates. COVID-19 has both known and not yet known linkages, including the outcomes of neoliberalism, globalisation, climate change, destruction of the natural habitat, the culture of comfort and consumption, and so on (Rana 2022). Societal institutions – politics, culture, and economy – have either stalled or transformed into a new sociality (bluntly termed new normal), yet remain an existential shock on all humanity. The globe is also under what sociologists call 'manufactured uncertainty,' recognised by the fact that they are outcomes of human decisions, created by society itself, collectively imposed and inevitably individually unavoidable (Beck 2009).

However, there is also great optimism to behold. The scientific community came to stand out in civil society, the media, and in the public imagination. The advances with vaccine production for COVID-19 are unprecedented. Novel medical technologies are discovering applications for other epidemics. The realisation that future pandemics are imminent has motivated scientific work in these areas. Crucially, a global public health policy that is inclusive, equal, and accessible has gained prominence.

Science has never been without optimism. In this line, we are assured that humanity undergoes alternate periods of 'rest' and 'unrest,' of 'weal' and 'woe,' and goes on advancing at a slow pace towards 'greater perfection' (Meek 2010). The permanent progression towards 'greater perfection' is indeed a great human tendency if it is that. However, alongside this observation by Turgot, writing during the 1750s during his ecclesial career, Turgot also warns us that 'circumstances' will either 'increase' or 'decrease' the 'rate of progress.' The transposing sides of 'greater perfection' and 'circumstances' appears inauspicious, where certainty on

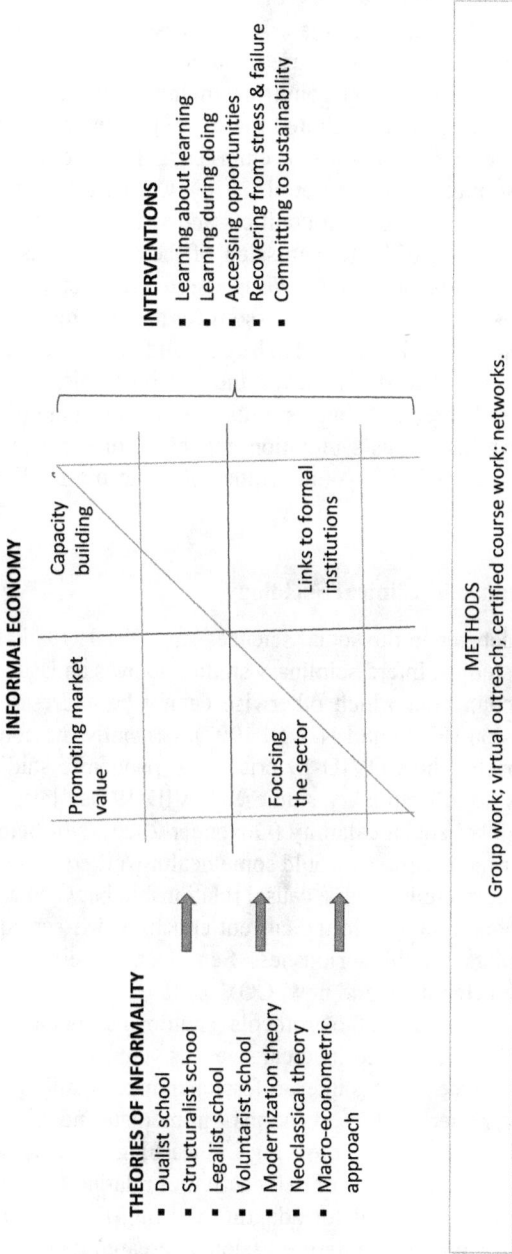

THEORIES OF INFORMALITY
- Dualist school
- Structuralist school
- Legalist school
- Voluntarist school
- Modernization theory
- Neoclassical theory
- Macro-econometric approach

INFORMAL ECONOMY

Promoting market value

Capacity building

Focusing the sector

Links to formal institutions

INTERVENTIONS
- Learning about learning
- Learning during doing
- Accessing opportunities
- Recovering from stress & failure
- Committing to sustainability

METHODS
Group work; virtual outreach; certified course work; networks.

Figure 19.1 Informal economy

the one hand affirms the human condition and uncertainty, influenced by known and unknown quantities, determines different destinies on the other hand. Turgot's dilemma cuts through the core sociological understanding of equality and social justice and, hence, the very idea of universalism.

Clinical sociology then provides the stretch and flexibility for a universal discipline, addressing the collective story of COVID-19 from the perspective of multiple lenses. For example, the Ebola crisis in West Africa led to a humanitarian crisis involving at first three countries, Guinea, Liberia, and Sierra Leone. Fear gripped the world, when other countries, including Mali, Nigeria, Senegal, Italy, Spain, United Kingdom, and United States, were affected. In attempting to explain this perfect storm, two main issues emerged, cultural context and a change in the epidemiology (Piot, Muyembe et al. 2014). Civil war, political trust, and weak health systems, combined with conflicts and risky traditional healing and funeral practices, accelerated the transmission of the Ebola virus. Accordingly, the high rates of communicability of the virus resulted from cultural practice and human mobility. There are similar sets of lessons for the high rates of infections of COVID-19 across the world. These need to be consolidated into a systematic body of clinical and non-clinical work. However, the added complexity of COVID-19 is not only the scale of infections but its mutation given change of contexts and clinical interventions. The virus's mutation capability may transform COVID-19 into an endemic disease that would require ongoing bio-medical and social interventions.

Overlapping Relevance in Clinical Sociology

One of the intense debates in the social sciences since the 1970s is the relevance of interdisciplinary studies. Interdisciplinary studies address an issue that is broad, complex, and interconnected which otherwise cannot be addressed by a single discipline or profession (Klein and Newell 1997). Crucially the context calls for an integrated approach. The COVID-19 crises and pandemic studies qualify to be studied vis-à-vis interdisciplinary studies. COVID-19 has been described by Amartya Sen as a global social calamity (Govender 2020). Not being tempted to refer to COVID-19 as a disease, as would some health workers and scientists, Sen presents the human community with a causal relationship between a social calamity and an end to social relations in the current epoch. Sen is serious and indications from March 2020 prove his seriousness. Sen lifts the interconnecting veils of economic history, development, and now, COVID-19.

The COVID-19 pandemic and the protocols (shutdowns, social distancing, etc.) suggest challenges for science, bio-medical sciences, and social sciences. Clearly, managing the pandemic centralises interprofessional understanding, collaboration, and working to deliver a series of interventions – immediate and critical healthcare; basic hygiene practices such as face covering and washing of hands, social distancing; vaccination; and reorganisation of daily activities relating to work and domestic life. Crucially, there is a need for adapting existing research methodologies and new research. Accordingly, interprofessional research can make a valuable contribution towards informing global responses to COVID-19 and towards planning for future global health crises (Sy, O'Leary et al. 2020).

Intersectionality is a relatively recent form of investigation. It was adopted by scholars, policymakers, and activists in the early 21st century (Collins and Bilge 2020). Intersectionality attempts to understand how power relations influence social relations, therefore also making it popular among feminists (Phoenix and Pattynama 2006). The tool of analysis considers the categories of race, class, gender, ethnicity, ageism, and so on, as interrelated and influencing each other. Hence the tool is useful for explaining complex phenomena in the world.

Clinical sociologists assess systems (interpersonal, community, international) to assist with change and improvements (Fritz 1989). The science is influenced by characteristics of humanism. It adopts a multidisciplinary approach. A contemporary view of clinical sociology was proposed by Wirth (Wirth 1931). Attention is focused on a case, a real problem; professional cooperation and the theoretical and clinical procedure result in the formulation of an interventionist procedure that has immediate effect and adjustment (Bruhn and Rebach 2012).

Is Clinical Sociology Poised to Tackle Complexity and Social Issues at Global Scale?

Clinical sociology is not without its own limits and challenges. The various extent definitions, purviews, and methods address social problems of individuals and groups. However, social phenomena are wide-ranging. They are easily recognisable when they present in the physical, emotional, and existential categories. With regard to the total whole of social phenomena, which include natural disasters, pandemics, environmentally related global warming, and moving further into the realms of sociality, issues present according to type of actions, their motivations, and outcomes. These are connected to teleological, legal, moral, and value precepts, which indicate so-called societal consensus and a certain standard of cultural development. The point then is for clinical sociology to also consider social diseases, conditions that affect individuals and groups systemically.

Taking the complex example of inequality for instance, the literature is writ large as to what the best possible intervention is to bring balance to a particular society, and thereby ensure equality between individual and groups. According to the International Labour Organization (ILO 2015) and the Organisation for Economic Co-operation and Development (Cingano 2014), inequality weakens the crucial link between economic growth and employment, and between economic growth and the reduction of poverty. It must be remembered that inequality has not only material but also important non-material dimensions, including unequal power, agency, rights, social protection, and so on. Further, according to the ILO and OECD research, these dimensions of inequality are linked and reinforce each other. Additionally, the dimensions of gender, race, and sexual inequality must not be excluded from the analytical methods of clinical sociology. Alternatively, do practitioners and the discipline exclude from their concerns meta and meso issues such as inequality, poverty, discrimination, exclusion, and so on? If this were the case, then a significant method of clinical sociology, i.e., policy intervention or policy programme may be foregone?

Posing the meta and meso issues differently, if no ideal society is possible, say a society whose public policy covers everybody; public resources are distributed; social justice is accessible to all; and the ideology of governmentality prevails, how does clinical sociology respond, given its interventionist and humane pursuits? This question overarches the concern for a new clinical sociology, which is addressed at the letter end of the chapter.

The COVID-19 Poly-pandemic

The world is used to waves of crises, usually normative cyclical financial crises of capitalism. When the world was battered by the 2007 financial crises, never mind that those during the crisis, i.e., the poor, hungry, and underprivileged, suffered more extensively and intensively, the rich and the powerful (countries of Northern America and Western Europe) were bearing gargantuan shock and dismay because theirs was crises of profitability (Pillay 2010). Other systems were affected as well, including the ecology through degradation, pollution, and loss of endangered species. The rich and wealthy were forced to momentarily leave their culture of comfort only because these crises affected production and consumption, eminently crucial for profitability. Only then, that is when the financial crisis brought on other effects, did it escalate to a poly crisis.

In a similar vein, the COVID-19 pandemic is a poly-pandemic (Eisentraut 2021). Covid-19 has exacted multiple pandemics, rather than just one, infecting over 418 million people with 5.87 million fatalities from causes of the virus (WHO 2022). COVID-19 has provoked a poly-pandemic that has stalled the world economy, locked in the people of the world in their homes, curtailed all forms of movements of people, banned all public cultural events and cancelled all levels of educational activities. The poly-pandemic has undermined developmental processes, enforced unfreedoms on people, and withdrawn the democratic processes and rights of people, allowed under emergency and disaster circumstances. The power of the state during the COVID-19 poly-pandemic was unprecedented in human history. The reactions of people, expressed in personal secular, religious, and democratic terms, have threatened the stability of the state and its functionality globally. The more powerful states turned inwards, protecting the interests of their citizens, leaving the developing world behind in their response to mitigate the spread and effects of the virus. Only when the science indicated that 'no-one is safe until everyone is safe' did the powerful states realise that vaccine nationalism would be a disaster, where the world of the future faces a choice: one of greater justice, abundance, and dignity; or one of conflict, insecurity, and poverty (UNICEF 2022).

COVID-19 has known and unknown origins, linkages, and consequences. Sorting through the muddle reveals a causal relationship between microcosmic and macrocosmic stages of society. At the microcosmic level, there was localised emergence, followed by spill-over, followed by pandemic spread. The analysis indicates that the pandemic spread is driven by underlying ecological, political, and socio-economic factors, including climate change, urbanisation, international travel and trade, land use change, and the breakdown or lack of public health procedures (Bogich, Chunara et al. 2012). These factors are indicative of a polyhedron of inequality.

The experience of COVID-19 is contradictory irrespective of the divide of wealthy and poor countries. In wealthy countries, like the United States, the vaccine was treated with mistrust by certain sections of the population. Historical prejudice vis-à-vis the US campaign to eradicate syphilis remains a sore reference for many African American people (Freimuth, Quinn et al. 2001) (Green, Maisiak et al. 1997). Similarly, in South Africa, the Depo-Provera injections forced on Black women to prevent unplanned pregnancies also remains etched as an apartheid memory (Brown 1987). The conquests and brutal treatment of first peoples and indigenous populations of the Americas, Canada, Latin America and social engineering of aborigines of Australia may be thought of as belonging in the historical past, or even erased by other accounts. However, lineages of first peoples, indigenous populations and aborigines have maintained their animistic courage to demand their rights and recognition from states that have not cared enough to redress and reconcile with them. For these categories of people, how then does the state and science reconcile with such historical realities of injustice?

Tragically, the transmission of infections is attributed to poverty, filth, and class to maintain a false sense of assurance and safety for the wealthier sections of society (Curtis and Biran 2001) (Idoiaga Mondragon, Gil de Montes et al. 2017). The episodes of bubonic plague, Asiatic flu, cholera, Middle East respiratory syndrome, and Ebola outbreaks in West Africa have been associated with polarisation, poverty, and racial and ethnic groups.

Contrast the so-called educated populations in the countries of the Atlantic regarding what is plainly scientific knowledge. Heterogeneous groups are articulating scientific, political, and philosophical objections to the COVID-19 vaccine. Activists and ordinary people have contributed to a body of toxic public opinion around the universal application of very advanced biological products. It is therefore not hard to dismiss people's suspicions when the structure of biologics is understood. Biologics are powerful medications that can be made of tiny components like proteins, DNA, parts of cells or tissues extracted from genetic material of living sources, including animals, bacteria, and even viruses (Shire 2009) (Thomas Morrow 2004). Accordingly, rather than viewing the vaccines from the perspective of personal protection from severe illness and fatality, the vaccines conflict with religious beliefs, philosophies, freedom to choose, and even freedom to decide about their children being injected with the COVID-19 vaccines. These moralisms and activisms have escalated to public protests and political challenges targeted at governments in Northern America and some parts of Europe.

The COVID-19 vaccines were not the only intervention under attack. Social distancing, face coverings, hygiene measures, shutdowns, travel bans, and border closures came under severe criticism. These prevention measures clashed in every sense of how people lived their lives. The measures had brought differential experiences of physical, mental, social, and financial consequences (Park, Russell et al. 2020). People were required to change their social behaviour through state declaration of protocols. However, these measures were not evaluated for their countervailing effects on people. There was no immediate realisation that the measures will lead to maladaptive behaviours to cope with increased stress and anxiety. Only after periods of home confinement was it possible for studies to gather information on how families and individuals coped under these radically changed living conditions.

Ironically indeed, it took the scientific and medical community some time to realise the effects of COVID-19 on health care professionals. Studies have shown that health workers risked infection, experienced psychological distress, and anxiety, suffered sleep disorders and fear of infecting family members (Teixeira, Soares et al. 2020). In developing countries, health workers were burdened by challenges of the work environment, poor, if not lack of, facilities, insufficient intensive care units, personal protection equipment, etc.

In South Africa, while the government was hard at work with interventions to curtail the pandemic, some public officials used this as an opportunity for self-enrichment by very devious and unconscionable means. They interfered with procurement processes, hired corrupt service providers, inflated prices, spread misinformation, and almost failed to secure vaccines for the population. Therefore, the government suffered setbacks to contain the pandemic. Crucially, the corruption, combined with an unsophisticated public service exerted tremendous pressure on the country's public finances, which had to secure loans from the IMF, African Development Bank, and the BRICS bank (Mlambo and Masuku 2020).

The COVID-19 pandemic presents the human community with a radical uncertainty on several fronts, including the possibility of it becoming globally endemic (Hunter 2020). Yet, there is cause for optimism. The scientific community triumphed in its grasp of studying the virus and its mutations. The production of scheduled vaccines in such a short space of time, whereas vaccines take several years to be available, is an unprecedented achievement by the world's leading scientists. In the process of developing the COVID-19 vaccines, other applications have become possible, including the treatment of HIV/AIDS. Crucially, technology platforms are diversifying, allowing for new-generation approaches to pandemics and other human diseases (Andreadakis, Kumar et al. 2020).

Also, on the positive side, the post-COVID-19 picture calls for transformation in the global health policies, interdisciplinary approaches to public health, investments in research and new technologies, addressing asymmetries in health services, and a systematic new approach to managing poly-pandemics in the future. The post-COVID-19 discourse also calls for discussions about culture. The lessons of previous pandemics must be studied and referenced for a post-COVID-19 world. A new focus on and relationship with public health and the environment must be imagined and forged. Crucially, a post-COVID-19 discourse must address the asymmetries of inequality and ensure that a system of medical capitalism does not confound what is a humanitarian issue. In the process, human consciousness must be transformed, which embraces a new philosophy of science, undergirded by a meta-methodology relevant for a human future within the matrix of the 4th

Industrial Revolution, growing conservatism, religious dogma, and deepening class stratification. Accordingly, the discourse requires the crossover of disciplines in the sciences, bio-medical sciences, and the social sciences. In this pursuit, new possibilities need to be imagined for the discipline of clinical sociology.

Capitalism in Crises during COVID-19

According to the World Economic Forum, today's capitalism faces a triple crises: (1) the pandemic has produced a global economic crisis, and piled up with the climate crisis, 'business as usual' is no longer possible; (2) the pandemic is exposing structural flaws in the global economy as more workers take on multiple and precarious jobs given the rise of the gig economy; and (3) the self-employed and entrepreneurs are left shocked by the sudden withdrawal of their participation in the formal economy (Mazzucato 2020).

Murshed (2020) elaborates on existential threats, such as the COVID-19 pandemic. They have forced intellectual paradigm shifts, transformed the economy, and adjusted the polity. Through the lens of the COVID-19 poly-pandemic, current global capitalism has exposed the deepening economic inequality and the decline of liberal democracy in both developed and developing countries. Financialisation and monopoly power have greatly skewed the distribution and share of wealth globally. The rich are getting richer, and the poor are getting poorer. COVID-19 has had a reciprocal relationship with socio-economic status (Binns and Low 2021). It is more likely to infect, and to have more severe consequences in, those who are socially disadvantaged. A structural perspective of the political economy indicates the COVID-19's disparate response to different people. It has exposed failures in public health care systems, working conditions, supply chains, vertical and horizontal inequality, racism, ethnicity, and how the unevenness of globalisation has created negative outcomes for the world's poor.

The unintended consequences of COVID-19 were remarkable (Govender 2020). The global capitalist engine stopped. People bought and consumed much less prior to the pandemic. Far lesser fossil fuels were retrieved and burnt. Far lesser plastics and associated garbage were dumped in the river systems and oceans. When people were forced into isolation, other species took up people's former spaces, probably resolving coexistence between humans and other species. Crucially, humans in general, not only the scientists, have realised the appreciation for the sameness of human destiny. If the ecology benefitted from COVID-19's unintended consequences, education, technology, and science grew in response to radically changed circumstances. In the broader sense, in the post-pandemic world, ideologies, systems, and technologies must be harnessed for those positive dimensions of the current capitalist system to undo inequality and build a newer world. There is the opportunity to re-think basic structures of current capitalism and re-imagine a more compassionate future. Possibly there is some hope for Arundhati Roy's dream: 'Another world is not only possible; she is on her way. Maybe many of us won't be here to greet her, but on a quiet day, if I listen very carefully, I can hear her breathing' (Roy 2003).

If dreams have failed, science has never been without optimism. In this line, we are assured that humanity undergoes alternate periods of 'rest' and 'unrest', of 'weal' and 'woe', and goes on advancing at a slow pace towards 'greater perfection' (Meek 2010). The permanent progression towards 'greater perfection' is indeed a great human tendency if it is that. However, alongside this observation by Turgot, writing during the 1750s during his ecclesial career, Turgot also warns us that 'circumstances' will either 'increase' or 'decrease' the 'rate of progress.' The transposing sides of 'greater perfection' and 'circumstances' appear inauspicious, where certainty on the one hand affirms the human condition, and uncertainty, influenced by known and unknown quantities, determines different destinies on the other hand. Turgot's dilemma cuts through the core sociological understanding of equality and social justice and, hence, the very idea of universalism. This universalism opens the opportunity for the social sciences; for a meta-methodology for a post-COVID-19 world; and a new clinical sociology to study the current poly-pandemic and such future social calamities.

Return to the Status Quo or Advance to the New Normal

The COVID-19 pandemic is a consequence of human action in this epoch (Rana 2022). This epoch dawns the 4th Industrial Revolution, promising a better world for all, reducing inequality, meeting the needs of all people, and consolidating global cohesion. Missing from these promises are peace, end to global warming, retarding rising sea levels and the submersion of islands and port cities across the world, retarding deforestation, and an end to ecological degradation. The possibilities of the 4th Industrial Revolution are therefore divided. On the one hand, the dialectical relationship between the 4th Industrial Revolution and ecological crises is not well understood at best or ignored at worst.

On the other hand, others are of the view that COVID-19 further promotes the development of the 4th Industrial Revolution (or Industry 4.0) and which will lead to the 5th Industrial Revolution (also known as Society 5.0). There is evidence from the vast medical and vaccine literature that artificial intelligence and big data have contributed to advances in understanding and addressing COVID-19. A key feature of the 5th Industrial Revolution is the super-smart society (Sarfraz, Sarfraz et al. 2021). In such a society, artificial intelligence, smart digital information, and manufacturing technologies will devise solutions to COVID-19 and control the rate of transmission of COVID-19 globally.

Therapeutics and treatment processes for COVID-19-infected patients will be based on detailed patient information and a smart healthcare environment. These technologies can also provide remote healthcare monitoring systems. The smart healthcare system will raise the levels of personalisation to meet the specific demands of patients and medical workers. The key is appropriate information provided to medical workers to deliver better treatment in real time. The new technologies can also critically help with medical training during the pandemic (Javaid, Haleem et al. 2020).

Judging from the above perspectives, then, some believe that the post-COVID-19 world will make life worse for most people due to extant and growing inequality, rising authoritarianism by the state and policy institutions, and unbridled misinformation arising from conservative campaigns and the social media. Conversely, others believe life will be better because of the contributions of the internet of things, transforming workplaces, health care, and social activity (Anderson, Rainie et al. 2021).

New Methods in Clinical Sociology

The old profession needs renewal. The current strengths of clinical sociology do not stand up to sociological theories and reliable methods and techniques for progress and change. It needs to redefine its role as a change agent. It also needs to refine the self, social group, and the situation. To achieve this project, a thorough historical study must be undertaken.

One aim of a new clinical sociology must be an international clinical sociology. The origins, prevalence, and dominance of clinical sociology in the United States, Europe, and some parts of Asia are well known. Global development denotes the idea that societies and countries have differing levels of economic and human development on an international scale. The key themes in today's international development include the impacts and implications of global warming, migration, strengthening the local, the 4th Industrial Revolution, growing the private sector where informality dominates, and new methods in development discourse. The quest for new methods in development discourse may become evident by examining the state of informality in Africa. According to the World Bank, Africa's informal sector accounts for 80.8% of all jobs, dominated by 95.8% urban youth (ages 15–24) and 92.1% women (Guven and Karlen 2020). This means that youth and women play a significant role in poverty alleviation in Africa and are deserving of developmental support towards a better future. Accordingly, different understandings and interventions are essential.

While it is not expected that the new clinical sociology addresses these global social diseases, it is possible to delineate interventions by category and scale. The diagram below provides certain interventionist possibilities in the case of the informal sector.

Like any social issue, there are differing theories that seek to explain an issue based on empirical studies and other forms of evidence. The informal economy is understood here according to schools of thought based on the intentions of the actors. Other approaches frame the informal sector within broader sociological theory, since the informal sector is part of larger society. Yet other approaches prefer to understand the informal economy as strictly economic theory.

The intersecting lines in the middle of the diagram indicate what needs attention in the informal economy. Promoting market value, capacity building, focusing the sector, and links to formal institutions are assumptions here. Empirical and clinical sociology studies will reveal actual needs.

The interventions must be framed according to the needs of an actual study. The list of interventions indicated in the diagram are examples, like the assumptions around what the needs are. The interventions in the diagram take the form of capacity building among those involved in the informal economy. Empirical and clinical sociology studies will indicate appropriate interventions.

Finally, the methods are the processes towards realising the needs vis-à-vis the interventions. The concept 'tools' are another way of thinking about the methods.

To summarise the diagram, first, the clinical sociologist must develop a conceptual understanding of the study based on an appropriate theory (and the literature study). Choosing an appropriate theory depends on rationalising (justifying) a phenomenon through observable data or experimentation (i.e., through a clinical sociology study). Secondly, the clinical sociologist must develop an understanding of the gaps or needs that will address the phenomenon or situation based on the findings of the study. Thirdly, the clinical sociologist must decide on what interventions are needed to close the gaps or meet the needs. Fourthly, the clinical sociologist must decide on what methods, tools, and processes to adopt, which will be best suited to correct the phenomenon or problem. This process is also understood as interventions in clinical sociology. Interventions may take the form of specific corrective measures, models, programmes, and policies. Interventions range from short-term, to medium term, to long-term, depending on the complexity of the phenomenon, problem, or social disease to be addressed.

The practical impact of the clinical approach can be applied from micro to macro levels. It may be applied meaningfully to issues of individuals and families, social groups, and communities, and to a state. Clinical sociology is relevant locally and internationally, vis-à-vis, for example, international non-governmental organisations working in the areas of climate change, disaster, children welfare, human rights, etc., as well as multilateral organisations working in the interests of peoples of the world such as the United Nations, the World Bank, African Union, and so on.

Clinical sociology must aim to 'make the world a better place,' i.e., imaginatively, and ontologically. The idea is to bring positive change for individuals and society through research-based best practices and sound sociological theory to address social diseases. Social diseases have multiple dimensions and structural causes, including history, contradictions, societal forces, unequal relationships, and other socio-cultural reasons.

The approach taken in the chapter clearly indicates a distinctive shift from the curative treatment of a pathology or abnormality. Rather clinical sociology is understood as scientific practice, reaching meaningfully and deeply into social relations and structures of society. Good scientific practice involves principles and capabilities. The principles of good scientific practice are concern for knowledge; framing proper questions; model-building; well-planned investigations; analysing and interpreting data; reasoning; mathematical and computational thinking; constructing descriptions, explanations, and arguments based on evidence; communicating information through scientific reports, seminars, and conferences.

Good scientific capabilities include reliability in research methods; maintaining objectivity; duty of care to subjects, cultures, beliefs, etc.; impartial and independent thinking and action; ethical practice; strictly follow referencing practices;

honesty, openness, and accessibility to other researchers; and supporting scientific endeavours in the future.

There is good evidence of successful clinical sociology studies on several social diseases. They include mixed race theory in everyday life (Rocha 2022); critical race theory (Yosso, Smith et al. 2009); crime among Black men (Glynn 2013); race, class, gender, and disability in education (Gillborn 2015); clinical sociology models in Africa (Khan and Ehiane 2021); in-service training approaches (Hall 2000); correctional counselling (Kennedy 1984); and so on. These and other clinical sociology studies assert the view that a new clinical sociology has taken off and is on the rise. This development confirms its relevance for the future.

Conclusion

This chapter examined the depth of poly-pandemic crises and the global response to it. The focus was on two aspects: the first is how the state, economy, the public health system, and people responded to COVID-19. This aspect was concerned about a return to the status quo, rather than a dramatic leap into the new normal. The second aspect pursued by the chapter was the possibility for a new clinical sociology, adopting a multidisciplinary approach supported by new meta-methodology and theorising to understand and address extant COVID-19 and a world where future poly-pandemics will occur.

Regarding the first aspect, the chapter is divided about both possibilities, that is, the world may retreat to an unequal, authoritarian, and misinformed status quo experienced prior to COVID-19. This is the approach of the critic. Alternatively, there is the belief that the 4th and 5th Industrial Revolutions will solve the challenges of the poly-pandemic vis-à-vis artificial intelligence, big data, and the super-smart society. This is the approach of some experts and scientists.

The second aspect attempted at a new clinical sociology application to the poly-pandemic. This idea included a multidisciplinary approach, supported by a meta-methodology and theorising. The opportunity exists during this experience of COVID-19 to frame such a new social science, in preparation for similar poly-pandemics of the future, obviating better breakthroughs as well as paving the way to a more equal and just world.

References

Anderson, J., et al. (2021). Experts say the 'new normal' in 2025 will be far more tech-driven, presenting more big challenges. *Pew Research Center*.

Andreadakis, Z., et al. (2020). The COVID-19 vaccine development landscape. *Nature Reviews Drug Discovery* 19, pp. 305–306.

Beck, U. (2009). World risk society and manufactured uncertainties. *Iris: European Journal of Philosophy & Public Debate* 1(2), pp. 291–299.

Binns, C. and Low, W. Y. (2021). *The rich get richer and the poor get poorer: The inequality of COVID-19*. 33, pp. 185–187: SAGE Publications, Sage CA: Los Angeles, CA.

Bogich, T. L., et al. (2012). Preventing pandemics via international development: A systems approach. *PLoS Medicine* 9(12), p. e1001354.

Brown, B. B. (1987). Facing the 'Black Peril': The politics of population control in South Africa. *Journal of Southern African Studies* 13(2), pp. 256–273.

Bruhn, J. G. and Rebach, H. M. (2012). *Handbook of Clinical Sociology.* Springer Science & Business Media.

Cingano, F. (2014). Trends in income inequality and its impact on economic growth. *OECD Social, Employment and Migration Working Papers,* No. 163, Paris: OECD Publishing. https://doi.org/10.1787/5jxrjncwxv6j-en.

Collins, P. H. and Blige, S. (2020). *Intersectionality.* John Wiley & Sons.

Curtis, V. and Biran, A. (2001). Dirt, disgust, and disease: Is hygiene in our genes? *Perspectives in Biology and Medicine* 44(1), pp. 17–31.

Eisentraut, S. (2021). *The "Polypandemic" Threat: Impacts on Development, Fragility, and Conflict.* FPRI: Foreign Policy Research Institute. Retrieved May 22, 2023, from https://policycommons.net/artifacts/1501559/the-polypandemic-threat/2160496/.

Freimuth, V. S., et al. (2001). African Americans' views on research and the Tuskegee Syphilis study. *Social Science & Medicine* 52(5), pp. 797–808.

Fritz, J. M. (1989). The history of clinical sociology. *Sociological Practice* 7(1), p. 11.

Gillborn, D. (2015). Intersectionality, critical race theory, and the primacy of racism: Race, class, gender, and disability in education. *Qualitative Inquiry* 21(3), pp. 277–287.

Glynn, M. (2013). *Black Men, Invisibility and Crime: Towards a Critical Race Theory of Desistance.* Routledge.

Govender, J. (2020). *Covid – 19, Capitalism and Science. Reflections during the Pandemic.* Spain: International Sociological Association.

Green, B. L., et al. (1997). Participation in health education, health promotion, and health research by African Americans: Effects of the Tuskegee Syphilis Experiment. *Journal of Health Education* 28(4), pp. 196–201.

Guven, M. and Karlen, R. (2020). Supporting Africa's urban informal sector: Coordinated policies with social protection at the core. World Bank Blogs: Africa Can End Poverty.

Hall, C. M. (2000). Clinical sociology in service learning. *Sociological Practice* 2(1), pp. 33–39.

Hawksbee, L., et al. (2022). Don't worry about the drug industry's profits when considering a waiver on covid-19 intellectual property rights. *BMJ* 376, p. e067367.

Hunter, P. (2020). The spread of the COVID-19 coronavirus: Health agencies worldwide prepare for the seemingly inevitability of the COVID-19 coronavirus becoming endemic. *EMBO Reports* 21(4), p. e50334.

Idoiaga Mondragon, N., et al. (2017). Understanding an Ebola outbreak: Social representations of emerging infectious diseases. *Journal of Health Psychology* 22(7), pp. 951–960.

ILO. (2015). Decent work country diagnostics – Technical guidelines to draft the diagnostics report. Report. Geneva: ILO.

Javaid, M., et al. (2020). Industry 5.0: Potential applications in COVID-19. *Journal of Industrial Integration and Management* 5(4), pp. 507–530.

Kennedy, D. B. (1984). Clinical sociology and correctional counseling. *Crime & Delinquency* 30(2), pp. 269–292.

Khan, M. S. and Ehiane, S. (2021). Clinical Sociology Models: Interventions and Analysis in Africa. *Alternation Special Edition* 37, pp. 1–10. https://doi.org/10.29086/2519-5476/2021/sp37a1

Khan, M. S. and Ehiane, S. (2021). Clinical sociology models: Interventions and analysis in Africa. Alternation Special Edition 37, 1–10. 1 Print ISSN 1023-1757; Electronic ISSN: 2519-5476. https://doi.org/10.29086/2519-5476/2021/sp37a1.

Klein, J. T. and Newell, W. H. (1997). Advancing interdisciplinary studies. In J. Gaff and J. Ratcliff (eds.), *Handbook of the Undergraduate Curriculum: A Comprehensive Guide to Purposes, Structures, Practices, and Change* (pp. 393–415). San Francisco, CA: Jossey-Bass.

Le, T. T., Andreadakis, Z., Kumar, A., Román, R. G., Tollefsen, S., Saville, M. and Mayhew, S. (2020). The COVID-19 vaccine development landscape. *Nature Reviews Drug Discovery*, 19(5), 305–306.

Mazzucato, M. (2020). Coronavirus and capitalism: How will the virus change the way the world works? W. a. P. Syndicate.

Meek, R. L. (2010). *Turgot on Progress, Sociology and Economics: A Philosophical Review of the Successive Advances of the Human Mind on Universal History Reflections on the Formation and the Distribution of Wealth.* Cambridge University Press.

Mlambo, V. H. and Masuku, M. M. (2020). Governance, corruption and COVID-19: The final nail in the coffin for South Africa's dwindling public finances. *Journal of Public Administration* 55(3-1), pp. 549–565.

Murshed, S. M. (2020). Capitalism and COVID-19: Crisis at the crossroads. *Peace Economics, Peace Science and Public Policy* 26(3), pp. 20200026. https://doi.org/10.1515/peps-2020-0026

Park, C. L., et al. (2020). Americans' COVID-19 stress, coping, and adherence to CDC guidelines. *Journal of General Internal Medicine* 35(8), pp. 2296–2303.

Phoenix, A. and Pattynama, P. (2006). Intersectionality. *European Journal of Women.* 13(3), pp. 187–192.

Pillay, D. (2010). The eco-logic of the global capitalist crisis. GLU conference, Berlin.

Piot, P., et al. (2014). Ebola in West Africa: From disease outbreak to humanitarian crisis. *The Lancet Infectious Diseases* 14(11), pp. 1034–1035.

Rana, U. and Govender, J. (2022). *Exploring the Consequences of the COVID-19 Pandemic.* Canada: Apple Academic Publishers.

Rocha, Z. L. (2022). Clinical sociology and mixedness: Towards applying critical mixed race theory in everyday life. *Genealogy* 6(2), p. 32.

Roy, A. (2003). *War Talk.* South End Press.

Sarfraz, Z., et al. (2021). Is COVID-19 pushing us to the fifth industrial revolution (society 5.0)? *Pakistan Journal of Medical Sciences* 37(2), p. 591.

Shire, S. J. (2009). Formulation and manufacturability of biologics. *Current Opinion in Biotechnology* 20(6), pp. 708–714.

Sy, M., et al. (2020). Doing interprofessional research in the COVID-19 era: A discussion paper. *Journal of Interprofessional Care* 34(5), pp. 600–606.

Teixeira, C. F. D. S., et al. (2020). The health of healthcare professionals coping with the Covid-19 pandemic. *Ciência & Saúde Coletiva* 25, pp. 3465–3474.

Thomas Morrow, L. H. F. (2004). Defining the difference: What makes biologics unique. *Biotechnology Healthcare* 1(4), p. 24.

UNICEF. (2022). *No-one is Safe until Everyone is Safe – Why We Need a Global Response to COVID-19. N. Mekki.* New York: UNICEF.

WHO. (2022). COVID-19 vaccine tracker and landscape.

WHO. (2022). WHO COVID-19 dashboard: WHO (COVID-19).

Wirth, L. (1931). Clinical sociology. *American Journal of Sociology* 37(1), pp. 49–66.

Yosso, T., et al. (2009). Critical race theory, racial microaggressions, and campus racial climate for Latina/o undergraduates. *Harvard Educational Review* 79(4), pp. 659–691.

20 Reflections on COVID-19

Interventions and Changes

Mariam Seedat-Khan and Johanna O. Zulueta

The Gendered Pandemic World

An international scientific scholarship collection from geographically diverse women scholars and researchers living on the edge of COVID-19 is delivered. Global North and scholars from the South have measured, assessed, and examined COVID-19 gendered experiences with a clinical focus intersecting on family, work, and community. This edited book offers sociological insights and records the events and circumstances surrounding COVID-19's impact and subsequent effect. COVID-19 at the time of writing this book had penetrated every sector of human existence.

This edited book is undeniably sociologically astute, given its meticulous scientific methodology. Commencing with a clinical certified introduction, Seedat-Khan and Zulueta offer insight into how COVID-19 caused the worsening of gender, race, class, labour, and political and socio-economic conditions in the North and South. Seedat-Khan and Zulueta offer a profound interrogation of systemic institutional inequality which is as a matter of course an extension of the capitalist economy. This edited volume is innovative, offering diverse realities of human suffering.

Authors deliver sensitised and profoundly reverential psycho-social constructions of social realities in families, work, and communities. The penetrating revulsion for the incorrigible pandemic state juxtaposes indefinable challenges impacting human conditions adversely.

Intersecting Themes

The preceding 19 chapters emphasised significant interconnected themes, with distinctive lived contexts, in Malaysia, South Africa, Japan, India, Brazil, Australia, the United Kingdom, the United States, Nigeria, and Zimbabwe. The seven overarching themes include but are not limited to gender-based violence, health, work, education, migration, adversity and resilience and reflections on COVID-19 lessons from interventions and change. Family, work, and community intersect with global themes that consider gender, race, class, and geographic levels, made worse by the onset of COVID-19 and its subsequent devastation.

Part I Gender-Based Violence

This section emphasises gender-based violence with segments on intimate partner violence amid the pandemic. As argued in Chapter 2, COVID-19 experiences of

DOI: 10.4324/9781003267133-27

pregnant women in Ibadan North, Oyo State Nigeria, entrench inequality and exacerbate women's vulnerability to intimate partner violence (IPV). The focus on pregnant women highlights how the pandemic complicated women's experiences and coping mechanisms. While IPV existed pre-pandemic, the severity increased during lockdowns, hindering access to help. The need to develop innovative public health responses ensures continued unhindered access to medical and psycho-social support.

Chapter 3 shows how gender-based violence experiences of Zimbabwean flood victims are a flagrant human rights violation, systemic in disrupting rural women's safety and well-being. Women living at the Chingwizi temporary shelter in 2020 revealed systemic patriarchy, gendered typecasts, and socially constructed cultural realities that subjugate women, increasing gender-based violence (GBV) and vulnerability amid natural disasters and pandemics.

Part II Health

In Chapter 4, authors use an autoethnographic lens to understand women and COVID-19 care in South Africa. Experiences of women patients, family members, health care workers, and a clinical sociologist are delivered. The visibility and valuation of care work consider how a pandemic context has necessitated new public and professional relations and engagements for clinical sociologists.

Narratives from community health workers reflect COVID-19 experiences in Jharkhand, India, as illustrated in Chapter 5. Community health workers are the backbone of the health delivery system consisting of only women workers who played a key role in the COVID-19 pandemic. Researchers use secondary data, reports, documented responses, and narrative experiences from women workers to explore first-hand working experiences during a pandemic.

In Chapter 6, the association of people with sickle cell disease (APEDFI) and black women with sickle cell disease in Ilhéus-BA (Brazil) amid COVID-19 offers a sociological analysis. APEDFI's 25-year trajectory of mobilisation, addressing the combative journey of black women, is especially deepened amid COVID-19 in Brazil.

Chapter 7 shows that Filipina caregivers' mental health is influenced by COVID-19, considering the impacts of familial obligations and insecurity on migrants in the United States. Filipina caregivers contend with personal and familial health, well-being, and livelihood decisions about work. The authors consider complex transnational commitments, gender and identity, intersections, and psycho-social impacts on Filipina caregivers.

Part III Work

Supermarket cashiers closing social distancing gaps consider artificial affective labour. Chapter 8 focuses on interactions between cashiers and customers in a coastal town in South Africa in 2020; COVID-19 restrictions required 'social distancing' and restricted interaction.

Qualitative in-depth telephone interviews explored the experiences and perspectives of women cashiers. Findings suggest that women cashiers engaged in emotional and affective labour to mediate interactions.

In chapter 9 are the chronicles of Indonesian domestic helpers as agents of successful women and Malaysian households examined narratives activated, produced, organised, and transmitted via social constructivism. Situational and interactional narratives unearthed embedded ideologies and acculturation.

Meanwhile, Chapter 10 looks at the unspoken truth from Malaysian deaf women's COVID-19 experiences and challenges. Deaf women confront the following challenges:

1. Communication during the time of the pandemic,
2. Financial constraints and well-being,
3. Socialising and social support, and
4. Interpersonal conflict.

Part IV Education

Chapter 11 provides an African perspective of female academics' career progression and motivation during COVID-19 explores experiences in African HEIs. Since the pandemic, African female career progression, workload, and motivation have provided a snapshot of data in the HEI context.

The impact of COVID-19 on school policies on assistant language teachers in Japan discusses the impact of Japanese schools' responses to the occupational health of foreign teaching staff in the first six months of the pandemic. Chapter 12 looks at the important role of online platforms and digital media in addressing women migrant teachers' mental and emotional well-being as they navigate and mitigate pandemic risks.

The educational impact of COVID-19 on lone mothers in the Global South is the focus of Chapter 13. This chapter considers a unique separatist South African history that impacts work, family, and community, intersecting women's education and economic position exacerbated by the pandemic.

Part V Migration

In Chapter 14, it is argued that women migrants' memories and narratives in Brazil deliver experiences to reframe their histories. The pandemic educational perspective of Brazilian women educators and Haitian women students employ narratives that remember suffering.

The impact of COVID-19 on policy and support services for migrant women experiencing DV in semi-rural areas of the UK is emphasised in Chapter 15. The significant increase in rural migrant population in England has created challenges for services, limited resources, knowledge, and skills to support needs. The focus is on the Cheshire East region, the case study in which limited migrant women's needs are marginalised, with inadequate community support. The recommendations for policy and service providers effectively support migrant women experiencing domestic violence.

Vulnerable female migrants with no recourse to public funds (NRPF) during the COVID-19 crisis is the focus of Chapter 16. The impact of a health crisis in England explores the pervasive ramifications of policy in vulnerable female migrants' lives, including the risk of poverty, homelessness, illegal work, degradation in physical and mental health, exploitation, and violence. Locating the policy within the nexus of migration, race, and gender subordination, the NRPF policy entraps female migrants into interlocking systems and structures of oppression and violence reinforced by the pandemic.

Part VI Adversity and Resilience

Women behind bars in the United States expose a hidden, vulnerable pandemic population, as argued in Chapter 17. The United States has the highest number of incarcerated women and girls in the world. The impact of COVID-19 on this hidden population draws on limited reporting of women in American correctional institutions. Data is complemented by an analysis of ethnographic observations from a gardening programme for women in a residential corrections community in the American Midwest. The clinical, sociological intervention addressed women's complaints about poor food quality and idle time in the corrections facility. The findings suggest a perceived lack of protection from COVID-19, inconsistent and opaque responses from criminal justice personnel, limited access to social support, and deteriorating food quality during the pandemic.

Chapter 18 explores the realities of the COVID-19 online teaching transition in South Africa. Illustrating challenges and risks, the authors offer clinical responses.

Part VII Conclusion: Interventions and Change

New clinical sociology for a post-COVID-19 world considers training and professionalisation of clinical and applied sociology. Chapter 19 calls for the requirement for its urgent development among the world's marginalised. Change agent professionals have received traditional medical and sociological methodologies. Theoretical foundations rest on the socio-medical crisis interventions mandated by the World Health Organization and government-led task teams that executed COVID-19 protocol and practice. Therefore, the proposal for developing new clinical sociological methods and applications must serve programmes, governance, institutions, and policies for effective human change. Such an endeavour requires the collaboration of clinical sociologists globally.

Chapter 20, 'Reflections on COVID-19' concludes the edited volume; this offers a starting point towards constructing a new solution-driven clinical and applied process that mitigates risk, reduces social problems, and improves the human condition of women living on the edge of COVID-19. Interventions and change must become inherent in the role of the state. The postscript *considers* gendered clinical and applied reflections recognising casualties of COVID-19.

Index

For Product Safety Concerns and Information please contact our EU
representative GPSR@taylorandfrancis.com
Taylor & Francis Verlag GmbH, Kaufingerstraße 24, 80331 München, Germany

www.ingramcontent.com/pod-product-compliance
Lightning Source LLC
Chambersburg PA
CBHW052119230326
41598CB00080B/3860